CLINICAL
RHEUMATOLOGY

CLINICAL RHEUMATOLOGY

A Problem-Oriented Approach to Diagnosis and Management

ROLAND W. MOSKOWITZ, M.D.

*Professor of Medicine
(Division of Rheumatic Diseases)
Case Western Reserve University
School of Medicine
Cleveland, Ohio*

LEA & FEBIGER

Philadelphia

Library of Congress Cataloging in Publication Data

Moskowitz, Roland W.
  Clinical rheumatology.

  Includes bibliographical references and index.
  1. Rheumatism. I. Title. [DNLM: 1. Arthritis. 2. Rheumatism WE344 M911c]
RC927.M64   616.7′2   74-23701
ISBN 0-8121-0512-5

Published in Great Britain by Henry Kimpton Publishers, London

PRINTED IN THE UNITED STATES OF AMERICA

Print Number 3 2

To my wife, Peta,

for her encouragement and the hours spent alone; and to my parents,

who made this book possible.

Foreword

A distinct honor was extended to me by Dr. Moskowitz when he asked me to write a foreword for *Clinical Rheumatology*. This volume is a comprehensive and problem-oriented presentation of rheumatology, presenting clearly and completely what the clinician needs to know about all rheumatologic problems, not just the more common forms of arthritis. Starting with the symptoms and findings noted in each patient, through differential diagnosis and treatment, the approach is practical. The arrangement of chapters has been carefully planned with a few basic chapters describing the necessary clinical skills and how to develop them. This is followed by the most important section of the book: Clinical Presentations. These 14 chapters have been masterfully organized to deal with each type of clinical problem, discussing differential diagnostic points and objectives of therapy. The third section deals with specific management of various problems encountered in rheumatology, and special types of treatment such as physical and occupational therapy, local injection therapy, and proper use of steroids.

By writing the entire book himself, the author has avoided many of the difficulties encountered in editing a collection of contributor papers that present differing opinions. It was a tremendous task, but he has done it well. I congratulate Dr. Moskowitz on an excellent job.

JOSEPH LEE HOLLANDER, M.D., M.A.C.P.

Preface

Rheumatology, one of the youngest medical subspecialties, has seen a burgeoning growth over the past several decades. Clinical and basic investigations have been expanded and increased numbers of capable people attracted to the field of study. Pessimism has given way to optimism that much can be done to control many of the rheumatic disorders. Application of the basic scientific disciplines, particularly immunology and biochemistry, provides hope that prevention and cure are not unreasonable goals for the near future.

Intensified interest and study in the rheumatic disorders was necessary and warranted. A recent task force survey by the Arthritis Foundation demonstrated that in the United States alone, at least 20,230,000 people were suffering from arthritis and arthritis-like conditions. Among the commonest causes of disability, these diseases result in untold human suffering in addition to massive economic losses. Rheumatic diseases represent a major component of the patient population seen by practicing physicians. Provision of optimal care requires development of full training programs in rheumatology in all medical schools, and expanded programs of postgraduate education. It is toward this latter effort that this book is primarily devoted. Hopefully, it will provide a resource whereby additional education can be provided on a background of everyday practice and experience.

Several excellent textbooks on rheumatology are already available. They have been particularly helpful to physicians who have a primary interest in the rheumatic diseases, or as reference texts. This textbook represents an effort to provide the practicing physician with a new, additional dimension of information. The clinical discussions are based on a problem-oriented approach, paralleling the disease manifestations as they appear initially to the physician. It is designed to be a working text, to be kept close at hand for use on a day-to-day basis as a helpful guide in the management of problems as they appear.

Many of the chapters are based on material used by me in daily teaching discussions in clinics, at the bedside, or in small conferences, which has been expanded for completeness. Although this text was written primarily for the general practitioner and the internist, who provide the bulwark of care to arthritis patients, hopefully medical students, house officers, rheumatologists, orthopedists, pediatricians and other physicians who come into contact with patients with rheumatologic complaints will find it valuable.

My deep appreciation is extended to Drs. Beno Michel, Samuel J. Horwitz, Paul J. Vignos, Jr., Phillip I. Lerner, Victor M. Goldberg and Harvey M. Rodman for their review and comments on the sections related to laboratory diagnosis, dermatologic disorders, muscle disease, infectious arthritis, and steroid management in stress situations. Miss Betsy J. Fallon, R.P.T., M.A., Mrs. Charlotte Ryan, O.T.R., and Mrs. Maxine Landers, O.T.R., collaborated on the preparation of the chapter on physical and occupational therapy. I am indebted to Drs. Allen Mackenzie, Charles W. Denko, Beno Michel, Victor M. Goldberg, Mahmood Pazirandeh, Fred Bishko, Robert Gatter and the national office of the Arthritis Foundation* for making material available for illustrations. Their contributions are recognized in the legends where these illustrations are used. Dr. Sergio A. Murillo, Fellow in Rheumatology, and Miss Fallon were most helpful in the preparation of some of the illustrations relative to diagnosis. Mrs. Mary Lee Berman assisted in many administrative tasks of manuscript preparation.

Photography was performed by Mr. Donald Schad and his associates, Mr. Ken-Ichi Kondo and Mr. Joseph Molter, of the Department of Medical Photography, Case Western Reserve University School of Medicine. Typing of the manuscript through its inception and numerous revisions was done by Mrs. Carole Walters and Mrs. Sondra Patrizi. I am grateful to the publishers, Lea & Febiger, for advice and guidance throughout preparation of the text for publication.

To my former mentors, Dr. John Lansbury, formerly Professor of Medicine at Temple University, and Dr. Charles H. Slocumb and his colleagues at the Mayo Clinic, I owe a deep debt of gratitude for my basic training in rheumatology. The examples of excellence they provided have served as a continuing guide throughout my own career of study. To Dr. Joseph L. Hollander, whose textbook of rheumatology stands as an outstanding contribution to the study of the rheumatic diseases, I am grateful for the foreword to this text. The assistance of Dr. Michael G. Sheahan, Senior Fellow in Rheumatology, in proofreading the manuscript is gratefully acknowledged.

Manuscript preparation was supported in part through the Division of Research in Medical Education, Case Western Reserve University, Grant #LM 00673, National Library of Medicine.

Cleveland, Ohio   ROLAND W. MOSKOWITZ

Contents

INTRODUCTION

Medical textbooks are usually organized by topics based on specific disease entities. Most patients, however, do not come to the physician with a disease already diagnosed and given a name; rather, they more commonly have a complex of symptoms and physical abnormalities. This textbook is organized in a problem-oriented fashion on the basis of presenting signs and symptoms, in the way that medical problems are more likely to appear to the physician.

The text is divided into three major divisions. The chapters in *Part I* review clinical examination, laboratory studies and diagnostic techniques in specific relationship to rheumatic disorders. Special attention is given to synovial fluid analysis, an important study in the diagnosis of these disease states.

The chapters in *Part II* are devoted to common clinical presentations of rheumatic disorders. The chapters in this section have a common format, as follows:

A. Introduction. A brief general discussion of the problem at hand is presented.

B. Differential diagnosis. A listing of those entities most likely to provide the answer to the patient's problem is given. No attempt is made to list the diseases within this group according to frequency of occurrence. A clinical description of diseases to be considered in diagnosis follows. This information is designed to provide important clues to diagnosis and direction to further clinical and laboratory investigation necessary for accurate diagnosis. Some repetition of these clinical outlines is carried out in the various chapters; this repetition is deliberate. It allows variation in emphasis on salient features of the disease states, depending upon the nature of the problem under discussion. In addition, it lessens the need for the reader to move back and forth between chapters for clinical information. Hopefully, this aspect of the book, in which each chapter provides a relatively complete discussion of the problem under investigation, will prove especially valuable to the physician using the text on a day-to-day basis.

Additional possible diagnoses, to be considered after the more common causes have been excluded, are noted for completion, but are generally discussed in lesser detail. These latter entities are less likely to represent the diagnosis at hand, either because the diseases themselves or their symptomatic presentation as the type of problem under discussion are uncommon.

C. Diagnostic studies to be considered in the evaluation. A comprehensive discussion of diagnostic studies with a detailed discussion of their application for most appropriate and effective use is given.

D. Therapy. Discussion of therapy is directed toward two phases of management. In the first phase, therapeutic procedures directed toward *symptomatic* relief *prior* to specific diagnosis are outlined. Great care has been exercised to avoid those measures which, though providing symptomatic help, would interfere with further clinical and laboratory diagnostic measures. The use of the recommended agents and procedures for temporary relief of pain and disability allows time for further clinical observation and diagnostic study, as well as time to carry out appropriate literature research into the patient's problem if required.

The second phase of therapy relates to *specific* measures of management to be utilized *after the diagnosis* has been made. In some instances, these specific therapeutic programs are outlined in detail in the chapter itself. Additional details regarding specific management of the more common rheumatic diseases are given in more complete form in the chapters on therapy in Part III.

Following the material in each chapter of Part II, representative cases typifying some of the problems under discussion are presented. These cases, based on patients seen in practice, demonstrate the clinical and laboratory aspects of diagnosis and management both before and after diagnosis has been made.

The chapters in *Part III* describe specific detailed management of some of the more common rheumatic diseases to be used after the diagnosis has been made. In addition, special chapters are devoted to physical therapy, occupational therapy and supportive appliances, and to local injection therapy, extremely important adjuncts to rheumatic disease care. The final chapter describes the management of corticosteroid therapy in patients in stress situations, with particular reference to its use in surgery and obstetrics.

References to available textbooks and key articles in medical journals are provided for more detailed study after each chapter and in the Appendix.

This textbook is designed to provide practical information that will allow judicious and appropriate study and management of the more commonly seen rheumatic disease problems. The more difficult or uncommon problems may require more extensive reading or, when indicated, referral to specialists in the rheumatic diseases.

This text represents a distillate of prevailing diagnostic and therapeutic philosophies as viewed and practiced by a single author. There is always a danger that such an approach will be dogmatic regarding both methods of evaluation and therapy. Realizing this danger, an attempt has been made to avoid dogmatism insofar as possible. It is hoped that most authorities in the field will agree in general with the concepts of management and treatment outlined. Of course, individual variations and preferences are to be expected. Material of controversial nature is specifically described as such when discussed.

Part 1

CLINICAL EXAMINATION, LABORATORY STUDIES AND DIAGNOSTIC TECHNIQUES

Chapter 1

HISTORY AND PHYSICAL EXAMINATION

HISTORY OF PRESENT ILLNESS

Effective history-taking in patients with rheumatic disorders requires paying attention both to the usual general inquiries and to specific symptoms. Close attention must be paid to the location, nature and course of the joint involvement. Important determinations include the duration of joint symptoms, the location of the joints first involved, the pattern of progression to other joints, and the acute, subacute or chronic nature of the symptoms observed. Frequency and periodicity of attacks are other important considerations. The examiner should ask questions about anatomic areas other than the musculoskeletal system, because joint manifestations are similar, if not identical, in many of these disorders. Diagnosis often depends on the demonstration of important ancillary findings. The age, sex and race of the patient may influence the consideration of certain diseases. Fever, weakness, fatigue and weight loss indicate systemic disease. Fibrositis or stiffness is a characteristic manifestation of many of the rheumatic diseases; when generalized, it suggests a systemic disorder. The patient complains of gelling of the muscles and joints, which occurs most prominently in the morning upon awakening. Stiffness is also present following inactivity during the day, with improvement following increased physical activity. It is more pronounced preceding stormy weather, when the barometric pressure falls and humidity is high. Commonly, cool, damp weather accentuates the stiffness and heat relieves it. Raynaud's phenomenon with its typical color changes is likely to herald the presence of a serious systemic disorder; cold is the most common precipitating factor. A suspected diagnosis of systemic lupus erythematosus is strengthened by the presence of sun sensitivity, pleurisy, drug allergy, or hair loss. Photophobic reactions, or a long history of nausea and dizziness on sun exposure, do not have the import of sun sensitivity reactions characterized by rash, fever, or arthritis. Skin rash is an important clue to the diagnosis of such entities as psoriatic arthritis, systemic lupus erythematosus, scleroderma and dermatomyositis, to name only a few. Gastrointestinal symptoms of chronic diarrhea and bleeding, when associated with joint symptoms, suggest a diagnosis of ulcerative colitis or regional enteritis. Frequent aphthous ulcers, commonly called canker sores by the patient, are seen in Behçet's and Reiter's syndromes. Renal stones may be the first manifestation of gout. Eye findings including conjunctivitis, episcleritis, and iritis are common in a number of systemic rheumatic disorders. Urethritis suggests the presence of gonococcal arthritis or Reiter's syndrome.

A complete rheumatologic history should include current and past details regarding dose, effectiveness and toxicity of antiarthritic agents used in the management of the patient's symptoms. In particular, specific information regarding the use of aspirin, analgesics, indomethacin, phenylbutazone, oral, intramuscular and intra-articular corticosteroids, antimalarials, gold and immunosuppressive agents should be obtained. Medications that the patient may be taking for unrelated illnesses should be noted for several reasons: Firstly, contraindicated drug combinations can be avoided. Secondly, certain drugs such as oral contraceptive agents, hydralazine, anticonvulsant medications and procainamide may be precipitating or causative factors in the patient's connective tissue disease symptoms.

SYSTEMS REVIEW

A complete review of systems is required. However, certain points of information command particular interest in this group of patients. Headaches and tenderness in the temporal area suggest a diagnosis of temporal (cranial) arteritis. The importance of eye symptoms characteristic of conjunctivitis, episcleritis or iritis was previously noted. Persistent dryness of the eyes and mouth should lead to a consideration of Sjögren's syndrome. Dysphagia as a result of esophageal dysfunction is a common manifestation of several connective tissue disorders, such as dermatomyositis and scleroderma. Symptoms of peptic ulcer disease are important to note because many of the medications commonly considered in the treatment of arthritis may be contraindicated. Symptoms of colitis are a clue to the diagnosis of enteropathic arthritis, such as the arthritis associated with ulcerative colitis. Dysuria and urinary frequency may indicate urethritis, a prominent manifestation of gonococcal infection and Reiter's syndrome. Cutaneous lesions on the genitalia are seen in Reiter's and Behçet's syndromes. Sensory symptoms such as burning and paresthesia of the extremities are common manifestations of neurologic complications associated with arthritic disorders. Specific muscle weakness should direct attention to the presence of either a primary myopathy or neurogenic atrophy secondary to involvement of the nervous system.

PAST MEDICAL HISTORY

In addition to the usual review of the patient's medical history, a history of acute rheumatic fever, other forms of arthritis, or trauma is often helpful in delineating the patient's problem. Detailed information regarding past surgery or fractures should be elicited. Knowledge of prior x-rays and their availability is useful, because they can be obtained for review if necessary. Drug allergies should be noted.

FAMILY HISTORY

A number of articular disorders such as gout, ankylosing spondylitis and osteoarthritis of the distal interphalangeal joints (Heberden's nodes) have an hereditary background. Their presence in other family members is supportive in diagnosis.

SOCIOECONOMIC HISTORY

Questions regarding the ability of the patient to perform the usual activities of daily living such as bathing, dressing, toileting, transfer and feeding provide information about the impact of the disease in limiting daily function. In addition, these parameters of function can be used as a guide to the progress of the disease. The patient's emotional response to the disease and the presence of complicating premorbid psychiatric disturbances should be ascertained. The effect of the disease on the family and on financial stability should be noted. Knowledge of the patient's occupation may have etiologic importance. In addition, limitations resulting from the patient's arthritis may require consideration of job alteration or total job retraining.

PHYSICAL EXAMINATION

One of the most serious errors a physician can commit in the diagnosis of rheumatic disorders is to look only at the principal site of complaint or at a limited number of joints. An evaluation of all components of the locomotor system is necessary to assess disease affecting any one joint. A complete examination of other systems is also required, since many of the rheumatic disorders have associated general findings. The patient should be fully undressed except for a short gown. Joint assessment includes observations related to erythema, increased warmth, swelling, tenderness on direct palpation, pain on movement, joint range of motion, instability and deformity. *Erythema* of the skin commonly occurs over acutely inflamed joints but is frequently absent in the presence of chronic inflammation. *Increased skin warmth* is a sensitive indicator of inflammation, but

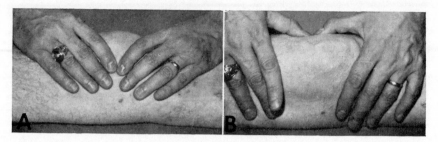

Figure 1-1. Bulge sign. (A) Fluid is compressed to one side of the knee. (B) Pressure on the opposite aspect of the knee produces a small fluid wave or bulge.

changes may be subtle. Comparing the same joint on the opposite side of the body is helpful when changes are minimal. *Swelling* reflects a number of joint abnormalities, including synovial inflammation, increased amounts of synovial fluid or proliferation of cartilage and bone. Inflamed synovium has a boggy edematous feel. Increased mobility of articular structures, such as the patella in the knee, suggests the presence of fluid. The patella can often be ballotted when fluid is present. Using one hand to compress the suprapatellar pouch in order to concentrate the fluid in the main compartment of the knee, the patella is then forcefully directed downward to demonstrate the sensation of bone riding on fluid. Small amounts of fluid in the knee can be detected by the "bulge sign." Fluid is compressed with the hands to one side of the knee (Fig. 1-1,A). This side is then gently tapped or compressed, following which a small fluid wave or bulge can be detected on the opposite aspect of the knee (Fig. 1-1,B). Small amounts of fluid can be detected by this simple maneuver. Bony enlargements are palpated as hard, irregular swellings. They occur most commonly in osteoarthritis and reflect the presence of proliferating spurs of cartilage and bone.

Tenderness, an important sign of joint disease, is tested by direct pressure. Mild tenderness may require a significant amount of pressure to elicit an abnormal response. Comparing the findings with joints on the opposite side of the body is important in determining the significance of the response when changes are mild. Tenderness can be graded in a gross fashion according to the degree of pressure required to elicit pain. More accurate grading can be performed by the use of an instrument called a dolorimeter, which numerically determines the amount of pressure required to bring on pain. The degree of tenderness parallels the severity of the inflammation. Localization of findings is extremely important, because disease of para-articular structures such as tendons or bursae may be misinterpreted as evidence of primary articular disease. Certain joints may not be tender to palpation but will be painful on *active or passive motion.*

Measurement of joint *range of motion* is important not only in defining the presence of joint disease, but also in providing an important parameter of disease progression or response to therapy. Familiarity with normal range of motion is essential to evaluate the significance of measurements in the presence of joint pathology. Comparison with similar opposite joints is helpful in differentiating abnormal from normal findings. The preferred system for joint measurement is based on the neutral zero method, whereby the normal anatomic position of the joint is defined as zero. For example, the flat position of the wrist would be defined as zero degrees. From this position, motion is recorded as the number of degrees of flexion or extension. When extension is an unnatural movement for a given joint, the term hyperextension is used and appropriately recorded. Accurate measurement or range of motion requires the use of a goniometer. This instrument is a hinged device with a scale showing the angle formed between two linear arms.

The presence of *instability* is usually demonstrated most readily by various stress maneuvers. These abnormalities in stability may reflect intra-articular changes, such as loss of cartilage and bone substance, or loss of integrity of supporting joint structures, such as capsule and ligaments. Instability may be obvious on joint use, but it is most readily demonstrated by fixing one component of the joint and testing for increased motion in various planes. Fixed joint *deformity* is usually obvious on inspection.

Completion of the musculoskeletal examination requires evaluation of the muscles for both atrophy and weakness. In patients in whom pathologic changes are located primarily in joints, atrophy and weakness are usually localized to those muscles associated with the affected joints. Erroneous misinterpretations of muscle atrophy may be made when joint swelling is present and the associated muscles look smaller in size by comparison. Generalized atrophy and weakness reflect primary muscle disorders. Muscle tenderness is uncommon except in patients with inflammatory muscle disease.

As noted earlier, proper examination of the patient with arthritis requires evaluation not only of the musculoskeletal system but of other systems as well. The following is a description of a suggested routine for examination in patients with musculoskeletal complaints. The procedure can be varied to suit the individual examiner, but I have found it useful as an effective routine.

The examination is begun as the patient enters the room. Abnormalities in gait and the ability to perform certain activities such as undressing, sitting and rising from a chair, and getting up on the examining table are observed. Direct study begins with an examination of the hands. The nails are examined for evidence of anemia, paronychial rash, psoriasis and subungual infarcts. The presence or absence of clubbing is noted. Tapering of the distal phalanges is characteristic of scleroderma. Observation of the palms may reveal rash, palmar erythema, subcutaneous nodules, and thickenings due to tenosynovitis or Dupuytren's contracture. Muscle atrophy should be noted. Ruptured tendons may be revealed by loss of active motion. The extent to which the patient can make a complete fist bilaterally is recorded. Grip strength is evaluated by having the patient attempt to squeeze the examiner's second and third fingers. At the same time, crepitus due to tenosynovitis may be observed. Each joint should be specifically evaluated for erythema, heat, swelling, tenderness, instability and deformity. Carpal and wrist joints are similarly examined. The primary motions at the wrist are flexion and extension, but radial and ulnar movement should also be evaluated. Elbow motion should normally allow movement from full extension (0°) to 150° flexion. Swelling is most readily palpated in the regions between the medial and lateral epicondyles and the olecranon process (Fig. 1-2). Tenderness over the epicondyles themselves reflects epicondylitis with inflammation of tendon attachments, as occurs in patients with tennis elbow. When examining the elbow joint, special note should be taken of the presence of rheumatoid nodules, gouty tophi or other subcutaneous swellings. Rheumatoid nodules may be truly subcutaneous and mobile, but they are frequently fixed to periosteum. Nonspecific bony irregularities may cause diagnostic confusion, but they usually can be readily differentiated, especially if they are present bilaterally. Rheumatoid nodules most often occur on the extensor surface of the

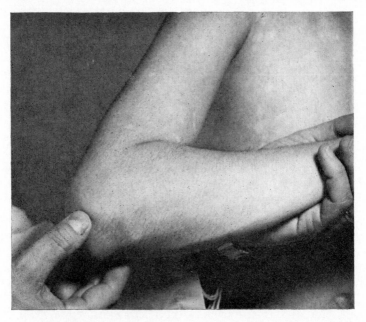

Figure 1-2. Rheumatoid arthritis, right elbow. Swelling is readily palpated between the lateral epicondyle and the olecranon process.

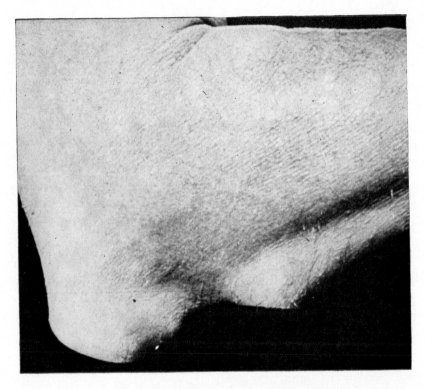

Figure 1-3. Subcutaneous nodules, rheumatoid arthritis. Lesions appear in both the subolecranon and the olecranon areas. (Courtesy, the Arthritis Foundation)

ulna in a subolecranon distribution (Fig. 1-3). Localization here is usually related to pressure exerted on arm rests while sitting. Later, nodules may occur over the olecranon area itself. In contrast, gouty tophi usually occur first in the olecranon area; later, tophi develop distally in the subolecranon area as well. Nodules of other origin, such as xanthomata, amyloid deposits, granuloma annulare, epidermoid cysts and subcutaneous nodules of rheumatic fever may be present. Olecranon bursitis may be observed as a swelling at the posterior aspect of the elbow, over the tip of the olecranon process (Fig. 1-4).

Swelling of the shoulder joint is often difficult to detect. It is seen most readily at the anterior aspect of the joint. Tenderness may be due to intrinsic joint disease, bursitis or tendonitis. Shoulder motions are a combination of glenohumeral and scapulothoracic motions. Glenohumeral motion is tested after first fixing the scapula by downward pressure. Motions to be evaluated include abduction, adduction, flexion, extension, and internal and external rotation. Abduction is tested by moving the shoulder away from the body with the elbow in 90° flexion (Fig. 1-5). Movement

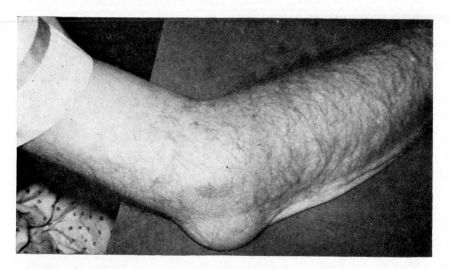

Figure 1-4. Olecranon bursal swelling in a patient with rheumatoid arthritis.

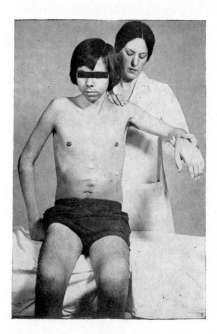

Figure 1-5. Shoulder abduction. The examiner fixes the left scapula of the patient with downward pressure. Abduction at the glenohumeral joint was limited to 70°.

to 90° abduction is normal. Rotation upward measures external rotation (normal, 80° to 90°); rotation downward measures internal rotation (normal, 80° to 90°). Pure adduction is obstructed by the thorax but can be measured by bringing the arm across the front of the chest. Swinging the arm forward and backward measures flexion and extension respectively. Following the examination for glenohumeral motion, total functional shoulder motions of flexion, extension, abduction and hyperabduction are tested without scapular fixation. Palpation of the acromioclavicular and sternoclavicular joints is performed for evidence of tenderness and swelling. Disease of the acromioclavicular joint is often misinterpreted as disease of shoulder origin, due to its proximity to the latter joint. Atrophy and strength of the deltoid muscles are determined as a screening maneuver for the presence of myopathy (Fig. 1-6).

Following these studies, the attention of the examiner is directed to the area of the head. The ears are evaluated for the presence of gouty tophi (Fig. 1-7) and scalp for rash or hair loss. Early small tophi may be difficult to differentiate from localized thickenings of ear cartilage. Differentiation is aided by use of transillumination, during which tophi are opaque. Eyes, ears, nose and throat are examined as part of the routine general exam. The neck is palpated for evidence of thyroid enlargement and lymphadenopathy. Cervical spine motion is tested for flexion, extension, rotation and lateral bending. The posterior cervical and upper trapezius muscles are palpated for the presence of tenderness, spasm or nodules. Cardiorespiratory examination and blood pressure readings follow. The

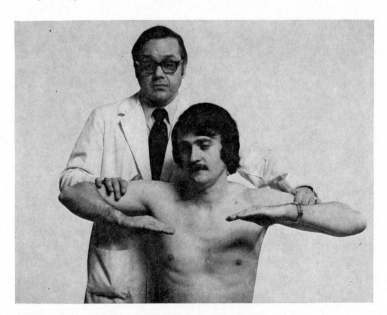

Figure 1-6. Screening maneuver for testing deltoid muscle weakness.

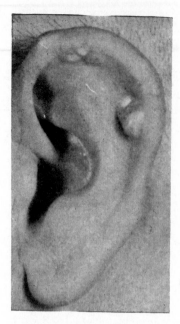

Figure 1-7. Multiple tophi in a patient with gout. Deposits were opaque to transillumination. (Courtesy, Dr. A. Mackenzie)

patient is then asked to lie down, following which abdominal examination and evaluation of the lower extremities can be carried out.

Hip motions to be tested include flexion, extension, abduction, adduction, and internal and external rotation. Hip flexion is measured by moving the flexed knee toward the abdomen. Fixed flexion deformities of the hip may be masked if the patient tilts the pelvis to the affected side. Accurate testing can be accomplished by holding the opposite hip in full flexion while attempting full extension of the hip being examined. Lack of full extension is a measure of the fixed deformity (Fig. 1-8). Extension is tested by drawing the leg backward as the patient lies on the opposite side. To test abduction, the leg is moved laterally. Adduction is evaluated by moving the leg medially in front of the opposite leg. Rotation may be measured with the leg extended or with the knee flexed to 90°. The limb is rolled outward to test for external rotation and inward for internal rotation. Abnormalities in hip motion can be rapidly screened by asking the patient to place the heel on the opposite knee while rotating the hip outward, in an attempt to bring the ipsilateral knee horizontal to the examining table (Fabere-Patrick maneuver). Normal hip rotation should allow the knee to be brought almost completely horizontal (Fig. 1-9). Tests of hip motion may be somewhat invalidated by disease of the knee, since pain in the latter joint may prevent full hip movement. Interpretation of the findings requires caution. Similarly, inflammation of the greater trochanteric bursa may limit hip motion due to pain, despite the absence of

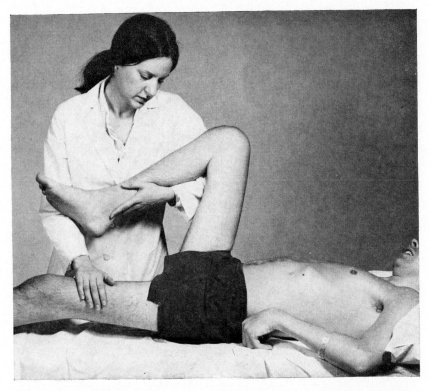

Figure 1-8.   Flexion deformity of left hip in a patient with rheumatoid arthritis. The right hip is
held in full flexion to avoid compensatory pelvic tilt.

intrinsic hip pathology. Tenderness on pressure applied over the bursa at
the trochanteric area is characteristic.

Measurements of leg length are important. The distance between the
anterior-superior iliac spine and the medial malleolus reflects true leg length.
Apparent leg length is measured from the umbilicus to the medial malleolus. Differences in true leg length occur in disease in or near the hip joint;
differences in apparent leg length alone may reflect pelvic tilt or scoliosis.
The strength of the iliopsoas muscle is determined to complete the screening for proximal muscle weakness. This is evaluated by applying downward pressure on the anterior aspect of the thigh as the patient holds the
knee and hip at 90° angles.

The knee lends itself readily to full examination. Obvious deformities
such as genu varus (bowleg) or genu valgus (knock knee) are readily
noted. The knee should be inspected for erythema and palpated for increased warmth, tenderness and swelling. Early swelling is often most obvious in the suprapatellar extension of the joint beneath the quadriceps
tendon. As noted earlier, joint swelling may be due to synovial inflamma-

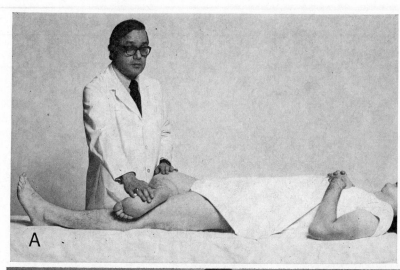

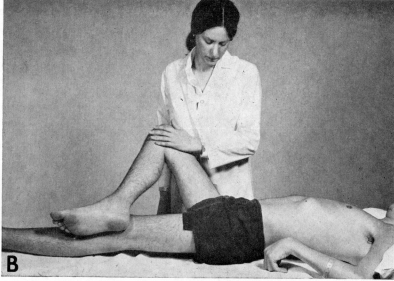

Figure 1-9.   Fabere-Patrick maneuver. (A) Normal. The right knee can be brought almost to the horizontal position. (B) Rheumatoid arthritis. Hip disease prevents rotation of the right knee toward the horizontal position.

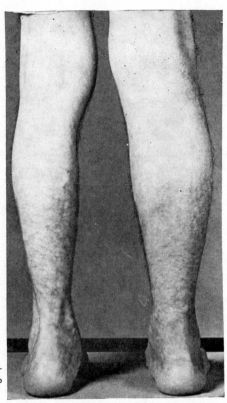

Figure 1-10. Popliteal cyst, right knee. Swelling behind the knee extends into the calf.

tion, increased amounts of joint fluid, or bony proliferation. Palpation at the posterior aspect of the knee is important to detect the presence of popliteal cysts (Fig. 1-10). Circumferential measurement of the thigh at a specific distance above the knee and at the knee joint itself is valuable in patient follow-up. Patellofemoral disease is suggested by pain and crepitus produced when the patella is moved forward over the femur. Abnormal patellar motion is detected by attempts at medial and lateral displacement. Instability of the collateral ligaments is tested by forcing medial and lateral motion with the knee slightly flexed; abnormal findings are accentuated with the patient in a standing position. Cruciate ligament instability is tested by moving the tibia forward and backward on the femur, which is held fixed (Fig. 1-11). Excessive forward motion reflects disease of the anterior cruciate ligament; excessive backward motion, disease of the posterior cruciate ligament. Quadriceps atrophy, common in the presence of knee arthritis, should be noted.

Swelling of the ankle may be difficult to detect. It is most commonly seen at the anterior aspect of the joint only. Swelling of tendons due to tenosynovitis in this area is not uncommon. The Achilles tendon should

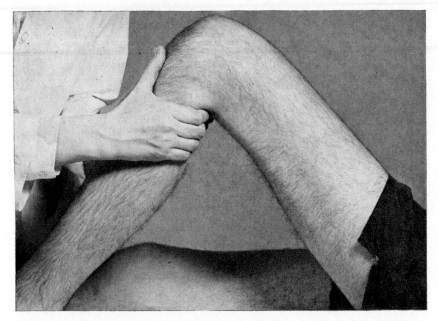

Figure 1-11. Firm anterior pull on the tibia tests instability of the anterior cruciate ligament.

be examined for the presence of tenderness; it is a common site for rheumatoid nodule formation. Flexion and extension motions at the ankle are tested. Subtalar disease is indicated by pain and limitation of inversion and eversion. Tarsal disease may lead to swelling and tenderness. The latter can be readily tested by firm compression of the entire tarsal area in the palm of the examiner. The tarsal joints are usually considered en masse since they do not lend themselves to separate examination. Heel tenderness should be noted. The metatarsophalangeal joints are each examined separately by palpation and pressure. The interphalangeal joints should be similarly observed for swelling and tenderness, and the toenails examined.

The musculoskeletal examination is completed by evaluation of the dorsolumbar spine and sacroiliac joints. The latter are tested for tenderness by direct pressure. Pain on sacroiliac motion may be elicited by having the patient lie on the back in a supine position near the edge of the examining table. Each leg is then separately moved off to the side and below the surface of the table. This maneuver distorts the pelvis and causes pain in the affected joint. Straight leg raising is an important maneuver to test for nerve root irritability in patients with suspected back disorders. The spine itself is examined with the patient in a standing position. Postural abnormalities including kyphosis (forward curvature), lordosis (backward curvature), or scoliosis (lateral curvature) are noted. Local-

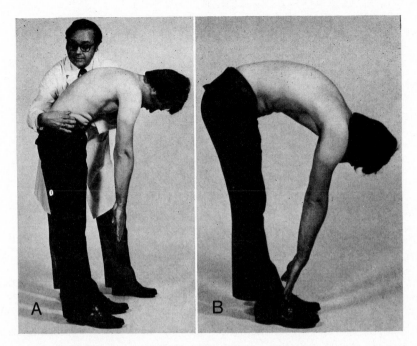

Figure 1-12. Examination of lumbar spine motion. Fixation of hips by the examiner (A) eliminates hip flexion. Compare motion with hips free (B).

ized angulations may be seen. Tenderness over the spine is tested by direct
percussion, using either the side of the fist or a percussion hammer. Flexion, extension, rotation and lateral motions are tested. In testing for flexion
motions, it is important to fix the hips by grasping the patient from behind
over the hip area. Otherwise, flexion limitations may be obscured by bending forward at the hip joints (Fig. 1-12, A and B). Chest expansion
measured at the nipple line is an index of costovertebral joint motion.

In addition to the screening procedures for proximal muscle strength
outlined previously, all muscles should be evaluated for weakness and
atrophy. Neurologic examination includes evaluation of deep tendon reflexes, pathologic reflexes such as the Babinski sign, and evaluation of
pain, touch, vibration, and position senses. The state of the vascular system is evaluated by palpation of radial, ulnar, temporal, carotid, femoral,
popliteal, and pedal pulses. Temporal artery examination is of particular
interest, because tenderness and nodularity support a suspected diagnosis
of temporal (cranial) arteritis. Rectal and pelvic examination completes
the over-all evaluation.

Forms utilized by me for the initial history and physical examination
appear in the Appendix. I have found these helpful as a guide for inter-
viewing the patient and recording physical findings.

Chapter 2

LABORATORY STUDIES AND DIAGNOSTIC
TECHNIQUES: INDICATIONS
AND INTERPRETATIONS

GENERAL STUDIES

A number of routine general laboratory tests are helpful and indicated in the diagnosis of patients with rheumatic disorders. Baseline studies should include a white blood cell count and a differential cell count, hematocrit, erythrocyte sedimentation rate and urinalysis. Leukopenia suggests a diagnosis of systemic lupus erythematosus. The presence of a severe anemia militates against a benign localized disorder, and the patient should be scrupulously studied for serious systemic disease. Similarly, an elevated erythrocyte sedimentation rate is strong evidence for the presence of a more generalized disorder. Abnormal findings on urinalysis favor a diagnosis of systemic lupus erythematosus, vasculitis or scleroderma rather than rheumatoid arthritis.

When suggested by clinical findings, other studies to be considered are serum protein electrophoresis, immunoelectrophoresis, calcium, phosphorus, alkaline phosphatase, creatinine, antistreptolysin O (ASO) titer, protein-bound iodine, cholesterol, triglycerides, lipoprotein electrophoresis, serum glutamic oxaloacetic transaminase, and hepatitis-associated antigen (HB Ag). Chest x-rays should be obtained if systemic disease is suspected. Roentgenograms of involved joints are indicated.

Certain diagnostic studies are particularly important in the study of rheumatic disorders. These are discussed in greater detail.

URIC ACID STUDIES

Serum Uric Acid

Routine determination of the serum uric acid is valuable in patients with articular symptoms. The study is important in determining whether symptoms are due to gout. In addition, many medications affect the serum

22

uric acid level. Determining the true baseline serum uric acid level is cumbersome and often difficult at a later time after such medications have been begun.

Serum uric acid determinations are usually made by the colorimetric method. A more accurate study is obtained using the enzymatic spectro-photometric method in which uric acid levels are determined both before and after uricase digestion. The latter method eliminates the effect of non-urate substances, which produce a spuriously high reading. Normal values vary, depending on the technique used. It is important for the physician to know the normal values obtained by the laboratory in which the test is conducted. Normal levels also differ in males and females. In our labora-tory, using a colorimetric method, the normal value for males is 4 to 6 mg/100 ml; for postmenopausal females, 3.5 to 5.5 mg/100 ml; and for pre-menopausal females, 3 to 5 mg/100 ml. Normal values tend to be higher with Auto-Analyzer techniques, and standardization of normal levels at 7 to 8 mg/100 ml is not uncommon. There is a mild to moderate varia-tion in serum uric acid levels throughout the day and at various times of the year. Although these variations are not marked, it is worth rechecking several uric acid determinations obtained at a similar time each day if the initial study is only slightly abnormal.

Table 2-1. Drugs and Disease States Associated with Secondary Elevation of Serum Uric Acid

Drugs

    Diuretics (e.g., chlorothiazide, hydrochlorothiazide, chlorthalidone, furosemide, triamterene, ethacrynic acid)

    Low dose salicylate therapy

    Pyrazinamide

    Ethambutol[1]

    Levodopa[2]

Disease states

    Chronic hemolytic anemia

    Myeloproliferative and lymphoproliferative disorders (lymphomas, multiple myeloma, polycy-themia vera)

    Lead intoxication (saturnine gout)[3]

    Psoriasis

    Glycogen storage disease (type I)[4]

    Hyperlactacidemia (acute ethanol ingestion, toxemia of pregnancy)

    Increased blood levels of beta hydroxybutyrate and acetoacetate (diabetic ketoacidosis, star-vation)

    Chronic renal failure

    Essential and renal hypertension[5]

    Postadrenalectomy for hypertension[6]

    Hyperparathyroidism[7]

    Hypoparathyroidism[8]

    Myxedema[9]

    Paget's disease[10]

Table 2-2. Drugs and Disease States that Lower Serum Uric Acid

---

Drugs
  Probenecid
  Sulfinpyrazone
  Allopurinol
  High dose salicylate therapy
  Coumarin derivatives
  Phenylbutazone
  Adrenal corticosteroids
  Radiocontrast agents[11]

Disease states
  Wilson's disease[12]
  Fanconi's syndrome
  Xanthine oxidase deficiency
  Neoplasms (carcinoma,[13] Hodgkin's disease[14])

Hyperuricemia may indicate primary gout or may represent an elevation secondary to various medications or disease states (Table 2-1).[1-10] A low or normal serum uric acid, on the other hand, may indicate (1) a normal state, (2) patients with an early stage of gout in which the serum uric acid is normal between attacks, or (3) patients in whom the uric acid has been lowered by certain drugs or disease processes (Table 2-2).[11-14]

Urinary Uric Acid

Information regarding the quantitative daily excretion of uric acid has diagnostic and therapeutic importance. In patients whose clinical symptoms suggest gout but whose serum uric acid is high normal or only slightly elevated, an increase in urinary uric acid excretion supports the diagnosis. In patients with a confirmed diagnosis of gout, the quantitative urinary uric acid determination is helpful in deciding the most appropriate drug to use in an interval therapy program. In those patients with a definitely elevated urinary uric acid, allopurinol is usually the drug of choice, since this agent lowers both serum and urinary uric acid and diminishes the hazard of kidney stone formation. In contrast, uricosuric agents such as probenecid and sulfinpyrazone increase urinary uric acid output and may increase the tendency to develop stones. Since less than 40% of all gouty patients are urinary overexcretors of uric acid, a normal excretion level does not exclude the diagnosis. On a purine-free diet, the mean daily excretion should not exceed 600 mg. In patients on an average normal daily diet, the daily uric acid excretion should not exceed 900 mg.

RHEUMATOID FACTORS

Abnormal proteins are found in the sera of many patients with rheumatoid arthritis. These circulating proteins, heterogeneous in type, have been classified as antibodies on the basis of their physical, chemical and behavioral characteristics. They have been named rheumatoid factors because they were first described in rheumatoid arthritis. Most rheumatoid factors are the IgM (19S macroglobulin) type. Less commonly, rheumatoid factors are the IgG or IgA variety. In the test tube, rheumatoid factor reacts with IgG (7S) gamma globulin. This reaction is the basis of most tests for rheumatoid factor. The technique most commonly used to identify the presence of rheumatoid factor uses agglutination of latex particles to demonstrate that the rheumatoid factor–IgG interaction has occurred. Specifically, latex particles are coated with IgG, which has been denatured to increase the sensitivity of the reaction. Sera to be tested are heated to eliminate prozone reactions, and then added to the suspension of globulin-coated latex particles. If rheumatoid factor is present, it will react with IgG and cause agglutination of the latex particles. The results can be observed macroscopically. The test for rheumatoid factor is considered positive if agglutination occurs in a serum dilution of 1:40 or higher. Rheumatoid factor is seen in approximately 40 to 50% of patients with rheumatoid arthritis during the early stages of the disease. In later stages, a positive rheumatoid factor test is seen in 80 to 90% of cases. Once present, the factor usually persists.

Although the presence of rheumatoid factor supports a diagnosis of rheumatoid arthritis, rheumatoid factor may be associated with many other disease states (Table 2-3).[15-24] In these other conditions, titers are usually low, but not always.

Table 2-3. Conditions Other than Rheumatoid Arthritis Associated with Rheumatoid Factor

---

Normal persons (2 to 4% of the population)
Relatives of rheumatoid arthritis patients
Aging (10 to 20% positive over age 65 years)[16]
Systemic lupus erythematosus
Scleroderma
Dermatomyositis
Sarcoidosis[17]
Leprosy
Dysproteinemias and paraproteinemias
Liver disease (infectious hepatitis, cirrhosis)
Syphilis
Idiopathic pulmonary fibrosis
Pneumoconiosis
Acute pulmonary tuberculosis[18]
Acute viral infections
Parasitic diseases
Following prophylactic vaccinations[19]
Subacute bacterial endocarditis[20]
Diabetes mellitus patients on insulin therapy[21]
Psychiatric disorders (schizophrenia, endogenous depression)[22]
Following multiple blood transfusions[23]
Parenteral narcotic addiction[24]

ANTINUCLEAR ANTIBODIES AND LE CELL STUDIES

· Antinuclear antibodies are abnormal circulating proteins that react with nuclei and with individual constituents of nuclei such as nucleoprotein, DNA and histone. Antinuclear antibodies are usually IgG (7S) in character, but IgM (19S) antibodies also occur. They are a heterogeneous group of antibodies with varying specificities for various nuclear constituents and for different sites on a particular nuclear constituent. To detect the presence of antinuclear antibody, the fluorescent antibody technique has been utilized. The test is performed as a two-stage procedure. The test serum is first applied to tissue sections containing nucleated cells. If antinuclear antibody is present, it will bind with the nuclei. Following this, fluorescein-labeled antiserum to human gamma globulin is applied to the cells. This anti-human gamma globulin will react with the antinuclear antibody and result in fluorescence of the nuclei. Patterns of localization of fluorescent stain may be helpful in diagnosis. Homogeneous patterns (Fig. 2-1) are least specific. A peripheral rim pattern (Fig. 2-2) suggests the presence of systemic lupus erythematosus. Staining of nucleoli or a speckled pattern suggests a diagnosis of scleroderma or Sjögren's syndrome. A speckled pattern also occurs in mixed connective tissue disease. Qualitative reactions overlap, however, and diagnoses made on this basis should be done with caution.

The anti-DNA antibody, one of the antinuclear antibodies, can be identified by complement fixation or agglutination reactions. It is more

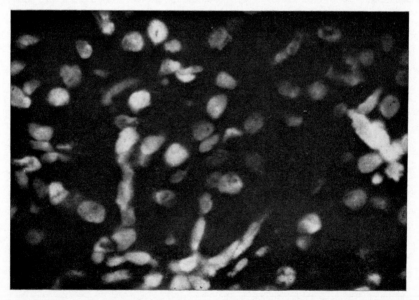

Figure 2-1. Antinuclear antibody, homogeneous stain. (Courtesy, the Arthritis Foundation)

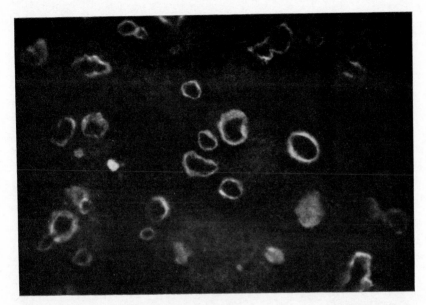

Figure 2-2. Antinuclear antibody, peripheral rim pattern. (Courtesy, the Arthritis Foundation)

specific for lupus and occurs less frequently and to much lower titer in other connective tissue diseases. The syndrome of mixed connective tissue disease, characterized by clinical features of systemic lupus erythematosus, polymyositis and scleroderma in the same patient, is associated with the presence of antibody to extractable nuclear antigen (ENA).

The LE cell test is based on an interaction between antinuclear antibody, nuclear material, and phagocytic white cells. The LE cell phenomenon results when antinuclear antibody (LE cell factor) reacts with nuclear material from damaged white cells. The nuclear material undergoes a change in structure, so that on staining it assumes a completely homogeneous ground-glass appearance and a basophilic color. This altered nuclear material (the hematoxylin body) is chemotactic for polymorphonuclear leukocytes, which proceed to surround the material in the form of rosettes (Figs. 2-3, 2-4). The nuclear material is then ingested by one of the polymorphonuclear leukocytes, in which it forms an inclusion body. The latter usually fills the cell and compresses the nucleus to the periphery (Fig. 2-3). At times, altered nuclear material will remain free (Fig. 2-4). When present, it has the same diagnostic significance as fully formed LE cells.

Since the LE cell reaction requires the presence of viable leukocytes, it may be negative in patients with severe leukopenia. LE cells must be differentiated from tart cells which result from ingestion of nuclear material by leukocytes as a normal phagocytic process.[25] In the latter cells,

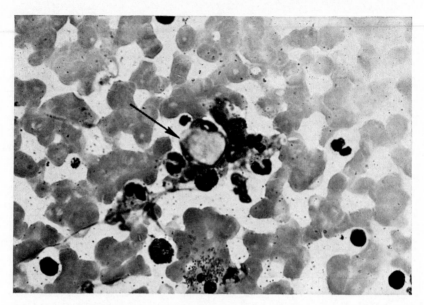

Figure 2-3.   LE cell (arrow) surrounded by polymorphonuclear leukocytes in form of rosette.

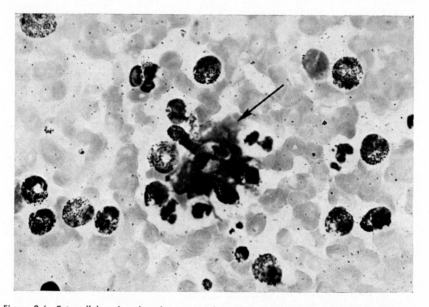

Figure 2-4. Extracellular altered nuclear material (arrow), with beginning rosette formation.

Table 2-4. Conditions Other than Systemic Lupus Erythematosus (SLE) Associated with Antinuclear Antibodies

---

Other connective tissue diseases (rheumatoid arthritis, scleroderma, dermatomyositis)

Sjögren's syndrome

Relatives of patients with SLE

Aging (antinuclear antibodies seen in up to 25% of normal females over 60 years; anti-DNA and LE cell studies normal)[26]

Chronic liver disease, infectious hepatitis

Idiopathic pulmonary fibrosis[27]

Pneumoconiosis[28]

Drug-related SLE (certain drugs may induce formation of antinuclear antibodies and a clinical syndrome similar to spontaneously occurring SLE):

    Hydralazine[29]
    Procainamide[30]
    Isoniazid[31]
    Anticonvulsant drugs (e.g., diphenylhydantoin, mephenytoin, trimethadione)[32]
    Antibiotics (penicillin, sulfonamides, tetracycline)
    Propylthiouracil[33]
    Methyl dopa[34]
    Oral contraceptive pills[35]
    Phenothiazines[36]
    D-penicillamine[37]
    Quinidine[38]
    Clofibrate[39]
    Oxyphenisatin[40]
    Griseofulvin

---

the chromatin structure of the enclosed nuclear material retains its fine fibrillar pattern.

Antinuclear antibodies are present in almost all patients with acute active systemic lupus erythematosus. In patients with subacute or chronic disease, the antibodies may be absent or present only in low titer. Anti-DNA antibody parallels lupus disease activity more closely than other antinuclear antibodies. More specific for lupus, it rarely occurs in other connective tissue diseases. It is particularly likely to be elevated in lupus patients with active nephritis. LE cells are seen in up to 80 to 85% of patients with systemic lupus erythematosus. They are more likely to be seen with acute disease activity and may completely disappear during disease remissions.

Although antinuclear antibodies are seen most frequently and to highest titer in systemic lupus erythematosus, they are associated with a number of other disease states (Table 2-4).[26–40]

SKIN BIOPSY

Routine histopathologic study of material obtained on skin biopsy is helpful in the diagnosis of a number of rheumatic disorders, such as sys-

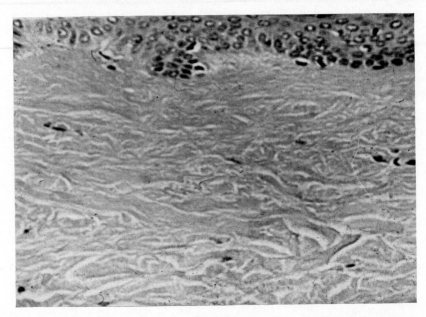

Figure 2-5. Skin biopsy, scleroderma. Characteristic changes include thinning of the epidermis, loss of rete pegs, atrophy of dermal appendages, and a marked increase in dermal collagen. (Hematoxylin and eosin) (Courtesy, Dr. A. Mackenzie)

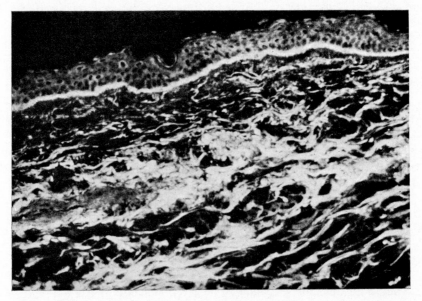

Figure 2-6. Skin, systemic lupus erythematosus. A band of immunofluorescence appears at the epidermal-dermal junction. (Courtesy, the Arthritis Foundation)

temic lupus erythematosus, scleroderma (Fig. 2-5), vasculitis, sarcoid arthritis and psoriatic arthropathy. Specimens for study can be obtained readily by use of a punch biopsy needle under local anesthesia. Further aid in differential diagnosis can be obtained by immunofluorescent staining techniques to identify immunoglobulins and complement in the area of the basement membrane at the epidermal-dermal junction.[41] The immunoglobulin deposits may be either antinuclear antibody or antibasement membrane antibody. Immunofluorescent study requires the use of skin that has been frozen rather than fixed, or that has been preserved in a special solution.[42] The skin sample is placed on a glass slide, over which is placed a solution containing fluorescein-labeled anti-human gamma globulin antibody. Positive tests reveal a band of immunofluoresence at the epidermal-dermal junction (Fig. 2-6). A positive reaction is seen in 90 to 95% of biopsies taken from the site of clinical rash in patients with systemic lupus erythematosus. A positive test occurs in 60% of SLE patients in biopsies from normal skin. In patients with chronic discoid lupus, a positive reaction occurs similarly in 85% of patients when areas of clinical involvement are studied. Normal skin, however, yields negative findings. Basement membrane immunofluorescence occurs in only a few other diseases, including bullous pemphigoid and lepromatous leprosy.

COMPLEMENT

The complement system consists of at least nine discrete protein substances (C1 to C9), and is related to both the immune and inflammatory mechanisms. Although the system was described classically as being activated by antigen-antibody complexes at the C1 site, more recent studies have demonstrated that later components may be directly activated. Changes in serum complement level are seen in certain connective tissue diseases and their study is helpful both in diagnosis and in evaluation of disease activity. Low serum complement levels are characteristic of active systemic lupus erythematosus, particularly when lupus glomerulonephritis is present. Low serum complement levels occur sometimes in patients with rheumatoid arthritis when the titer of serum rheumatoid factor is high.[43]

Techniques for determining the complement level vary. Most frequently, the whole hemolytic complement activity, CH^{50}, is measured. The result reflects the interaction of all nine components of the system. Specific components of the complement system can also be determined; they may be selectively abnormal in the presence of a normal total complement. Synovial fluid complement has some value in differential diagnosis. Low synovial fluid complement levels occur in systemic lupus erythematosus. In rheumatoid arthritis, synovial fluid complement levels are low, normal or slightly elevated. Synovial fluid complement is characteristically elevated in many patients with Reiter's syndrome.

SEROLOGIC TEST FOR SYPHILIS

Serologic studies for syphilis have some diagnostic value, because a false positive serologic test for syphilis (STS) is seen in as many as 10 to 15% of patients with various forms of connective tissue disease.[44] A false positive test is most often associated with systemic lupus erythematosus, but it also occurs in the presence of rheumatoid arthritis, scleroderma and sarcoidosis. The routine serologic test for syphilis (STS) is performed first. If positive, the fluorescent treponema antibody absorbed test (FTA-ABS) should be carried out. A negative FTA-ABS study excludes the presence of luetic infection in almost all cases. A positive study characterized by a *uniform treponemal fluorescence* indicates syphilis in all but rare instances. Positive fluorescence may be seen in patients with rheumatoid arthritis and systemic lupus erythematosus but the treponemal fluorescence in these connective tissue disorders has a *nonuniform beaded pattern.*[45] The treponema pallidum immobilization test (TPI) is utilized when the interpretation is still in doubt. This latter test, though more costly and difficult to perform, is highly specific for treponemal disease.

In some patients, a positive STS is noted by chance as part of the routine physical examination of otherwise healthy persons. If follow-up studies reveal a false positive test, the patient should be carefully evaluated for clinical evidence of one of the connective tissue diseases. Further studies helpful in clarifying the issue include a white blood cell count and differential cell count, hematocrit, urinalysis, erythrocyte sedimentation rate, serum studies for rheumatoid factor and antinuclear antibodies, LE cell determination, and serum protein electrophoresis. If all findings are negative, the clinical examination and laboratory studies should be repeated at periodic intervals. The underlying systemic disease, if present, may take years to become apparent.

DIAGNOSTIC STUDIES FOR MUSCLE DISEASE

Serum Muscle Enzymes

Measurement of serum muscle enzymes is important in the diagnosis of muscle disorders.[46,47] Elevated values commonly occur in the primary myopathies, but are unusual in neurogenic atrophy. In the latter, elevations when present are usually mild. The three serum muscle serum enzymes most commonly employed for study are serum glutamic oxaloacetic transaminase (SGOT), aldolase and creatine phosphokinase (CPK). Although all three enzymes may be elevated simultaneously in patients with primary myopathy, elevation of only one or two enzymes is not uncommon. Thus, diagnostic accuracy is enhanced if all three enzymes are routinely studied.

The CPK is the most sensitive and SGOT the least sensitive determination. CPK is the most specific for muscle disease, but all may be elevated by a number of causes.[48-53] The SGOT is increased in patients with myocardial disease or hepatic cell breakdown. Serum aldolase may be elevated if hepatic cell damage is present. In addition, a rise in serum aldolase occurs in the presence of a hemolytic anemia or if a hemolyzed blood specimen is sent to the laboratory, due to enzyme release from erythrocytes. CPK elevations occur in the presence of myocardial disease and following frequent intramuscular injections,[48] and it may be significantly elevated following prolonged strenuous exercise.[49] Elevated blood levels have been noted in association with strokes and subarachnoid hemorrhage.[50] Elevated levels have been described in patients with acute psychosis.[51] Other nonmyopathic causes of a rise in serum CPK include pulmonary infarction and acute pneumonia. Patients with hypoparathyroidism may have elevated CPK levels,[52] even in the absence of overt muscle symptoms. Finally, elevated levels of CPK may be associated with large muscle mass in heavy-framed normal individuals.[53] Recent techniques capable of measuring CPK isoenzymes produced by different tissues will allow more accurate utilization of this study as a diagnostic procedure.

Elevation of these enzymes occurs as a result of either the release of enzyme from degenerating muscle fibers or the escape of enzymes from muscle with increased membrane permeability. Although elevated levels support a diagnosis of myopathy, normal levels may occur in the presence of active muscle disease.

Creatine-Creatinine Ratio

Creatine is formed primarily in the liver and is converted into creatinine by muscle. In the presence of muscle disease, creatine conversion decreases and its urinary excretion subsequently increases. In studies of the creatine-creatinine ratio, the 24-hour urinary creatinine excretion is first determined. Urinary creatine is then converted to creatinine and the analysis repeated. The resulting value represents total urinary creatine plus creatinine. The original creatinine value is subtracted from the total to provide an absolute measure of creatine excreted. The creatine value divided by total creatine plus creatinine yields percent creatinuria:

$$\% \text{ Creatinuria} = \frac{\text{creatine (mg/24 hrs)}}{[\text{creatine} + \text{creatinine}] \text{ (mg/24 hrs)}} \times 100$$

The values for percent creatinuria in both males and females should not exceed 6%. Excretion is somewhat higher in pregnant females. Children have a physiologic creatinuria, with values up to 40% at age three years, 20% at age eight years, and normal adult values at age 15. Patients on androgen therapy may demonstrate an elevated excretion of urinary creatine due to stimulation of creatine formation in the liver. Two 24-hour urine determinations of creatine-creatinine ratio should be obtained routinely in order to confirm results and also because slight variations in the amount of creatinine excreted occur from day-to-day. The two daily values should not vary by more than 10% if accurate urine collections have been obtained. Creatine-creatinine ratios are increased not only in primary myopathies but also in disuse and neurogenic atrophy. Elevations generally appear earlier in the primary myopathies. The study is valuable not only as a diagnostic tool, but also in disease follow-up during therapy.

Electromyogram

The electromyogram is utilized to study the electrical activity of skeletal muscle. Abnormalities appear both in primary myopathic disorders and in neurogenic atrophy. In patients with primary myopathy, the size of the individual motor unit potentials associated with voluntary contraction is decreased, and a relative increase occurs in the number and rate of firing. Polyphasic potentials of decreased size and short duration are characteristic. In lower motor neuron disease, the number and rate of unit firings are decreased. Low-voltage, long-duration polyphasic potentials during voluntary contraction are characteristic. Fibrillations at rest, although sometimes seen in myopathies, are most often associated with neurogenic atrophy. Electromyography is helpful not only in diagnosis but also in defining involved muscles most likely to provide positive biopsy results.

Muscle Biopsy

Muscle biopsy studies are important in the diagnosis of muscle disorders. These studies are most likely to provide informative findings if performed on muscles that demonstrate involvement either by clinical symptoms or by positive electromyographic study. The physician should direct the surgeon to the specific muscle desired for biopsy and the surgeon should be well-trained in the proper handling of the muscle specimen. All too often, specimens are so damaged in handling that a proper pathologic analysis of the tissue cannot be made. Frozen sections and sections fixed in formaldehyde should be obtained. Frozen sections are utilized for detailed enzymatic studies. Electron microscopic examination is valuable when one of the more unusual disorders is suspected.

ROENTGENOLOGIC EXAMINATION

Roentgenologic examination of the joints is an important aid in differential diagnosis. In addition, it is valuable in the study of disease progress.

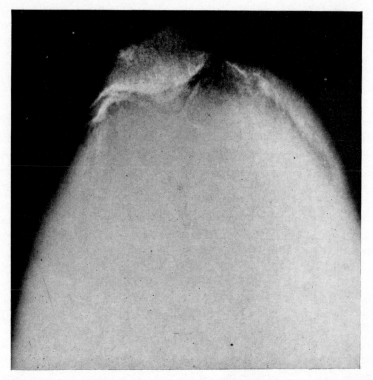

Figure 2-7. Skyline view, patellofemoral joint. Joint space narrowing and spur formation clearly show in this patient with degenerative joint disease.

Views other than the usual PA and lateral may be necessary to delineate subtle abnormalities. For example, skyline views of the knee will show pathologic changes in the patellofemoral joint more clearly than routine views (Fig. 2-7). Tunnel views taken with the knee in flexion outline abnormalities of intra-articular joint structure more clearly. Special techniques, such as spot films, laminograms, cineradiograms and myelograms, should be used when indicated. Cervical and lumbosacral spine studies require PA, lateral and oblique views for complete examination. Chest x-rays should be obtained from patients with any type of systemic disorder. X-rays of other areas such as the gastrointestinal tract and kidneys should be ordered as the clinical picture dictates.

RADIOISOTOPE SCAN

Although not used in routine diagnosis, radioactive isotope scans are sometimes useful.[54,55] They have been used to demonstrate the presence of early inflammation in symptomatic joints that are negative to objective clinical examination. Bone scans are especially useful when metastatic bone disease is suspected but not otherwise proved. Technetium scans of the parotid glands aid diagnosis in patients with suspected Sjögren's syndrome.

ARTHROGRAMS

Roentgenologic examination of joints following the instillation of contrast material, or air plus contrast material, helps to delineate a number of joint disorders. These procedures are particularly useful in the diagnosis of tears of the meniscus or capsule of the knee, and in the demonstration of synovial cysts (Fig. 2-8). Ruptures of the rotator cuff of the shoulder can often be delineated. Double contrast arthrograms with air and contrast media generally provide more information than those using contrast media alone. False positive or false negative interpretations are not uncommon, especially in inexperienced hands.

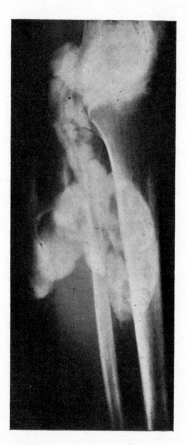

Figure 2-8. Arthrogram of knee. A large popliteal cyst extends well into the calf.

SYNOVIAL BIOPSY

Synovial biopsy has its greatest value in the differential diagnosis of monoarticular or oligoarticular arthritis. In patients with more diffuse articular disease, the biopsy is likely to be nonspecific and less helpful, due to similarities in pathologic findings in these disorders. Special needles for closed synovial biopsy are available; their use is attended with minimal morbidity and complications. The knee is the most commonly biopsied joint because it lends itself easiest to this procedure. Closed biopsy should be strongly considered before open biopsy whenever possible. The Parker-Pearson needle (Fig. 2-9, A) is the smallest needle available and is usually utilized first. The Polley-Bickel needle (Fig. 2-9, B), a large-bore needle, requires a small skin incision and suture. It may be used initially or for repeat biopsy if the material obtained with the Parker-Pearson needle is inadequate. Strict adherence to aseptic technique is vital. Syno-

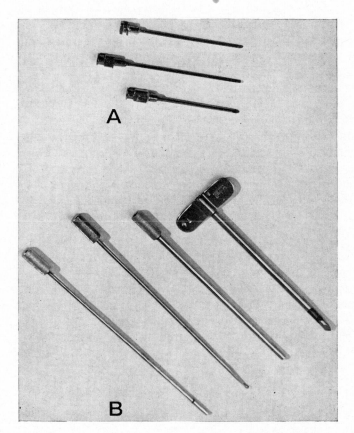

Figure 2-9. Synovial biopsy needles. (A) Components of Parker-Pearson needle. (B) Components of Polley-Bickel needle.

vial fluid is removed for analysis at the time of biopsy. Sufficient local anesthesia with 1% lidocaine is important to prevent discomfort. In addition, it is helpful to give meperidine, 50 to 75 mg IM, 20 to 30 minutes before biopsy. Specimens are obtained for culture and pathologic study. Tissue is taken from a number of sites to avoid missing localized isolated lesions. Following the biopsy, a compression bandage is placed around the knee and the patient is cautioned to avoid activity other than going to the bathroom or sitting quietly in a chair. Analgesics are prescribed to relieve postbiopsy pain. After a period of 24 hours, the compression bandage is removed and the patient may resume normal ambulation. Biopsy can be performed as an outpatient procedure when appropriate facilities are available. Complications of biopsy include infection and hemorrhage. These are rare when close attention to proper technique is carried out.

ARTHROSCOPY

Intra-articular examination can be performed by inserting an arthroscope through a small joint incision. The instrument is similar to instruments utilized for cystoscopy. The technique has advanced over the past decade to the point where it is a useful procedure in experienced hands. Studies thus far have been limited mostly to the knee, which lends itself best to this procedure on the basis of size and accessibility. Inspection of joint morphology, biopsy of synovium or cartilage and, if feasible, removal of loose bodies can be performed. The procedure is done in a regular operating room under spinal or general anesthesia. Diagnostic information obtained with this technique may prevent the need for exploratory arthrotomy in some patients. On the other hand, although postoperative morbidity is greater, open arthrotomy is still preferred by many because it allows the opportunity for more definitive treatment as well as diagnosis.

THERMOGRAPHY

Thermography, which measures external joint temperatures, can be used to assess joint involvement in inflammatory arthritis.[56] It is useful in defining the presence of inflammation in minimally involved joints and in quantitating response to therapy. Close control of ambient temperature is essential for accurate serial readings. Although it is an interesting diagnostic technique, facilities for its use are not generally available.

REFERENCES

1. Postlethwaite, A. E., Bartel, A. G. and Kelley, W. N.: Hyperuricemia due to ethambutol. N Eng J Med 286:761, 1972.
2. Honda, H. and Gindin, R. A.: Gout while receiving levodopa for Parkinsonism. JAMA 219:55, 1972.
3. Ball, G. V. and Morgan, J. B.: Chronic lead ingestion and gout. Southern Med J 61:21, 1968.

4. Alepa, F. P., Howell, R. R., Klinenberg, J. R. and Seegmiller, J. E.: Relationships between glycogen storage disease and tophaceous gout. Am J Med 42: 58, 1967.
5. Cannon, P. J. et al.: Hyperuricemia in primary and renal hypertension. N Eng J Med 275:457, 1966.
6. Itskovitz, H. D. and Sellers, A. M.: Gout and hyperuricemia after adrenalectomy for hypertension. N Eng J Med 268:1105, 1963.
7. Mintz, D. H. et al.: Hyperuricemia in hyperparathyroidism. N Eng J Med 265: 112, 1961.
8. Kirschner, D.: Hyperuricemia in hypoparathyroidism. Metabolism 5:703, 1956.
9. Leeper, R. D. et al.: Hyperuricemia in myxedema. J Clin Endocrinology 20: 1457, 1960.
10. Franck, W. A. et al.: Rheumatic manifestations of Paget's disease of bone. Am J Med 56:592, 1974.
11. Postlethwaite, A. E. and Kelley, W. N.: Uricosuric effect of radiocontrast agents. Ann Int Med 74:845, 1971.
12. Bishop, C., Zimdahl, W. J. and Talbott, J. H.: Uric acid in two patients with Wilson's disease (hepatolenticular degeneration). Proc Soc Exp Biol Med 86: 440, 1954.
13. Cooper, D. S.: Oat-cell carcinoma and severe hypouricemia. N Eng J Med 288:321, 1973.
14. Bennett, J. S. et al.: Hypouricemia in Hodgkin's disease. Ann Int Med 76:751, 1972.
15. Bartfeld, H.: Distribution of rheumatoid factor activity in nonrheumatoid states. Ann N Y Acad Sci 168:30, 1969.
16. Moskowitz, R. W., Benedict, K. J. and Stouffer, R.: Serum antibodies to gamma globulin: inter-relationships of aging, disease and geography. J Chron Dis 20:291, 1967.
17. Oreskes, I. and Siltzbach, L. E.: Changes in rheumatoid factor activity during the course of sarcoidosis. Am J Med 44:60, 1968.
18. Singer, J. M. et al.: Presence of antigamma globulin factors in sera of patients with active pulmonary tuberculosis. Ann Int Med 56:545, 1962.
19. Aho, K. et al.: Transient appearance of the rheumatoid factor in connection with prophylactic vaccinations. Acta Path Microbiol Scan 56:478, 1962.
20. Williams, R. C., Jr. and Kunkel, H. G.: Rheumatoid factor, complement, and conglutinin aberrations in patients with subacute bacterial endocarditis. J Clin Invest 41:666, 1962.
21. Oreskes, I. and Spiera, H.: Diabetes and rheumatoid factor. Ann Rheum Dis 32:431, 1973.
22. Oreskes, I. et al.: Rheumatoid factors in an acute psychiatric population. Ann Rheum Dis 27:60, 1968.
23. Vierucci, A.: Gm groups and anti-Gm antibodies in children with Cooley's anemia. Vox Sang 10:82, 1965.
24. Spiera, H., Oreskes, I. and Stimmel, B.: Rheumatoid factor activity in heroin addicts on methadone maintenance. Ann Rheum Dis 33:153, 1974.
25. Hargraves, M. M., Richmond, H. and Morton, R.: Presentation of two bone marrow elements. The "tart" cell and the "LE" cell. Mayo Clin Proc, 1948.
26. Svec, K. H. and Veit, B. C.: Age-related antinuclear factors: Immunologic characteristics and associated clinical aspects. Arth Rheum 10:509, 1967.
27. Nagayo, H., Buckley, E. and Sieker, H. D.: Positive antinuclear factor in patients with unexplained pulmonary fibrosis. Ann Int Med 70:1135, 1969.
28. Kang, K. Y., Yagura, T. and Yamamura, Y.: Antinuclear factor in pneumoconioses. N Eng J Med 288:164, 1973.
29. Hahn, B. H. et al.: Immune responses to hydralazine and nuclear antigens in hydralazine induced lupus erythematosus. Ann Int Med 76:365, 1972.
30. Blomgren, S. E., Condemi, J. J. and Vaughan, J. H.: Procainamide-induced lupus erythematosus. Am J Med 52:338, 1972.

31. Cannat, A. and Seligmann, M.: Possible induction of antinuclear antibodies by isoniazid. Lancet 1:185, 1966.
32. Jacobs, J. C.: Systemic lupus erythematosus in childhood. Report of 35 cases with discussion of seven apparently induced by anticonvulsant medication and of prognosis and treatment. Pediatrics 32:257, 1963.
33. Amrhein, J. A., Kenny, F. M. and Ross, D.: Granulocytopenia, lupus-like syndrome, and other complications of propylthiouracil therapy. J Pediatr 76:54, 1970.
34. Sherman, J. D., Lover, D. W. and Harrington, J. F.: Anemia, positive lupus and rheumatoid factors with methyldopa. Arch Int Med 120:321, 1967.
35. Bole, G. G., Friedlander, M. H. and Smith, C. K.: Rheumatic symptoms and serological abnormalities induced by oral contraceptives. Lancet 1:323, 1969.
36. Fabius, A. J. M. and Gaulhofer, W. K.: Systemic lupus erythematosus induced by psychotropic drugs. Acta Rheum Scand 17:137, 1971.
37. Harpey, J. P. et al.: Lupus-like syndrome induced by D-penicillamine in Wilson's disease. Lancet 1:292, 1971.
38. Kendall, M. J. and Hawkins, C. F.: Quinidine-induced systemic lupus erythematosus. Postgrad Med J 46:729, 1970.
39. Howard, E. J. and Brown, S. M.: Clofibrate-induced antinuclear factor and lupus-like syndrome. JAMA 226:1358, 1973.
40. Reynolds, T. B. et al.: Chronic active and lupoid hepatitis caused by a laxative, oxyphenisatin. N Eng J Med 285:813, 1971.
41. Grossman, J., Callerame, M. L. and Condemi, J. J.: Skin immunofluorescence studies on lupus erythematosus and other antinuclear-antibody positive diseases. Ann Int Med 80:496, 1974.
42. Michel, B., Milner, Y. and David, K.: Preservation of tissue-fixed immunoglobulins in skin biopsies of patients with lupus erythematosus and bullous diseases—a preliminary report. J Invest Derm 59:449, 1973.
43. Franco, A. E. and Schur, P. H.: Hypocomplementemia in rheumatoid arthritis. Arth Rheum 14:231, 1971.
44. Tuffanelli, D. L.: False positive reactions for syphilis. Arch Derm 98:606, 1968.
45. McKenna, C. H. et al.: The fluorescent treponemal antibody absorbed (FTA-ABS) test beading phenomenon in connective tissue diseases. Mayo Clin Proc 48:545, 1973.
46. Vignos, P. J. and Goldwyn, J.: Evaluation of laboratory tests in diagnosis and management of polymyositis. Am J Med Sci 263:291, 1972.
47. Munsat, T. L. et al.: Serum enzyme alterations in neuromuscular disorders. JAMA 226:1536, 1973.
48. Cacace, L.: Elevated serum CPK after drug injections. N Eng J Med 287:309, 1972.
49. Demos, M. A. and Gitin, E. L.: Acute exertional rhabdomyolysis. Arch Int Med 133:233, 1974.
50. Schiavone, D. J. and Kaldor, J.: Serum CPK in brain damage. N Eng J Med 285:753, 1971.
51. Alias, A. G.: Serum transaminase and alkaline phosphatase in schizophrenia. Biological Psychiatry 4:89, 1972.
52. Hower, J. et al.: CPK activity in hypoparathyroidism. N Eng J Med 287:1098, 1972.
53. Garcia, W.: Elevated creatine phosphokinase levels associated with large muscle mass. JAMA 228:1395, 1974.
54. McCarty, D. J., Polcyn, R. E. and Collins, P. A.: [99m]Technetium scintiphotography in arthritis. II. Its nonspecificity and clinical and roentgenographic correlations in RA. Arth Rheum 13:21, 1970.
55. Dick, W. C.: The use of radioisotopes in normal and diseased joints. Seminars in Arth and Rheum 1:301, 1972.
56. Collins, A. J. et al.: Quantitation of thermography in arthritis using multi-isothermal analysis. Ann Rheum Dis 33:113, 1974.

Chapter 3

SYNOVIAL FLUID ANALYSIS

Synovial fluid analysis in the diagnosis of connective tissue disease should be considered equivalent to the use of urinalysis in the study of kidney disease. Studies may prove diagnostically specific as, for example, in septic or crystal-induced arthritis. In other cases, findings may be nonspecific but

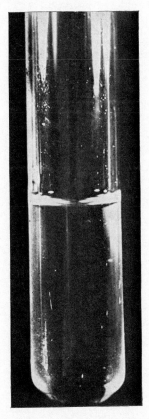

Figure 3-1. Normal synovial fluid. (Courtesy, Dr. R. Gatter)

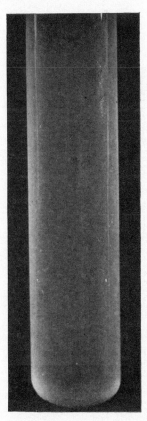

Figure 3-2. Synovial fluid, rheumatoid arthritis. The fluid is slightly cloudy. (Courtesy, Dr. R. Gatter)

are still valuable in differentiating noninflammatory joint disease from inflammatory disorders. Complete examination of the fluid involves not only gross studies but also detailed microscopic, biochemical and bacteriologic evaluations.

GROSS ANALYSIS

Normal synovial fluid is a light yellow straw color and sufficiently clear that large print can be read through it (Fig. 3-1). Turbidity increases with inflammation (Figs. 3-2, 3-3). The presence of gross blood or xanthochromia suggests a possible diagnosis of fracture, capsular or ligamentous tears, tumor or blood dyscrasias. Bleeding may also be seen sometimes in patients with rheumatoid arthritis, osteoarthritis and pseudogout. Normal fluid has a high viscosity similar to that of motor oil. It flows slowly from an inverted test tube and, when placed between the fingers, can be spread apart several inches before the fluid stream ruptures. In the presence of inflammation, the fluid becomes less viscous and more watery.

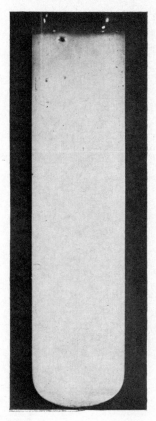

Figure 3-3. Synovial fluid, septic arthritis. The fluid is grossly purulent. (Courtesy, Dr. R. Gatter)

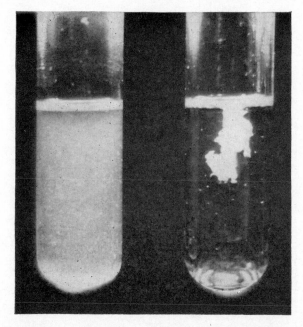

Figure 3-4. Mucin clot test. A tight ropy clot forms when glacial acetic acid is added to osteo-arthritic synovial fluid (right). In contrast, a flocculent precipitate forms when the acetic acid is added to rheumatoid synovial fluid (left). (Courtesy, Dr. R. Gatter)

When normal synovial fluid is mixed with glacial acetic acid, a tight ropy mucin clot, white in color, is formed (Fig. 3-4). In the presence of inflammation, the clot becomes friable and flocculent in increasing proportion to the degree of inflammation (Fig. 3-4).

DETAILED ANALYSIS

Detailed studies of synovial fluid involve a total leukocyte count, a differential white blood cell count, sugar and protein determinations, obtaining smears and culturing for organisms, and analysis for crystals (Table 3-1). The white cell count should be performed using saline as a diluent, because the usual white count diluent contains acetic acid, which will cause the synovial fluid to clot. The differential white blood cell count, performed after staining with Wright's stain, provides information about the relative number of monocytes and polymorphonuclear cells. Normally, the total leukocyte count is usually less than 200 cells per cubic mm, and the differential white cell count will reveal less than 25% polymorphonuclear cells. As inflammation increases, the total leukocyte count and percentage of polymorphonuclear cells progressively increase. Levels of 100,000 white cells per cubic mm with a differential count of 95% poly-

Table 3-1. Synovial Fluid Analysis in Arthritis

	Disease	Color	Clarity	Viscosity	Mucin Clot	WBC/mm^3	% Polys	Sugar	Protein	Crystals	Bacteria, Fungi
Normal (Fig. 3-1)		Yellow	Clear	High	Good	< 200	25	± 10% of blood	2 Gm%	0	0
Group 1 Noninflammatory	Osteoarthritis Traumatic arthritis	Yellow*	Clear	High	Good	< 2,000	25	± 10% of blood	2 Gm%	0	0
Group 2 Mild to moderate inflammation (Fig. 3-2)	Rheumatic fever Rheumatoid arthritis Systemic lupus erythematosus Tuberculous and fungal arthritis	Yellow	Slightly cloudy	Variably decreased	Variably decreased	5,000 to 30,000	50 to 80†	20 to 50% less than blood	2.5 to 3.5 Gm%	0	0 (Except in tuberculosis or fungal infection)
	Gout Pseudogout	Yellow to milky	Slightly cloudy to cloudy	Low	Poor	20,000 to 80,000	60 to 90	20 to 50% less than blood	2.5 to 3.5 Gm%	+	0
Group 3 Severe inflammation (Fig. 3-3)	Gonococcal arthritis Septic arthritis	Yellow to purulent	Turbid to purulent	Low	Poor	50,000 to >100,000‡	75 to 100	More than 50% less than blood	3.0 to 4.0 Gm%	0	+

* May be bloody to xanthochromic if traumatic.
† 30 to 50% in rheumatic fever.
‡ May be lower in mild or early infection.

morphonuclear cells are not unusual in septic arthritis. Somewhat lesser elevations are seen in patients with crystal-induced inflammation.

Synovial fluid sugar determination is diagnostically important, especially if septic arthritis is suspected. The normal synovial fluid sugar varies within ± 10% of the fasting blood sugar. Synovial fluid and blood specimens should be drawn at the same time and with the patient in a fasting state, because it requires approximately four to six hours for the blood and synovial fluid sugar to equilibrate after food intake. Synovial fluid aspiration and analysis should not be delayed, however, if the clinical situation dictates the need for more immediate evaluation of other diagnostic synovial fluid studies. A very low absolute value for synovial fluid sugar is diagnostically important regardless of when the specimen was obtained. Very low synovial fluid sugar values are characteristic of severe septic arthritis. However, low values may also occur in patients with chronic rheumatoid or tuberculous arthritis that has been present for a long period of time.

Normal synovial fluid protein varies between 1.5 and 2.5 Gm%. The value progressively increases in proportion to the degree of inflammation.

Obtaining smears and culturing for organisms should be routinely performed if infection is suspected. In patients in whom gonococcal infection is a consideration, the fluid should be plated immediately directly on blood agar and chocolate agar and taken at once to the laboratory for incubation. Repeated cultures of synovial fluid may be required for accurate diagnosis in any of the septic arthritides.

Analysis of synovial fluid for crystals is important in the diagnosis of gout and pseudogout. Initial studies are performed using an ordinary light microscope. Although studies may be performed immediately on undiluted fluid, it is preferable to add an anticoagulant so that the fluid can be re-examined later if necessary. Heparin, EDTA (ethylenediamine tetra-acetic acid) or sodium citrate in solution can be used for this purpose. Oxalate powder is to be avoided because it provides a confusing source of crystal contamination. One or two drops of synovial fluid are placed on a glass microscope slide that has been thoroughly washed with alcohol and dried to remove contaminating particulate matter. A similarly washed cover slip is placed on top of the fluid and the edges of the slip are sealed with nail polish or Permount. The use of a sealant keeps the preparation from drying while under observation and also prevents motion of the fluid field. The crystals can often be seen at a magnification of 100×, but the 430× magnification is usually required. In acute attacks of gout or pseudogout, crystals are generally numerous and both intracellular and extracellular in location. These findings, properly interpreted, establish a diagnosis of crystal-induced synovitis.

Initial identification of crystals can be made on the basis of morphology. Monosodium urate (MSU) crystals are linear and needle-shaped (Fig.

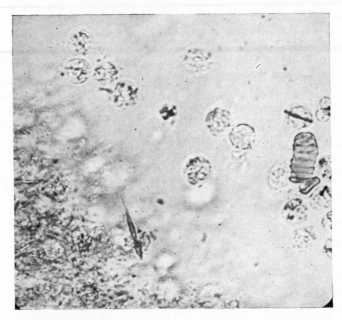

Figure 3-5. Linear and needle-shaped monosodium urate crystals in synovial fluid. (Courtesy, Dr. A. Mackenzie)

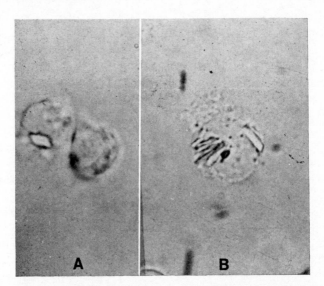

Figure 3-6. Calcium pyrophosphate dihydrate crystals. (A) Rhomboid crystal, light microscopy. (B) Linear and rhomboid crystals, compensated polarized light microscopy. The large crystal lying at right angles to the axis of slow vibration is yellow, in contrast to the blue color of the crystals lying parallel to the axis. (Courtesy, the Arthritis Foundation)

3-5). Calcium pyrophosphate crystals are linear or rhomboid (Fig. 3-6, A). The linear form of the latter crystal is rod-like with blunt ends, in contrast to the more sharply pointed ends of urate crystals. Although the morphologic characteristics seen with ordinary light microscopy are helpful in differentiating the two types of crystals, polarizing microscopy is required for more specific diagnosis.[1,2] MSU crystals are strongly birefringent, in contrast to calcium pyrophosphate crystals, which are weakly or nonbirefringent. More specific identification can be obtained by using a first-order red plate compensator in the polarizing system. With this technique, urate crystals exhibit a strong negative birefringence. The crystals appear yellow when lying parallel to the axis of the line of slow vibration of the compensator and blue when lying at right angles to it. Calcium pyrophosphate dihydrate (CPPD) crystals, on the other hand, are nonbirefringent or weakly positively birefringent. They appear blue when lying parallel to the axis of the line of slow vibration of the compensator, and yellow at right angles (Fig. 3-6, B). For practical purposes no further differential studies are usually necessary. Absolute identification of crystals requires more specialized techniques, such as x-ray or electron diffraction.

Crystals other than urates or calcium pyrophosphate may sometimes occur in synovial fluid. Calcium oxalate crystals may be present if oxalate anticoagulant has been used. Dusting powders of starch used on sterile rubber gloves may be a contaminant. These crystals are ovoid-shaped and strongly birefringent. Steroid crystals are seen in fluid from joints recently injected with corticosteroid preparations for therapeutic purposes.[3] The appearance of these crystals varies, depending on the agent used. Some are identical in appearance to MSU crystals. Cholesterol crystals are not uncommon in chronic effusions. They have a characteristically flat plate-like appearance with notched corners. Other crystal populations related to arthritis have been described. Occasional cases have demonstrated the presence of dicalcium phosphate dihydrate crystals. These are strongly birefringent in a positive direction. Strongly birefringent negatively-directed crystals have been described in the absence of gout.[4] The exact nature of these crystals has not yet been defined.

Some of the foregoing procedures for crystal identification can be performed in the physician's office with ordinary light microscopy. Studies of birefringence require polarizing disks, which are readily available and can simply be added to the ordinary microscope. Although a first-order red plate compensator requires a special microscope attachment, a reasonable substitute has been described that uses simple adhesive transparent cellophane tape.[2] One piece of tape is applied to the top of a glass slide, and then another piece of tape is applied over this. The cellophane-taped slide is placed over the polarizing disk and carefully rotated until the background is red. The long axis of the taped slide substitutes for the axis of

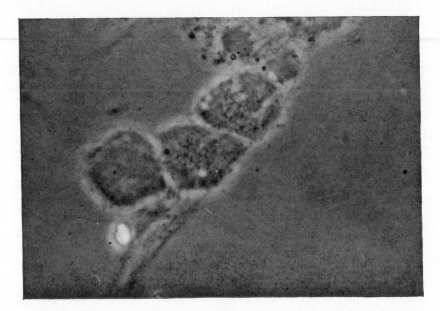

Figure 3-7. "RA cells," with protein inclusion bodies. (Courtesy, Dr. R. Gatter)

slow vibration of the first-order red plate compensator. Not all adhesive cellophane tape is equally effective and trials with various positions of tape may be required.

In addition to crystals, microscopic analysis may reveal protein inclusion bodies in the cytoplasm of polymorphonuclear cells (Fig. 3-7). These cells with their inclusions are called "RA cells," because they were first described in rheumatoid synovial effusions. Although they are seen most consistently and in highest number in rheumatoid arthritis, they are nonspecific and may occur in other rheumatologic disorders. Fragments of cartilage debris are not uncommonly observed during synovial fluid analysis. Although initially thought to be diagnostic of osteoarthritis, these fragments are a nonspecific finding associated with cartilage breakdown in many of the arthritides.

The presence of rheumatoid factor in synovial fluid tends to parallel positive findings in serum. Its presence in synovial fluid has limited diagnostic value, however, because a positive test may be seen in other rheumatic disorders.[5] Synovial fluid complement determinations may provide some help in differential diagnosis. Low levels occur in systemic lupus erythematosus. Levels are characteristically high in many patients with Reiter's syndrome. In rheumatoid arthritis, synovial fluid complement is low, normal or slightly elevated.

REFERENCES

1. Gatter, R. A.: The compensated polarized light microscope in clinical rheumatology. Arth Rheum 17:253, 1974.
2. Fagan, T. J. and Lidsky, M. D.: Compensated polarized light microscopy using cellophane adhesive tape. Arth Rheum 17:256, 1974.
3. Kahn, C., Hollander, J. and Schumacher, R.: Corticosteroid crystals in synovial fluid. JAMA 211:607, 1970.
4. Moskowitz, R. W. and Katz, D.: Chondrocalcinosis and chondrocalsynovitis (pseudogout syndrome). Am J Med 43:322, 1967.
5. Huskisson, E. C., Hart, F. D. and Lacey, B. W.: Synovial fluid Waaler-Rose and latex tests. Ann Rheum Dis 30:67, 1971.

Part II
CLINICAL PRESENTATIONS

Chapter 4

ACUTE MONOARTHRITIS

Acute monoarthritis is a common form of joint disease. This problem frequently represents a medical semiemergency because pain and swelling can be severe and disabling, and also because infection, a common cause of this symptom, can result in rapid destruction of the involved joint.

DIFFERENTIAL DIAGNOSIS

Most likely causes to be considered:
Septic (infectious) arthritis
Gonococcal arthritis
Osteomyelitis
Gout
Pseudogout
Trauma
Mechanical internal derangement
Hemorrhage
Episodic rheumatoid arthritis
Palindromic rheumatism
Intermittent hydrarthrosis
Migratory osteolysis

Septic (infectious) arthritis due to acute infection is the most threatening cause of acute monoarthritis.[1,2] Gram-positive organisms such as streptococcus, staphylococcus and pneumococcus are most frequently implicated in pathogenesis; gram-negative organisms such as the coliforms and salmonella are less frequently involved. Hemophilus influenzae is a common invader in infants and children up to age three years. Hematogenous spread from infections elsewhere, such as the skin, genitourinary tract and lungs, is the most common mechanism of infection. Septic arthritis may result, however, from direct spread of organisms from structures contiguous to the joint or by direct penetration of the joint itself. Joints that are already the site of prior disease, such as rheumatoid arthritis or osteoarthritis, are

3

particularly susceptible to secondary infection, much in the way that damaged heart valves are prone to develop subacute bacterial endocarditis. Septic arthritis is commonly seen in debilitated elderly patients, or in patients with chronic illness with low general resistance to infection. A diagnosis of septic arthritis should be strongly considered in patients with a disorder of the immune mechanism such as lymphoma and multiple myeloma. Clinically, large joints are more frequently involved. The joint becomes symptomatic over a relatively short period of time, usually measured in days. Pain, swelling, heat, redness and tenderness, the hallmarks of the inflammatory process, are present and increase in severity as the disease process advances.

Gonococcal arthritis, a form of septic arthritis, is discussed separately because it has characteristic clinical features not commonly seen in infectious arthritis due to other organisms.[3,4] Younger individuals are usually affected and a history of sexual exposure can often be obtained. In males, symptoms of urethritis are frequently present prior to or at the time arthritis develops. Interestingly, gonococcal arthritis is now more frequent in females than males, probably because genitourinary gonococcal infection in the male is usually more obvious clinically than in the female and therefore more likely to be treated before joint infection develops.

Gonococcal arthritis occurs in two major clinical forms, systemic and localized. The systemic form is characterized initially by polyarthritis, high fever, rash and general malaise. Later, joint symptoms may become localized to one joint with persistent acute inflammation (Fig. 4-1). This clinical sequence can be likened to a burlesque show, in which the chorus girls step forth and then return to the line one at a time, after which the star finally comes out and stays! Large joints are more frequently involved, although small joints may be affected. The rash, usually seen best on the extremities, is the result of either hematogenous spread of infection to the skin with infectious angiitis, or a systemic hypersensitivity reaction. It is most commonly characterized by pustulovesicular lesions that proceed to hemorrhage, ulcerate and crust (Fig. 4-1). Bullous lesions sometimes occur. The localized form of gonococcal arthritis is characterized by acute monoarthritis without the associated systemic manifestations just described. Prior involvement of other joints and cutaneous manifestations are absent; fever, if present, is low-grade. In both forms of the disease, tendonitis is common and most frequently involves the tendons over the dorsum of the hands and feet.

Acute osteomyelitis, an infection of the bony metaphysis, produces symptoms very much like those seen in septic arthritis and should be considered in the differential diagnosis of acute joint infection. A rapidly destructive disease, it occurs most frequently in infants and children. Although the infection may be initiated by introduction of bacteria from outside through a wound or from a neighboring infection of joints or soft tissues, hematog-

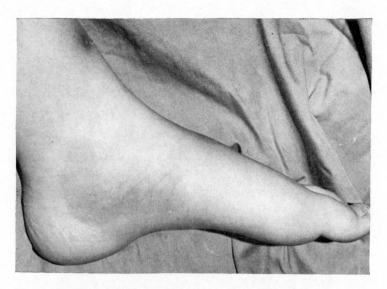

Figure 4-1. Acute gonococcal arthritis, left ankle. A typical pustulovesicular lesion of the skin appears in the lower tibial area. (Courtesy, Dr. F. Bishko)

enous spread from a focus elsewhere is the most common inciting cause. Staphylococcus aureus is the most frequent infecting organism. In the usual hematogenous type, infection begins in the metaphysis of a long bone, most commonly the tibia, femur or humerus. Bacteremia with septicemia are associated findings. Common constitutional manifestations include fever, chills, tachycardia, sweating and weakness. Locally, there is exquisite tenderness over the involved bone. The overlying skin is warm and the soft tissues are indurated. Laboratory studies reveal peripheral leukocytosis and an elevated erythrocyte sedimentation rate. Blood cultures are frequently positive. Roentgenograms may appear normal for several weeks. Later, bone destruction in the metaphysis is noted (Fig. 4-2). New bone formation is seen and the periosteum is elevated. Early diagnosis is important if severe bone destruction is to be avoided.

Most likely to be confused with monoarthritis of infectious origin are the crystal-induced arthritides, gout and pseudogout (chondrocalcinosis). *Gout* classically involves the metatarsophalangeal articulation of the great toes (podagra) (Fig. 4-3). Involvement of other areas, such as the tarsal joints, ankles (Fig. 4-3), and knees, is not uncommon, however. They may be the joints involved initially. Indeed, a significant number of patients may not show great toe involvement until after several years, if at all. Joint involvement is acute, often developing over a period of several hours. The average attack lasts three to five days, but prolonged symptoms lasting as long as several weeks may be present if the attack is untreated. The attack is related to precipitation of monosodium urate crystals with

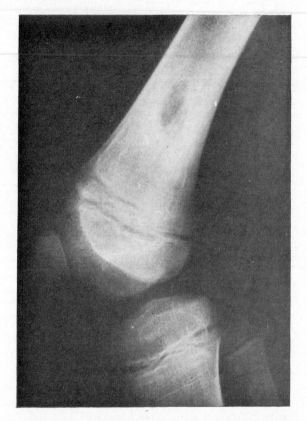

Figure 4-2. Acute osteomyelitis, femur. Bony destruction appears as a radiolucent area in the metaphysis. (Courtesy, Dr. V. Goldberg)

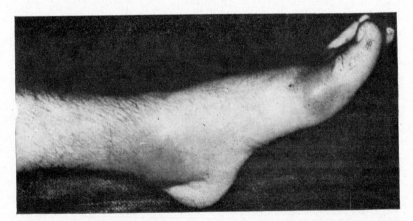

Figure 4-3. Acute gouty arthritis. Acute inflammation of the first metatarsophalangeal joint. Acute gouty arthritis of the ankle was also present. (Courtesy, the Arthritis Foundation)

subsequent release of inflammatory mediators. Although an elevated serum uric acid is a characteristic finding in patients with acute gouty arthritis, normal levels may be seen in the initial stages of the disease. In some patients, elevated levels are noted only if the serum for study is drawn during the height of the acute attack. In other patients, for unexplained reasons, serum uric acid is normal during acute attacks, with elevations occurring during asymptomatic interval periods.[5]

Pseudogout, also known as chondrocalcinosis or CPPD (calcium pyrophosphate deposition disease), is also characterized by an inflammatory synovitis induced in response to deposition of crystals.[6,7] In this disorder, calcium pyrophosphate dihydrate crystals are deposited in articular hyaline and fibrocartilage and synovium, in contrast to urate crystal deposits in true gout. Symptoms are most frequently characterized by acute attacks; however, subacute and chronic symptoms characterized by low grade arthralgia or persistent swelling may occur. The knees are the most frequently involved joints; podagra has been noted only infrequently. Other joints may be involved, including the wrists, elbows, shoulders and ankles. Joint involvement may be monoarticular or polyarticular. Radiologic examination reveals characteristic calcifications in articular hyaline and fibrocartilage, which are seen with highest frequency in the knees (Fig. 4-4) and the wrists (Fig. 4-5). Although symptoms and roentgenographic evidence of joint cartilage calcification frequently correlate, joint calcification may occur without symptoms. Conversely, symptoms may be present in the ab-

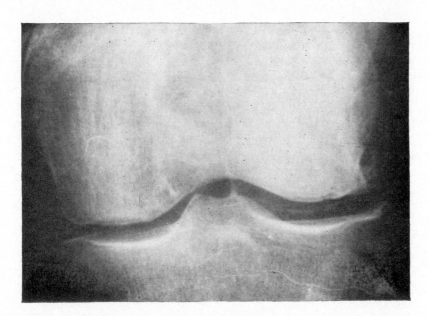

Figure 4-4. Knee, pseudogout syndrome. Meniscal calcification.

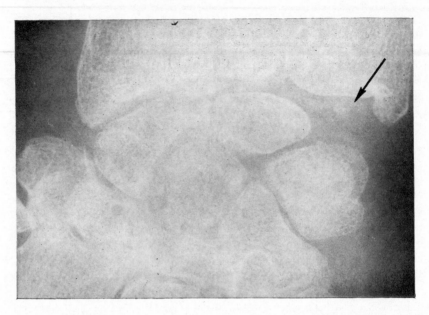

Figure 4-5. Wrist, pseudogout syndrome. Note calcification of triangular cartilage at ulnar-carpal articulation (arrow).

sence of calcification on routine radiologic examination. In such cases, a diagnosis of pseudogout depends on finding calcium pyrophosphate crystals in synovial fluid or in synovial tissue at biopsy.

In most patients, pseudogout syndrome is idiopathic. However, pseudogout has been described in association with other disorders, including hyperparathyroidism, hemochromatosis, Wilson's disease, gout and chronic renal disease. It has been suggested that inhibition of pyrophosphatase by calcium, ferrous and cupric ions may be related to the development of pseudogout in patients with hyperparathyroidism, hemochromatosis, and Wilson's disease respectively. Studies for serum calcium, phosphorus and alkaline phosphatase, serum uric acid, and serum iron studies should be performed in all patients with this syndrome.

Acute trauma may cause acute joint swelling, with or without associated hemarthrosis. Pain, swelling and tenderness follow the trauma almost immediately. This is in contrast to the relationship of trauma to the precipitation of acute attacks of gout. In the latter situation, joint symptoms are usually delayed by six to 12 hours following injury, and the severity of joint manifestations is out of proportion to the extent of trauma itself. *Internal derangements of the knee,* such as tears of the menisci or cruciate ligaments, or loose bodies in the joint, are often associated with acute pain, swelling and limitation of motion. A history of trauma can often be elicited. The medial meniscus is most frequently involved and "locking" is common.

Fracture in the area of a joint may simulate acute inflammatory arthritis as a result of tissue reaction to hemorrhage and damaged bone. A misdiagnosis of septic or gouty arthritis in patients with a fracture near a joint line is not uncommon!

Acute hemorrhage into a joint produces severe pain and tenderness. In addition to obvious swelling and warmth, the joint may become ecchymotic due to release of blood pigments. Joint hemorrhage may occur in normal persons following severe trauma. Patients with blood dyscrasias frequently develop hemarthroses, either spontaneously or following mild trauma.[8] Joint neoplasms such as synovial hemangiomas or malignant tumors must be strongly considered in diagnosis and appropriately excluded in patients who develop hemarthrosis in the absence of trauma or a known bleeding diathesis. Bleeding into the joint is a common complication of pigmented villonodular synovitis, a joint disorder of unknown etiology. Joint fluid in this disease is grossly bloody, or, more frequently, xanthochromic, as a result of previous hemorrhage. Pathologic study reveals a villous synovitis which, on histologic examination, shows synovial inflammation, distended synovial cells laden with lipid deposits, multinucleated giant cells and deposits of hemosiderin. Monoarthritis is the most common form of presentation, although sometimes two or three joints may be involved simultaneously.

Rheumatoid arthritis may occur as episodic attacks of acute monoarthritis (*episodic rheumatoid arthritis*). The patient's history reveals acute attacks of joint pain and swelling that begin abruptly and rapidly progress. Pain, often excruciating, is the initial symptom, and is followed in several hours by joint swelling, heat and redness. Interestingly, the pain may decrease in intensity as swelling ensues. The overall attack lasts several days to a week, and is followed by complete resolution. Small joints of the hands and feet, as well as larger joints, are involved. As the disease progresses, acute attacks become more frequent and prolonged, and complete remission no longer occurs. At this point, chronic joint changes characteristic of rheumatoid arthritis are noted. A similar clinical presentation occurs in patients with *palindromic rheumatism.*[9] Acute attacks of joint pain and swelling are similar to those described in episodic rheumatoid arthritis. Para-articular attacks of painful erythematous swelling of soft tissues is a frequent associated finding. Transient intracutaneous and subcutaneous nodules are seen. Chronic joint symptoms never develop, which differentiates this entity from episodic rheumatoid arthritis.

Intermittent hydrarthrosis, another form of intermittent joint disease, is characterized by acute, relatively painless, joint swelling.[10] This disorder usually involves one or both knees, although other joints may be affected. Attacks usually last two to four days. A true periodicity is noted, with attacks occurring at intervals of several weeks to months with almost clockwork repetitiveness.

An unusual cause of acute monoarthritis is *migratory osteolysis* (regional migratory osteoporosis, transient osteoporosis of the hip).[11] Patients are usually middle-aged men, and the hip, knee or foot is most frequently involved. Pain is often severe. Roentgenograms may be normal in the first several weeks, but osteoporosis becomes readily apparent later. Symptoms are self-limited, with symptoms disappearing and roentgenologic findings returning to normal after several months. Subsequent attacks in the same or other joints are not uncommon.

Although the foregoing disorders will account for the majority of patients with acute monoarthritis, almost any arthritic disease may occur in such fashion. Thus, in some patients, acute monoarthritis may be the initial manifestation of systemic lupus erythematosus, ankylosing spondylitis, the arthritis of ulcerative colitis or regional enteritis, Reiter's syndrome, necrotizing vasculitis and sarcoidosis. These latter illnesses are more likely to result in subacute or chronic polyarthritis, however, and associated clinical findings are usually sufficiently obvious to alert the physician to the correct diagnosis.

DIAGNOSTIC STUDIES

Synovial fluid analysis (see Chapter 3) is the most useful laboratory study available in the diagnosis of acute monoarthritis. Carefully performed, it often provides the diagnosis at the time of the first visit to the physician. Fluid from a septic joint is grossly opaque and cloudy and has a decreased viscosity. Frank pus is seen in severe cases. The addition of synovial fluid to acetic acid reveals a poor mucin clot, characterized by a loose flocculent precipitate. The white blood cell count is markedly elevated; counts of 90,000 to 100,000 white cells/mm^3 are almost diagnostic. Polymorphonuclear leukocytes are the most prominent cells, and comprise 75 to 100% of the cells seen on differential white count study. The offending organism may be seen on gram-stain study or will be identified by the next day following appropriate culture. If gonococcal arthritis is suspected, the fluid should be cultured onto blood agar and chocolate agar immediately at the time of arthrocentesis. Simultaneous determinations of synovial fluid and blood sugar are important aids in the diagnosis. In septic arthritis, the synovial fluid sugar is markedly lowered, with the disparity between synovial and blood sugar paralleling the severity of the joint infection.

The synovial fluid in acute attacks of gout and pseudogout has many similarities to changes that occur in septic arthritis; the differences are mainly ones of degree. The fluid appears grossly opaque and cloudy, with decreased viscosity. The mucin clot test with acetic acid reveals a loose flocculent precipitate. The leukocyte count is most likely to range from 20,000 to 80,000 white cells/mm^3, and the differential white count reveals 60 to 90% polymorphonuclear leukocytes. Characteristic crystals of monosodium urate or calcium pyrophosphate dihydrate can be seen, usually in large numbers (see Chapter 3). Although a specific definition of crystal type is obviously important in final diagnosis, light microscopy alone is usually sufficient to determine that the patient has a crystal-induced synovitis. This information allows the institution of appropriate therapy for relief of symptoms, because both diseases respond to several similar therapeutic agents. The analysis of synovial fluid for crystals is most accurate if it is performed within several hours of arthrocentesis. If coagulation of the specimen has been allowed to occur, crystals can be best seen in white cells in the clot rather than in the supernatant. Although the finding of large numbers of crystals reassures one that the diagnosis is acute gout or pseudogout, septic arthritis may also be present on rare occasions; it is well to carry out appropriate cultures to complete the study.

Radiologic examination of the involved joint should be performed in all patients with acute monoarthritis. Loss of cartilage and bone demineralization are characteristic of septic arthritis, especially if diagnosis and treatment are delayed. Osteomyelitis reveals characteristic osteoporotic changes in the area of the metaphysis. X-rays of the joint should be obtained at intervals of several days when osteomyelitis is suspected, because changes may not develop for a period of seven to 14 days following onset of the disease. Evidence of fracture or chondrocalcinosis are other findings of value in the radiologic study of patients with acute involvement of a single joint.

Although clinical, synovial fluid and roentgenographic findings will lead to the correct diagnosis in many patients with acute monoarthritis, other laboratory studies may be necessary for diagnosis. Blood cultures are often positive in the presence of septic and gonococcal arthritis, and in patients with osteomyelitis. Gram-stains of material aspirated from cutaneous lesions in patients with gonococcal arthritis may reveal typical organisms. Interestingly, cultures from the same lesions are often negative. Uterine cervical and urethral cultures should be routinely performed if gonococcal infection is suspected. Rectal swab and pharyngeal cultures may be positive, particularly in patients infected by homosexual contact. It is imperative that all materials for culture for gonococcus be plated on culture media directly at the bedside, because the organism is very sensitive to temperature changes. Blood agar, chocolate agar and Thayer-Martin media should be utilized routinely for cultures from nonarticular areas.

Serum uric acid levels are valuable if gout is suspected, not only to provide diagnostic support but also to determine the severity of the biochemical abnormality prior to treatment. A needle can be used to demonstrate monosodium urate deposits if tophi are present. A 22-gauge needle is inserted directly into the tophus and rotated several times. Upon withdrawal of the needle, a small amount of urate material will be present at the needle tip. This is transferred gently to a clean glass microscope slide and studied as described in the crystal study of synovial fluid (p. 45). The tophaceous areas are usually avascular and bleeding is not a problem. Pain is usually minimal to absent. Serum calcium, phosphorus and alkaline phosphatase determinations, serum uric acid, and serum iron, iron-binding capacity and saturation levels should be performed routinely in patients with pseudogout to exclude associated disease states.

Studies of coagulation factors such as the platelet count, prothrombin time and partial thromboplastin time should be routinely performed if hemarthrosis is present. An elevated erythrocyte sedimentation rate militates against a mechanical etiology. A positive test in high titer for serum rheumatoid factor supports a diagnosis of episodic rheumatoid arthritis. Additional laboratory studies directed toward the diagnosis of less common causes of acute monoarthritis should be performed when these are suspected.

THERAPY

Patients with acute monoarthritis are often best managed by admission to hospital, especially if infectious arthritis is suspected or confirmed. Obvious cases of gout or pseudogout can usually be managed on an ambulatory basis. Even in these cases, however, severe discomfort may require a short period of hospitalization until symptoms are brought under control. Hospitalization allows expeditious institution of appropriate diagnostic studies and treatment. This is vital not only for relief of discomfort, but also to avoid rapid destruction of the joint in cases of infectious etiology.

In all forms of acute monoarthritis, pain relief is markedly aided by temporary immobilization. This can be most conveniently carried out by appropriate splinting. If a weight-bearing joint is involved, ambulation with its attendant stresses should be avoided until symptoms are under control. As symptoms subside, gentle joint range-of-motion exercises and power-building exercises for muscles should be instituted. Superficial applications of local heat may provide symptomatic relief. They pose some therapeutic hazard in the management of infectious arthritis because they may augment the inflammatory process; cold applications may be useful. Analgesic agents should be used as required. Although milder analgesics such as propoxyphene hydrochloride (Darvon), ethoheptazine citrate (Zactane) and acetominophen may be sufficiently effective, temporary use of narcotic agents may be necessary.

The specific management of septic and gonococcal arthritis and osteomyelitis requires the use of appropriate antibiotic agents directed toward the offending organism (see Chapter 18).

Acute gouty arthritis may be treated with any of a number of effective agents, including colchicine, indomethacin, phenylbutazone, adrenocorticotrophic hormone and adrenal cortical hormone derivatives (see Chapter

18). Colchicine is the treatment of choice in patients whose diagnosis is questionable, since an excellent response supports the diagnosis. If the diagnosis based on clinical and laboratory findings is secure, the other agents outlined in management can be utilized. Acute pseudogout is similarly managed by one of several effective programs (see Chapter 18). Since the acute attack most commonly involves the knee, aspiration followed by intra-articular corticosteroid injection is feasible and effective. Symptoms in the knee and other joints also respond well to a short course of phenylbutazone.

Joint rest is important in the management of acute monoarthritis due to trauma or internal derangement. Cold applications are advisable in the early stages, both to provide symptomatic relief and to prevent swelling. Warm applications are indicated later to reduce joint swelling. Isometric exercises help to prevent muscle weakness; elastic compression bandages are helpful. Surgical intervention may be indicated if ligamentous or cartilage injury is present.

Acute joint hemorrhage secondary to trauma usually responds to bedrest, immobilization with splints to relieve pain, and appropriate analgesic agents. Cold applications used early help to diminish bleeding by inducing vasoconstriction. Warm applications are used later to speed resolution of swelling and resorption of clotted blood. The blood usually resorbs over a period of three to seven days and knee motion returns readily with appropriate physical therapy. In patients with blood dyscrasias, appropriate therapy for the underlying hemorrhagic disorder should be instituted to avoid further bleeding. If the hemorrhagic effusion is small, aspiration is not usually necessary. If there is a large, bulging effusion, aspiration is helpful to speed relief *after* the bleeding diathesis is systemically corrected.

Acute arthritides other than those of infectious, crystal-induced, traumatic or hemorrhagic origin can be treated initially with nonspecific antiinflammatory agents such as aspirin, indomethacin, or phenylbutazone. More definitive therapy is instituted after the specific diagnosis has been ascertained (see Chapter 18).

CASE HISTORIES

History 4-1. Septic Arthritis

R. W., a 61-year-old black female, was well until January, 1973, at which time she noted dyspnea on exertion. Shortly thereafter, she developed muscle weakness that involved the proximal muscles of the upper and lower extremities. Joint symptoms were limited to the left knee. The latter symptoms had been present for many years and were characterized by pain in the knee on use, without swelling. Laboratory studies, including open lung biopsy and biopsy of the left deltoid muscle, were consistent with a diagnosis of polymyositis with pulmonary fibrosis. Left knee symptoms appeared unrelated to her primary diagnosis and were consistent with severe osteoarthritic changes seen on x-ray. The patient was placed on therapy with prednisone, 15 mg

QID, to which both the muscle weakness and dyspnea responded well. Steroid therapy was gradually reduced to a maintenance dose of prednisone, 5 mg BID.

In June, 1973, the patient noted swelling and increased pain in the left knee. Symptoms became progressively worse over a two-week period. Analysis of synovial fluid aspirated from the knee revealed 55,000 WBC/mm³ with 78% polymorphonuclear leukocytes. Synovial fluid glucose/blood glucose values obtained with the patient in a fasting state were 30 mg%/96 mg%. No crystals were seen. Gram stain revealed gram positive cocci. A culture of synovial fluid grew Staphylococcus aureus, coagulase positive. Antibiotic therapy with intravenous oxacillin was begun. Therapy with this agent was continued when sensitivity studies revealed that the organism was penicillin resistant. Oral oxacillin was substituted after four days, when clinical examination showed marked improvement in swelling, and synovial fluid analysis revealed a decrease in total white cell count and polymorphs. Therapy was continued for a period of six weeks, with successful resolution of acute findings.

Discussion: This patient with polymyositis and interstitial pulmonary fibrosis developed septic arthritis of an osteoarthritic left knee while on steroid therapy. Septic arthritis is more likely to occur in joints damaged by other arthritic diseases. Not infrequently, symptoms are attributed to a flare of the underlying disorder, rather than septic arthritis. A diagnosis of septic arthritis especially should be considered in patients on steroid treatment, because resistance to infection is diminished.

History 4-2. Acute Gonococcal Arthritis

R. N., a 48-year-old white male, was first seen in consultation in hospital in September, 1973. He had been in good health until three weeks prior to admission, at which time he noted pain in the dorsum of the left foot while walking. After a period of one week, the pain became more severe and was associated with swelling and redness of the involved area. Studies performed elsewhere revealed a normal serum uric acid and complete blood count. Treatment with phenylbutazone, 100 mg QID and, subsequently, prednisone, 7.5 mg QID, had no symptomatic benefit. When seen, the patient gave no history of fever, chills, or joint symptoms elsewhere. System review revealed absence of skin rash, Raynaud's phenomenon, sun sensitivity, hair loss, dry eyes or mouth, or pleurisy. He denied recent sexual intercourse. Past history was unremarkable.

Physical examination revealed a temperature 38°C. There was no lymphadenopathy, and examination of the heart, lungs and abdomen was within normal limits. No urethral discharge was noted. Rectal examination revealed a nontender normal-sized prostate gland. Musculoskeletal evaluation showed marked tenderness, swelling and erythema over the dorsum of the tarsal area of the left foot and left ankle. There was associated muscle atrophy of the left quadriceps muscle. Laboratory studies revealed a hematocrit of 39%, a white blood cell count of 19,600/mm³ with a normal differential, and an erythrocyte sedimentation rate of 23 mm/hour (Wintrobe). Urinalysis, liver function studies, routine serum electrolytes, electrocardiogram and chest x-rays were normal. Studies for serum rheumatoid factor and antinuclear antibody were negative. X-rays of the left foot and ankle revealed no abnormal findings. Approximately 3 cc of synovial fluid were removed by aspiration from the left ankle. Synovial fluid white cell count was 21,000/mm³, with 25% polymorphonuclear cells. Gram stain and culture were negative. The patient continued to have temperature elevations up to 38°C daily. In the absence of confirmatory evidence of infection, a diagnosis of oligoarticular rheumatoid arthritis of acute onset was considered feasible, although the clinical findings were atypical. Blood, urethral and rectal cultures were reported negative.

The patient continued to be febrile during the second week of hospitalization and repeat studies of synovial fluid removed from the left ankle by aspiration were performed. Total white cell count in the synovial fluid was $10,000/mm^3$ with a normal differential. Gram stain and culture were once again negative. Repeat roentgenographic examination of the left foot and ankle at this time revealed severe osteoporotic changes in the bones of the tarsal area. Orthopedic consultation was requested and arthrotomy was advised. At surgery, purulent-appearing material was seen in the areas of the fifth metatarsal and cuneiform bones. Gram stain was negative but culture of this material was positive for Neisseria gonorrhoeae. The patient was treated with aqueous crystalline penicillin, 10 million units daily, intravenously. He had remarkable clinical improvement over the next several days and was discharged after one week, to continue oral antibiotic therapy. Interestingly, just prior to discharge from hospital, the patient admitted homosexual activities one week prior to onset of his present illness.

Discussion: Although a diagnosis of acute gonococcal or septic arthritis was considered early in the course of this patient's localized joint symptoms, the diagnosis was difficult to substantiate until relatively late. Synovial fluid abnormalities were not diagnostic and were consistent with several forms of inflammatory arthritis. The importance of serial x-ray determinations in a case of this type is demonstrated. A high clinical index of suspicion and persistence in diagnostic efforts are often required for accurate diagnosis of gonococcal arthritis.

History 4-3. Gout

W. L., a 50-year-old white male, was first seen in consultation in October, 1973. Joint symptoms had begun approximately four years previously, at which time he noted acute onset of pain and tenderness in the left first metatarsophalangeal (MTP) joint. Serum uric acid studies performed at that time were elevated and a diagnosis of gouty arthritis was made. Joint symptoms resolved without specific therapy. An interval therapy program was not initiated. The patient had recurrent attacks of pain and swelling which separately involved the first MTP joints of both feet. Attacks were sudden in onset and lasted three to four days. Initially, episodes occurred at approximately six-month intervals; later, attacks became more frequent. Several months prior to evaluation he had noted acute pain and swelling in the third proximal interphalangeal (PIP) joint of the right hand. There was no known family history of gout and the patient had no history of renal stones. Colchicine was used for treatment of his last attack in the right first MTP joint, with excellent relief of symptoms. Six weeks prior to consultation, the patient had been placed on hydrochlorothiazide, 50 mg daily, for treatment of hypertension. System review was otherwise negative and past medical history was unremarkable. Social review revealed a moderately high intake of alcohol, with the patient consuming 6 to 8 ounces of whiskey per day.

On physical examination, blood pressure was 160/82 mm Hg. The third PIP joint of the right hand was slightly tender to palpation. Slight tenderness was also noted over the lateral epicondyle of the right elbow. No other physical abnormalities were noted. Laboratory studies revealed normal urinalysis, a hematocrit of 44%, a white blood cell count of $8400/mm^3$, and an erythrocyte sedimentation rate of 26 mm/hour (Wintrobe). Serum creatinine was 1 mg/100 ml. Serum studies for rheumatoid factor and antinuclear antibody were negative. Serum uric acid was 10.2 mg/100 ml. X-rays of the chest, both hands and both feet revealed no abnormalities. A diagnosis of gouty diathesis with acute attacks of gouty arthritis was made. The patient was placed on colchicine, 0.6 mg BID. Laboratory studies were repeated several weeks later after hydrochlorothiazide therapy had been discontinued. Serum uric acid was 8 mg/100 ml and 8.6 mg/100 ml on repeat studies. Urinary uric acid excretion was 670 mg/24 hours. Creatinine clearance was normal. The patient was placed on probenecid, 0.5 gm daily, with instructions to increase his dose at weekly intervals to a total of 0.5 gm TID. Colchicine, 0.5 mg BID, was continued. Hydrochlorothiazide therapy was not reinstituted at that time. The patient was instructed to increase his daily fluid intake and to reduce or discontinue his alcohol consumption. On evaluation two months later, serum uric acid was 5.2 mg/100 ml on a dose of probenecid, 0.5 gm TID. Blood pressure was 140/82 mm Hg. No acute attacks of gout had occurred during the period of followup.

Discussion: This patient had a typical history of acute gouty arthritis characterized by recurrent acute attacks involving the first MTP joints. Laboratory confirmation of the diagnosis was complicated by his diuretic therapy. Accurate evaluation of baseline uric acid metabolism required discontinuation of hydrochlorothiazide therapy. Colchicine, which does not affect uric acid metabolism, was given as prophylaxis against acute attacks while baseline laboratory investigations were being completed.

Should therapy for his hypertension be required in the future, several therapeutic approaches may be utilized. Mild hypertension may be treated with agents such as methyldopa or reserpine, which do not elevate the serum uric acid. Therapy with thiazides or other diuretics that elevate the serum uric acid may be utilized if appropriate increases in probenecid therapy are made to control the serum uric acid level.

History 4-4. Gout

H. M., a 59-year-old black male, was first seen in the hospital emergency room for evaluation of acute painful swelling of the left knee which had begun suddenly earlier that day. Symptoms had become progressively more severe and the patient had difficulty with ambulation. There was no prior history of joint symptoms, and no history of recent trauma. On physical examination, the left knee was acutely inflamed with marked swelling, heat and tenderness. Synovial fluid aspirated from the left knee was cloudy with a moderate decrease in viscosity. The mucin clot test was very abnormal. Detailed analysis of the fluid revealed 60,000 WBC/mm^3 with 92% polymorphonuclear cells. No bacteria were seen on gram stain. Further study showed numerous needle-shaped crystals with strong negative birefringence, both intracellular and extracellular in location. Subsequent laboratory studies revealed a serum uric acid of 11 mg/100 ml and a negative synovial fluid culture. The patient was placed on phenylbutazone, 100 mg QID, with instructions to gradually decrease the dose over a period of one week. Response to therapy was excellent. Repeat serum uric acid was 12.6 mg/100 ml, and daily urinary acid excretion was 540 mg. Interval therapy with probenecid and colchicine was begun. Probenecid, 0.5 gm BID, was required to maintain the serum uric acid at a normal level. No recurrence of joint symptoms was noted during three months of followup evaluation.

Discussion: This case demonstrates the onset of acute gouty arthritis in a joint other than the great toe. Arthrocentesis and synovial fluid analysis allowed immediate diagnosis of the problem. Although the diagnosis of acute gouty arthritis appeared solid on the basis of synovial fluid findings, bacterial studies were performed to exclude septic arthritis, which may at times coexist. Phenylbutazone was used in the treatment of the attack, because side reactions are fewer than with colchicine. A trial of colchicine therapy would have been diagnostically valuable if the etiology of the patient's symptoms had been less certain.

History 4-5. Pseudogout Syndrome

W. T., a 62-year-old white male, was well until approximately six weeks prior to evaluation, at which time he noted acute onset of pain, swelling and tenderness of the left knee. There was no history of trauma or locking of the knee. Symptoms responded well to a short course of oral steroid therapy prescribed by his private physician. When seen at the time of referral, the patient was entirely asymptomatic. System review was essentially negative and past medical history was noncontributory. Specific inquiry revealed no prior history of joint symptoms. Physical examination was essentially normal with no evidence of joint swelling, tenderness or limitation. Presumptive differential diagnosis included gout, pseudogout, episodic rheumatoid arthritis or internal derangement of the knee. Laboratory studies revealed a normal complete blood count and urinalysis. Erythrocyte sedimentation rate was 23 mm/hour (Wintrobe). Serum studies for rheumatoid factor and antinuclear antibody were negative. Serum uric acid was 4.2 mg/ml. Serum calcium, phosphorus, and alkaline phosphatase values were normal. X-rays of the knees showed calcification of the medial meniscus of the right knee and calcification of the medial and lateral menisci of the left knee. Joint spaces were well preserved. X-rays of the wrist, feet and ankles were normal. A diagnosis of pseudogout syndrome as the probable cause of the patient's symptoms was made. No specific therapy was given and the patient was instructed to return for synovial fluid aspiration and analysis if acute joint swelling recurred.

The patient returned one month later when he had an acute onset of pain and swelling in the left knee similar to his initial episode. The left knee was grossly swollen; 50 cc of synovial fluid were removed. Analysis of the fluid revealed 32,000 white cells/mm^3 with 72% polymorphonuclear cells. Numerous linear and rhomboid-shaped crystals were noted, both intracellular and extracellular in location. Most of the crystals were nonbirefringent, but some crystals showed weak positive birefringence. The findings confirmed the initial diagnosis of pseudogout syndrome made earlier on the basis of clinical history and roentgenographic studies. The left knee was injected with local steroid and lidocaine, with good resolution of symptoms over several days. Colchicine, 0.6 mg BID, was begun. Recurrent acute swelling of the left knee occurred one month later. The patient had stopped colchicine intake because of loose stools. Repeat intra-articular injection of the left knee with steroids was performed and colchicine was restarted in a dose of 0.6 mg daily. The patient continues in followup.

Discussion: The clinical picture and laboratory findings in this patient were characteristic of pseudogout syndrome. Chondrocalcinosis of the menisci of the knees is not uncommon in older persons in the presence of few or no joint symptoms. It has also been described as a coincidental finding in patients whose joint manifestations are due to another underlying etiology, such as rheumatoid arthritis or gout. For this reason, pseudogout was initially considered a probable rather than definite cause of left knee symptoms in this patient when roentgenographic evidence of calcification was noted. Confirmation required demonstration of numerous crystals characteristic of calcium pyrophosphate in synovial fluid at the time of an acute attack.

In many patients with pseudogout syndrome, acute attacks are relatively infrequent and the disease can be managed effectively by joint aspiration and intra-articular injection of steroids at the time of an acute episode. When acute attacks are relatively frequent, prophylaxis may be attempted using various anti-inflammatory agents. Daily colchicine is sometimes effective.

Should the patient not respond to this agent, daily indomethacin or phenylbutazone therapy may be helpful.

History 4-6. Internal Derangement of the Knee

L. E., a 62-year-old white male, was in good health until 1964, at which time he sustained a twisting injury to the left knee when he fell from a golf cart. Slight swelling was noted and the patient was treated with ten days bed rest. Symptoms completely resolved. In 1967 and 1968 the patient had acute episodes of pain in the left knee associated with locking. Symptoms lasted for only several days each time and no swelling was noted. The patient was admitted to the hospital in November of 1972 for treatment of persistent locking of the left knee, which had developed two days previously. He was unable to achieve full extension of the knee without pain. No swelling was noted. System review was otherwise negative and the patient considered himself to be in good health. Past medical history was noncontributory.

Physical examination was completely normal except for findings involving the left knee. There was tenderness to palpation at the medial aspect of the joint line. Extension was limited to 15°. No swelling was noted. Laboratory studies revealed a hematocrit of 47%, a white blood cell count of 8100/mm³, an erythrocyte sedimentation rate of 4 mm/hour (Wintrobe), and a normal urinalysis. Serum uric acid was 4.9 mg/100 ml. Serum calcium, phosphorus and alkaline phosphatase determinations were normal. Routine serologic test for syphilis was nonreactive. Serum studies for rheumatoid factor and antinuclear antibody were negative. Chest x-ray was normal. X-rays of the knees revealed narrowing of the medial joint space of the left knee with marginal osteophyte formation on the tibia and femur. An ovoid ossicle, 5 by 10 mm in size, appeared posterior to the tibial plateau, and seemed to represent a loose body. The right knee was normal. A double contrast arthrogram of the left knee was performed. The lateral meniscus appeared normal. The medial meniscus was shorter than normal and had a slight irregularity consistent with a tear. Arthrotomy of the left knee was carried out. There was an anterior tear of the medial meniscus, and two cartilaginous loose bodies were found. The lateral meniscus was badly scarred. The loose bodies were removed and the medial and lateral menisci were excised. The joint was carefully irrigated many times and a careful search was made for more loose bodies, but none were found.

Discussion: Monoarthritis in this patient was related to the presence of loose bodies and damaged medial and lateral menisci. Degenerative joint disease characterized by joint space narrowing and spur formation are frequent associated findings in patients with internal derangement disorders of the knee. Symptoms of locking are highly suggestive of the presence of loose bodies or meniscus injury. Recurrent acute effusions and, later, chronic persistent swelling are commonly seen. Similar symptoms are seen in patients with tears of the cruciate ligaments.

REFERENCES

1. Argen, R. J., Wilson, C. H. and Wood, P.: Suppurative arthritis. Arch Int Med 117:661, 1966.
2. Kelly, P. J., Martin, W. J. and Coventry, M. B.: Bacterial (suppurative) arthritis in the adult. J Bone Joint Surg 52A:1595, 1970.
3. Keiser, H. L. et al: Clinical forms of gonococcal arthritis. N Eng J Med 274:234, 1968.
4. Partain, J. O., Cathcart, E. S. and Cohen, A. S.: Arthritis associated with gonorrhea. Ann Rheum Dis 27:156, 1968.

5. Hadler, N. M. et al: Acute polyarticular gout. Am J Med 56:715, 1974.
6. Moskowitz, R. W. and Katz, D.: Chondrocalcinosis and chondrocalsynovitis (pseudogout syndrome): Analysis of 24 cases. Am J Med 43:322, 1967.
7. Moskowitz, R. W. and Garcia, F.: Chondrocalcinosis articularis (pseudogout syndrome). Arch Int Med 132,87, 1973.
8. Kisker, C. T., Perlman, A. W. and Benton, C.: Arthritis in hemophilia. Seminars in Arth and Rheum 1:220, 1971.
9. Mattingly, S.: Palindromic rheumatism. Ann Rheum Dis 25:307, 1966.
10. Weiner, A. D. and Ghormley, R. K.: Periodic benign synovitis. Idiopathic intermittent hydrarthrosis. J Bone Joint Surg 38A:1039, 1956.
11. Duncan, H. et al: Migratory osteolysis of the lower extremities. Ann Int Med 66:1165, 1967.

Chapter 5

SUBACUTE AND CHRONIC MONOARTHRITIS

The diagnosis of subacute or chronic monoarthritis often represents one of the more difficult challenges in differential diagnosis in patients with rheumatic disease. This difficulty stems from the fact that subacute or chronic monoarthritis may be the presenting finding in a diverse number of rheumatic diseases, the clinical characteristics of which are often similar and at times indistinguishable. Fortunately, this form of arthritis usually does not represent a medical emergency. There is a reasonable period of time to elaborate the diagnosis, and nonspecific anti-inflammatory therapy is available for symptomatic relief until the diagnosis is made.

DIFFERENTIAL DIAGNOSIS

Most likely causes to be considered:

Rheumatoid arthritis
Degenerative joint disease (osteoarthritis)
Mechanical internal derangement
Osteochondritis dissecans
Avascular necrosis
Chronic infection with Mycobacterium tuberculosis or fungi
Sarcoidosis
Pigmented villonodular synovitis
Synovial chondromatosis and osteochondromatosis
Joint neoplasms

Rheumatoid arthritis frequently appears in the monoarticular form, particularly in the juvenile form of the disease, in which monoarticular or oligoarticular involvement is common. The knee is particularly prone to this type of involvement, although any peripheral joint may be so affected. Swelling results from synovitis and accumulation of joint fluid. Other signs of inflammation, such as increased heat, redness and tenderness, are often present. Pain, even at rest, is a prominent complaint. These clinical characteristics are nonspecific and do not allow ready differentiation from

70

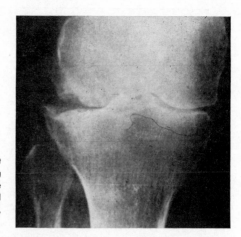

Figure 5-1. Rheumatoid arthritis, right knee. Joint space narrowing is present. Bony erosions are most marked at the lateral aspect of the knee. (Courtesy, The Arthritis Foundation)

other forms of monoarthritis. The erythrocyte sedimentation rate may be elevated only slightly; the test for serum rheumatoid factor is frequently negative. Roentgenographic examination reveals normal findings early in the disease. Later, osteoporosis, joint space narrowing and bony erosions appear (Fig. 5-1).

In *degenerative joint disease,* symptoms are slower and more insidious in onset. At first, pain occurs only with use; later, pain at rest is noted. Swelling, the result of proliferative changes in cartilage and bone, occurs late. Signs of inflammation are minimal unless an acute flare of disease is present. An exception to the usual lack of inflammation is seen in osteoarthritis of the hands. Here, osteoarthritis is often associated with a moderate inflammatory reaction in the distal and proximal interphalangeal joints. The erythrocyte sedimentation rate in degenerative joint disease is normal, and tests for serum rheumatoid factor are characteristically negative. Radiologic study reveals joint space narrowing, osteophytic spurs, subchondral bony sclerosis, and bony cyst formation (Figs. 5-2, 5-3).

Degenerative joint disease secondary to neuropathy, the so-called Charcot joint, produces marked distortion of joint structures (Fig. 5-4). This florid form of osteoarthritis is associated with such disorders as tabes dorsalis, diabetes mellitus and syringomyelia, in which neuropathic changes affect normal pain and proprioceptive sensations in the joint. The joint is readily overused, resulting in severe degeneration. The knee is involved most frequently, except in patients with diabetic neuropathy, in whom the joints of the feet are most frequently affected.[1]

Mechanical internal joint derangements most frequently involve the knee and usually result from tearing one of the menisci or cruciate ligaments. A history of trauma can usually be elicited, athough the trauma is often so minor as to be overlooked. Pain occurs primarily with use; a history of

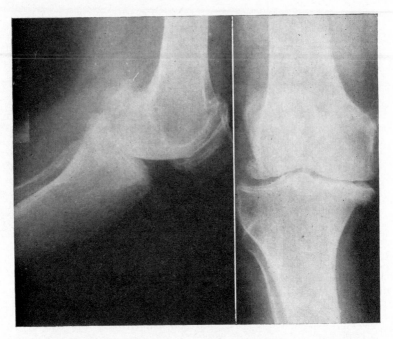

Figure 5-2. Degenerative joint disease, right knee, lateral and PA views. Note joint space narrowing, extensive osteophyte formation and subchondral bony sclerosis.

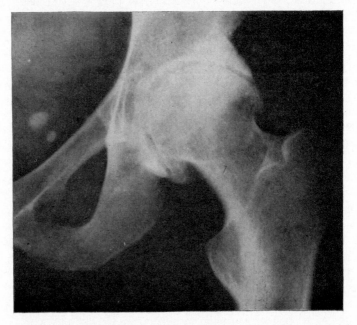

Figure 5-3. Degenerative joint disease, left hip. Joint space narrowing, spurs, and bony cyst formation is evident.

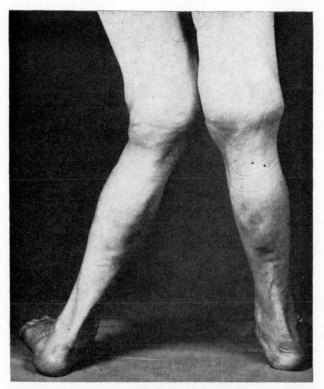

Figure 5-4. Charcot joint, left knee. Valgus formation is severe. (Courtesy, Dr. A. Mackenzie)

locking is common. In contrast to rheumatoid arthritis, swelling at first is usually intermittent; persistent swelling follows if the disorder is left untreated. Secondary degenerative joint disease is common. Loose joint bodies composed of fragments of cartilage, or cartilage and bone, produce similar symptoms.

Osteochondritis dissecans, a disease of unknown etiology, most frequently involves the knee and is usually monoarticular in distribution. This disorder is characterized by a separation of a section of cartilage and underlying bone from the larger bone to which it was attached. Necrosis of the separated fragment follows. Although the lateral aspect of the medial femoral condyle of the knee is the most common site of occurrence, any diarthrodial joint may be involved. Pain, recurrent swelling, and locking are typical clinical findings. X-rays reveal a separation between the involved segment of bone and cartilage and the bone to which it had been attached (Fig. 5-5). Early, the separated fragment lies in a relatively normal position within the bone. Later, there is a shallow excavation at the articular surface and a fragment of cartilage and bone may be seen lying free as a loose body. Although the etiology of the disorder is unknown, several

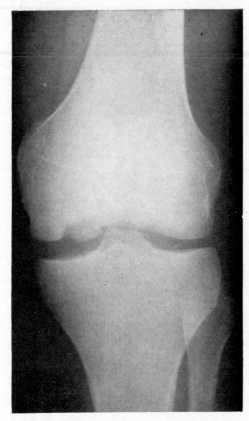

Figure 5-5. Osteochondritis dissecans, left knee. X-ray reveals separation of a fragment of cartilage and bone.

mechanisms of pathogenesis have been postulated. An endarteritis that affects the blood supply to a segment of bone may result in necrosis and subsequent detachment of the involved segment from its underlying bony structure. On the other hand, detachment of a segment of cartilage and bone may be a direct result of trauma, and ischemia of the fragment occurs as a secondary phenomenon once the segment has separated.

Avascular (aseptic, ischemic) necrosis of bone results when an interruption occurs in its blood supply. Pain and disability in the involved joint occur. Lesions are most commonly monoarticular but multiple joints may be involved. The head of the femur is a common site of involvement but the disease affects other joints as well. Symptoms of pain and joint limitation are slow in onset and localized. Roentgenograms reveal areas of bone resorption in association with areas of increased bone density and fragmentation (Fig. 5-6). Bone scans may demonstrate abnormalities prior to obvious roentgenographic change. Although the disorder may be idiopathic in origin, underlying diseases that compromise the vascular supply of bone are often related.[2-5] Vascular impairment may follow trauma or may be

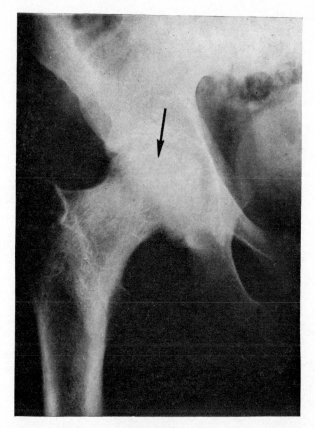

Figure 5-6. Avascular necrosis, hip. A wedge-shaped area of bone resorption (arrow) is surrounded by areas of increased bone density.

associated with hematologic disorders such as hypercoagulability, polycythemia vera and hemoglobinopathy.[2] It occurs as a clinical complication of vasculitis in patients with systemic lupus erythematosus.[3] An increased frequency of avascular necrosis in patients on adrenocorticosteroid therapy[4] may be related to lipid changes in the blood, to fatty emboli from a fatty liver, or to marrow infarction from an increased fat cell volume. It is seen frequently in patients following renal transplantation,[5] in alcoholics, and in patients with cirrhosis or pancreatitis. Increased occurrence recently has been described in patients with hyperuricemia. An uncommon underlying cause is Gaucher's disease. Conservative therapy is designed to relieve pain and limit disease progression. Overuse of joints or excessive weight-bearing should be avoided. Analgesic agents provide pain relief. Treatment of associated underlying disorders may prevent involvement of other joints. Surgical management, including intramedullary bone grafting, osteotomy, arthroplasty or prosthetic joint replacement, may be required as the disease advances.

Inflammatory monoarthritis due to *Mycobacterium tuberculosis* or various *fungi* may completely mimic that seen in rheumatoid arthritis. Pain and swelling are usually slow in onset. Systemic manifestations of the underlying disorder may be minimal or absent. Joint infection is usually secondary to primary infection elsewhere, such as in the lungs or genitourinary tract. Appropriate x-rays and culture studies directed to these common sites of primary involvement are essential in the complete evaluation of the patient. *Sarcoidosis* may similarly produce monoarthritis.[6] Synovial biopsy studies reveal either a nonspecific chronic inflammation that resembles that seen in rheumatoid arthritis, or may demonstrate noncaseating granulomas. Other manifestations of sarcoid, such as skin rash, parotid swelling and pulmonary symptoms, may be present.

A rare cause of monoarticular disease, but one that should be considered in every such differential diagnosis, is *pigmented villonodular synovitis*.[7,8] This disorder has characteristics of both an inflammatory process and a benign neoplasm. Gross examination reveals a characteristic villous nodu-

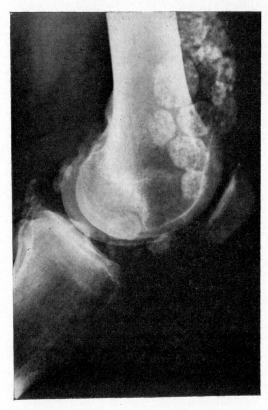

Figure 5-7. Synovial osteochondromatosis, knee. Florid ossification of synovium is apparent.

lar synovitis. Histologic study reveals multinucleated giant cells, hemosiderin and distended synovial cells laden with lipid deposits. Pain and swelling are the principal clinical findings. Recurrent hemorrhage into the joint is common and accounts for the presence of grossly bloody or xanthochromic synovial fluid. Large joints such as the knees are most commonly affected but small joints may be involved. *Synovial chondromatosis,* another interesting entity, is characterized by metaplasia of synovium with replacement of synovial tissues by normal-appearing hyaline cartilaginous tissue. Ossification frequently follows with development of synovial osteochondromatosis (Fig. 5-7). This disease also occurs most commonly in the knee and presents as a chronic monoarthritis. Hips, elbows and shoulders may also be involved, but to a lesser frequency.

Neoplasms of the joint, though relatively uncommon, must always be considered in the diagnosis of subacute or chronic monoarthritis. Lipomas and fibromas are seen, but are quite rare. Synovial sarcoma (malignant synovioma) is a highly malignant disease of synovium with a low survival rate. Roentgenograms reveal a para-articular soft tissue mass, foci of calcification, and osteolytic defects in contiguous bone due to secondary in-

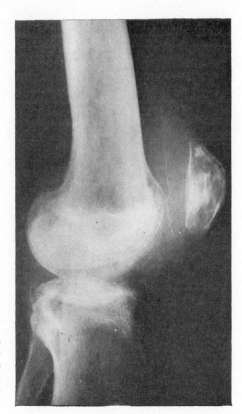

Figure 5-8. Synovial sarcoma. A soft tissue mass is interposed within the patello-femoral articulation. Lytic defects in the patella and femur are apparent. (Courtesy, Dr. V. Goldberg)

vasion (Fig. 5-8). Metastatic neoplasms that involve bony structures close to joints may simulate chronic arthritis and should be excluded in differential diagnosis.

The preceding disease states will account for a high percentage of diagnoses in patients with chronic monoarthritis. Other etiologies must be considered, however, when the diagnosis is still unexplained. Chronic monoarthritis may be the presenting or major manifestation of any of the other connective tissue diseases, such as systemic lupus erythematosus, scleroderma or ankylosing spondylitis. Similarly, chronic monoarthritis may occur in psoriatic arthritis, the arthritis of ulcerative colitis and regional enteritis, and Reiter's syndrome. Finally, symptoms due to inadequately treated septic or gonococcal arthritis, gout or pseudogout may persist for many weeks and be the cause of subacute monoarticular disease.

DIAGNOSTIC STUDIES

As in the diagnosis of acute monoarthritis, synovial fluid analysis is helpful in differentiating the various causes of subacute or chronic monoarthritis. Findings characteristic of an inflammation (see Chapter 3) generally exclude degenerative joint disease as the cause of symptoms. Gross findings of xanthochromic or bloody fluid suggest a diagnosis of pigmented villonodular synovitis or joint neoplasm. Smear and culture of fluid should be performed routinely to exclude tuberculosis or fungal infection. Synovial fluid sugar is characteristically low in the presence of these latter chronic infections, but it may be similarly reduced in the presence of long-standing rheumatoid arthritis.

Peripheral blood studies should include a leukocyte count, differential white blood cell count, erythrocyte sedimentation rate and hematocrit, because abnormalities in these laboratory parameters are a clue to the presence of systemic disorders. Positive results for serum rheumatoid factor and antinuclear antibody are characteristic findings in rheumatoid arthritis and other related connective tissue diseases. It must be remembered, however, that positive tests for serum rheumatoid factor and antinuclear antibody are frequently seen in other disease states (see Chapter 2). Serum anti-DNA and LE cell studies should be obtained if systemic lupus erythematosus is suspected. Although gout is not a common cause of subacute or chronic monoarthritis, a serum uric acid determination helps to exclude this diagnosis. Abnormalities in the serum protein electrophoresis pattern support a diagnosis of a systemic disorder such as rheumatoid arthritis, tuberculosis or sarcoid. A broad elevation of the gamma globulin band is the most characteristic change observed.

Roentgenograms of the joint often have diagnostic value and should always be performed. Rheumatoid arthritis in its early stages is associated with a normal roentgenologic appearance of the joint. Later, osteoporosis of bone adjacent to the involved joint is seen. Advanced disease reveals loss of joint space due to cartilage erosion, bone cysts, and gross deformity of joint structures. Degenerative joint disease is characterized by loss of joint space, osteophyte spur formation, sclerosis of subchondral bone and bone cysts. It is important to note that osteoarthritis is a ubiquitous disease; degenerative changes may be present as a "red herring" and not be related to the clinical problem. Mechanical derangements of the knee usually do not produce radiologic changes unless they are chronic, at which time mild to moderate degenerative changes are noted. Double contrast arthrograms with air and opaque media are helpful in the diagnosis of meniscal tears, but experience is required for accurate interpretation. False negative and false positive reports are common. Roentgenographic changes similar to those described for rheumatoid arthritis are seen in patients with tuberculous or fungal infection, and in sarcoid arthritis. Pigmented villonodular synovitis produces characteristic large cystic erosions of cartilage and bone. Synovial chondromatosis is not visible on x-ray unless ossification with osteochondromatosis is present. In the latter condition, multiple bony opacities are observed within the confines of the joint. Erosive changes due to neoplasms are obvious when bone destruction occurs. Chest x-ray is helpful in delineating the presence of tuberculosis, fungal infection, sarcoid or primary neoplasm.

Skin testing for tuberculosis should be performed routinely. A negative test is reassuring evidence against tuberculosis but is consistent with a diagnosis of sarcoid. Cultures of sputum and urine should be considered if tuberculosis is strongly suspected. Appropriate serum serologic studies and skin tests should be performed if fungal infection is suspected.

When the diagnosis is not readily apparent, synovial biopsy should be considered. Closed synovial biopsy is attended by minimal morbidity and disability. Although the study can be performed on an ambulatory basis, it is often preferable to admit the patient to hospital for one or two days. Complications, which include infection and hemorrhage, are rare when the study is done properly. Tuberculous and fungal infections are characterized histologically by the presence of granulomas. The inciting organisms themselves are frequently demonstrable with appropriate staining techniques. Sarcoidosis is characterized by noncaseating granulomas; more commonly, however, nonspecific inflammatory changes of less diagnostic help are noted. Nonspecific inflammatory changes appear in rheumatoid arthritis and associated connective tissue diseases. Synovial findings in pigmented villonodular synovitis include multinucleated giant cells, hemosiderin and lipid deposits. Replacement of synovium by islands of hyaline cartilage, or cartilage and bone, are typical of synovial chondromatosis and osteochondromatosis respectively. Culture of synovium is helpful in the diagnosis of tuberculosis and fungi, since synovial fluid cultures may be negative even though infection of the joint is present. Open biopsy is valuable in those patients in whom closed synovial biopsy is unsuccessful, or in whom too little tissue was obtained for accurate interpretation. This procedure allows exploration of the joint for internal derangements and allows more accurate localization of pathologic areas for biopsy. Open biopsy, however, is a major procedure. The patient is partially immobilized for several weeks, until healing and physical therapy allow restitution of joint function.

Arthroscopy is diagnostically helpful when disorders of internal derangement of the knee are suspected (see Chapter 2). This method also allows localization of pathologic lesions due to other disorders for biopsy. Extended experience in use of this technique is required for accurate interpretation of observations.

Unfortunately, the correct diagnosis of the cause of chronic monoarthritis may remain obscure even after extensive evaluation utilizing all the above procedures.

THERAPY

Treatment of subacute or chronic monoarthritis usually involves two phases: treatment *prior to diagnosis* and treatment *after diagnosis*. Treatment prior to diagnosis is symptomatic and directed toward relief of pain, swelling, and limitation of motion. Adequate rest of the involved joint is important. The use of a cane or crutch in the hand opposite the involved joint is particularly beneficial if a weight-bearing joint is involved. Aspirin given in full dosage lessens inflammation and relieves pain. Further pain relief is provided by use of mild analgesic agents such as propoxyphene HCl (Darvon), ethoheptazine citrate (Zactane), or acetominophen on a regular or as-needed basis. Heat reduces inflammation and lessens pain; isometric exercises maintain tone and strength of involved muscles. In patients requiring more vigorous therapy, indomethacin can be added to the above program in a dose of 100 mg daily in divided doses with food. Phenylbutazone, 100 mg four times a day, is also frequently effective. The latter agent is best used on a short-term basis only, because serious side reactions such as peptic ulceration, bone marrow depression, and salt and water retention are potential complications of prolonged administration. When infection has been excluded, treatment with intra-articular corticosteroids may be considered. Use of the latter agent should be attended with appropriate caution; repeated injudicious use may result in secondary degenerative changes due to joint overuse and a direct deleterious effect of steroids on cartilage. In general, systemic corticosteroids are to be avoided even after infection has been excluded because their strong anti-inflammatory effect may obscure the diagnosis as the patient is observed in followup evaluation.

Specific forms of management will vary depending on diagnosis. These measures can be instituted when the diagnosis becomes apparent (see Chapter 18).

CASE HISTORIES

History 5-1. Rheumatoid Arthritis

L.W., a 26-year-old white female, complained of left knee swelling beginning in August, 1972. Swelling and disability were gradual in onset. Pain was more severe in the morning and on stair-climbing. She was treated elsewhere with three intra-articular injections of local steroid into the knee, which gave relief for only short periods and was followed each time by recurrence of pain and swelling. There was no prior history of similar symptomatology and no history of trauma or locking. There were no joint symptoms elsewhere. System review and past medical history were noncontributory and she was in good general health. Physical examination at the time the patient was first seen in consultation in October, 1972 was negative except for moderate swelling of the left knee with slight limitation of flexion.

Laboratory studies revealed normal white blood cell count and differential, hematocrit, urinalysis, serologic test for syphilis and erythrocyte sedimentation rate. Latex fixation and antinuclear antibody studies of sera were negative, and serum uric acid was 4 mg/100 ml. Intermediate PPD and fungus skin tests were negative. Roentgenograms of the chest and left knee were normal. Synovial fluid aspiration studies of fluid from the left knee showed 3700 wbc/mm^3, with 43% polymorphonuclear leukocytes. Cultures for routine organisms, tuberculosis and fungi were negative. Initial diagnosis was monoarthritis of the left knee of indeterminate origin, possible monoarticular rheumatoid arthritis.

The patient was placed on therapy with aspirin, 960 mg QID, physical therapy, and avoidance of joint overuse. The patient had only moderate improvement and was admitted to hospital in January, 1973, for closed synovial biopsy. Repeat study of synovial fluid from the left knee showed no significant differences from the previous analysis. Tissue specimens obtained by closed synovial biopsy revealed mild synovial proliferation associated with a round cell inflammatory response and increased vascularity. No granulomas were seen. The patient was discharged on the same basic conservative program as previously outlined. Left knee swelling gradually improved, with only slight objective swelling noted nine months later.

Discussion: Findings in this case were consistent with monoarticular rheumatoid arthritis. No clinical or pathologic evidence of other causes of monoarthritis, such as tuberculosis, fungus infection, pigmented villonodular synovitis, osteochondromatosis, or internal derangement of the knee, were present. The patient did well clinically on a conservative program and showed no evidence of arthritis elsewhere. Roentgenographic examination and closed synovial biopsy were helpful in excluding other causes of monoarthritis.

History 5-2. Degenerative Joint Disease

R.K., a 74-year-old white female, was admitted to the hospital in December, 1973, for evaluation of pain and limitation of the left knee. Symptoms in the left knee had begun approximately ten years prior, when the patient noted onset of pain that was mild at first but became progressively more severe. Symptoms recently made ambulation difficult. Pain was aggravated by weight-bearing but was absent at rest. The patient complained of a grating sensation in the knee with use. There was no history of significant trauma or operative procedures to the knee. The patient denied symptoms in other joints and considered herself to be in generally good health. System review was otherwise negative and past medical history was noncontributory. Treatment with aspirin, indomethacin, physical therapy and use of a cane in the right hand gave only limited relief of symptoms.

On physical examination, there were no abnormal findings except for those noted in the left knee. Knee motion ranged from 5° extension to 100° flexion. There was no varus or valgus deformity. The knee was not tender and there was no evidence of effusion. A grating sensation was noted on palpation when the knee was moved through range of motion. Ligaments were stable. Laboratory studies revealed a hematocrit of 40%, a white blood cell count of 6400/mm³, an erythrocyte sedimentation rate of 16 mm per hour (Wintrobe), and a normal urinalysis. Serum electrolytes, fasting blood sugar and serum calcium, phosphorus and alkaline phosphatase values were normal. Routine serologic test for syphilis was negative, as were serum studies for rheumatoid factor and antinuclear antibody. Serum uric acid was 4.2 mg/100 ml. Serum protein electrophoresis was within normal limits. Chest x-ray was normal. Roentgenograms of the knees revealed marked narrowing of the medial and lateral compartments of the left knee joint. Cystic changes were seen in the medial femoral condyle. Spur formation on both femoral condyles of the left knee was marked. The right knee joint appeared normal. X-rays of the lumbosacral spine revealed moderately severe degenerative joint disease that involved the L1-2 and L2-3 intervertebral discs, and the apophyseal joints at L4-5. X-rays of the pelvis and the hips were within normal limits. A diagnosis of degenerative joint disease of the left knee and lumbar spine was made.

Due to the patient's severe pain and limitation of activity, a polycentric arthroplasty was performed on the left knee. At surgery, marked erosions of the cartilage of the medial plateau of the tibia and medial condyle of the femur were noted. The lateral femoral condyle revealed multiple small erosions. Large spurs were seen. Evidence of synovitis was minimal.

Discussion: In this patient, chronic monoarthritis was due to severe degenerative joint disease of the left knee. Treatment with aspirin, indomethacin, physical therapy and the use of a cane in the right hand was ineffective in controlling symptoms. The clinical features were consistent with a diagnosis of degenerative joint disease. Specifically, the patient had localized joint disease that was insidious in onset and slowly progressive. Systemic symptoms were absent. The pathologic findings noted on roentgenologic examination and at surgery were consistent with the degree of pain and limitation noted clinically.

History 5-3. Avascular Necrosis

J.M., a 37-year-old white male, was seen for evaluation in October, 1972. He had been well until a year prior, when he noted insidious onset of pain in the right hip. Symptoms gradually progressed, with increased pain and limitation of motion. Treatment with aspirin and short courses of phenylbutazone gave only mild relief. Crutch use was required to relieve increased distress associated with weight-bearing. No other joint symptoms were noted. System review was otherwise negative. Past medical history revealed a heavy intake of alcohol, up to 6 or 7 ounces of whiskey daily. On physical examination, the right hip was markedly limited and painful with motion. The remainder of his general physical examination and musculoskeletal system evaluation was negative.

Laboratory studies revealed a hematocrit of 46%, a white blood cell count of 6400/mm³ with a normal differential, an erythrocyte sedimentation rate of 8 mm per hour (Wintrobe), and a normal urinalysis. Fasting blood sugar, serum alkaline phosphatase and protein electrophoresis studies were normal. Serum uric acid was consistently elevated with values ranging from 7.5 to 9 mg/100 ml. Twenty-four-hour urinary uric acid excretion on a normal diet was 830 mg. Creatinine clearance was normal. Serum studies for rheumatoid factor and antinuclear antibody were negative, as were LE cell determinations. Chest x-ray was normal. X-rays of the hips showed flattening of the right femoral head with preservation of joint space. The left hip appeared normal. Changes in the right hip were consistent with early avascular necrosis. Varus osteotomy and placement of a fibular bone graft into the right upper femur was performed.

Discussion: Avascular necrosis of the right hip developed over a relatively short period of time in this otherwise generally healthy male. Underlying etiologic factors that might have been related to the development of avascular necrosis in this patient included heavy alcohol intake and hyperuricemia. The patient was instructed to discontinue alcohol intake and was placed on an interval therapy program with probenecid for treatment of his hyperuricemia. No further evidence of avascular necrosis in other joints has been noted in subsequent followup.

History 5-4. Pigmented Villonodular Synovitis

S.D., a 73-year-old white female, first noted joint symptoms at age 72, at which time she developed intermittent pain and swelling of the right knee. Onset of attacks was subacute and symptoms lasted for periods of 7 to 21 days. There was no history of trauma or locking. Synovial fluid study during one of these clinical episodes revealed a grossly bloody effusion. The patient was in otherwise good health and no other joint symptoms were noted. Physical examination was unremarkable except for the right knee, which was moderately swollen, slightly warm, and tender to palpation. Flexion was limited to 90°. Laboratory studies revealed a hematocrit of 36%, a white blood cell count of 6200/mm^3 with a normal differential, and an erythrocyte sedimentation rate of 28 mm per hour (Wintrobe). Urinalysis, prothrombin time, partial thromboplastin time and platelet count were normal. Serum rheumatoid factor and antinuclear antibody studies were negative. Serum uric acid was 4.3 mg/100 ml. Skin test with intermediate strength PPD was minimally positive. Analysis of synovial fluid from the right knee showed normal color and viscosity. White cell count was 800/mm^3 with 28% polymorphonuclear cells. Cultures for routine organisms, tuberculosis and fungi were negative. Chest x-ray was normal. Roentgenograms of the right knee showed degenerative spur formation and moderate narrowing of the femoral-tibial articulation. Severe narrowing and spur formation of the patellofemoral joint were also seen. Persistent severe symptoms were attributed to degenerative joint disease. Surgery of the knee was performed. Gross examination revealed moderate thickening of the synovial membrane and multiple erosions of joint cartilage. Histopathologic studies revealed changes characteristic of pigmented villonodular synovitis. A patellectomy and partial synovectomy were performed. The patient had moderate relief of symptoms and improvement in knee function.

Discussion: Pigmented villonodular synovitis most frequently presents as monoarticular arthritis. Xanthochromic or grossly bloody effusions are common. Etiology of this interesting entity is unknown. Symptoms may simulate those seen in monoarticular rheumatoid arthritis, severe degenerative joint disease, chondrocalcinosis, tuberculous arthritis, osteochondromatosis, internal derangements of the joint, or hemorrhagic blood dyscrasias. Definitive diagnosis depends on the demonstration of characteristic histopathologic findings on closed or open synovial biopsy.

REFERENCES

1. Sinha, S., Munichoodappa, C. S. and Kopak, G. R.: Neuro-arthropathy (Charcot joints) in diabetes mellitus: Clinical study in 101 cases. Medicine 51:191, 1972.

2. Tanaka, K. R., Clifford, G. O. and Axelrod, A. R.: Sickle cell anemia (homozygotes) with aseptic necrosis of the femoral head. Blood 11:988, 1956.
3. Ruderman, M. and McCarty, D. J.: Aseptic necrosis in systemic lupus erythematosus. Report of a case involving six joints. Arth Rheum 7:709, 1964.
4. Heinmann, W. G. and Freiberger, R. H.: Avascular necrosis of the femoral and humeral heads after high-dosage corticosteroid therapy. N Eng J Med 263:672, 1960.
5. Harrington, K. D. et al: Avascular necrosis of bone after renal transplantation. J Bone Joint Surg 53A:203, 1971.
6. Spilberg, I., Siltzback, L. E. and McEwen, C.: The arthritis of sarcoidosis. Arth Rheum 12:126, 1969.
7. Smith, J. H. and Pugh, D. G.: Roentgenographic aspects of articular pigmented villonodular synovitis. Am J Roentgenol Radium Ther Nucl Med 87:1146, 1962.
8. Granowitz, S. P. and Mankin, H. J.: Localized pigmented villonodular synovitis of the knee. J Bone Joint Surg 49A:122, 1967.

Chapter 6

ACUTE POLYARTHRITIS

Acute polyarthritis is a common manifestation of many rheumatic diseases. Relatively rapid diagnostic and therapeutic decisions are required by the physician to relieve the acute pain and limitation imposed on the patient. Hospitalization is frequently necessary to carry out appropriate diagnostic studies and to institute appropriate therapeutic measures for symptomatic relief.

DIFFERENTIAL DIAGNOSIS

Most likely causes to be considered:

Acute rheumatic fever
Rheumatoid arthritis
Systemic lupus erythematosus
Gonococcal arthritis
Reiter's syndrome
Rubella arthritis
Arthritis associated with ulcerative colitis or regional enteritis
Sarcoidosis
Erythema nodosum
Hepatitis-associated arthritis
Serum sickness
Sickle cell anemia
Palindromic rheumatism

The arthritis of *acute rheumatic fever* is a characteristic prototype of acute polyarthritis. Classically, the arthritis is migratory, although a number of joints may be involved at one time. Although almost any peripheral joint may be affected, the rarity of involvement of the temporomandibular joints is a key diagnostic point. Fever, almost regularly present, may be as high as 103 to 104° F and is most frequently remittent in type. Clinical evidence of carditis as manifested by congestive heart failure, pericarditic chest pain and murmurs secondary to endocarditis is common. Subcu-

4

taneous nodules occur primarily over bony surfaces, such as the subolecranon area of the elbow. Erythema marginatum, an evanescent nonpruritic pink or red rash, is a major manifestation of the disease. Lesions are characterized by peripheral erythema with central clearing. The margin of the rash frequently forms a ring, the so-called erythema annulare lesion. The rash usually affects the trunk and sometimes the limbs, but never involves the face. Individual lesions appear and disappear rapidly over a period of a few hours. Evidence of prior streptococcal infection should be sought.

Rheumatoid arthritis may also begin as an acute polyarthritis. Onset may be strikingly abrupt with immobilizing joint manifestations developing over a period of 12 to 24 hours. More often, however, polyarthritic symptoms develop over a period of days. Systemic symptoms such as stiffness, fever, sweats and fatigue are prominent. Acute polyarthritis commonly occurs as the initial symptom in juvenile rheumatoid arthritis (JRA). Fever, a characteristic associated symptom, is high and intermittent in type; daily swings of 5 to 6° F are not unusual. At times, a remittent fever indistinguishable from that seen in rheumatic fever occurs. In contrast to the migratory arthritis seen in rheumatic fever, the arthritis in the JRA patient is persistent. Clinical diagnosis of JRA is aided by the presence of a typical rash that occurs in approximately one-third of patients. The eruption consists of pink or salmon-colored macular or maculopapular lesions that are rarely pruritic. Large lesions often exhibit central fading. Lesions tend to be evanescent and migratory and frequently develop concomitant with fever

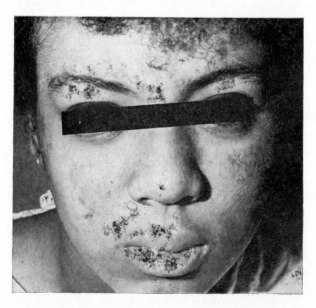

Figure 6-1. Facial butterfly rash, systemic lupus erythematosus. (Courtesy, Dr. B. Michel)

spikes. Involvement occurs chiefly on the limbs and trunk, but lesions may appear on the face, palms and soles.

Systemic lupus erythematosus may also begin as an acute polyarthritis. Other acute systemic manifestations such as fever, pleurisy and the characteristic facial butterfly rash (Fig. 6-1) are common associated symptoms. Additional symptoms, such as Raynaud's phenomenon, sun sensitivity and hair loss, may occur. Other of the so-called connective tissue diseases, such as polyarteritis nodosa, scleroderma, and dermatomyositis, may occasionally be associated with acute polyarthritis and simulate the joint manifestations of rheumatoid arthritis. In most of these diseases, however, the joint symptoms are limited and are overshadowed by other clinical manifestations.

Gonococcal arthritis often causes polyarthritis prior to localization to a monoarticular form of the disease. Low-grade fever and chills are frequently present. Tenosynovitis, although seen in other rheumatic disorders, is especially characteristic. A distinctive skin rash occurs: early, it is characterized by small maculopapular and vesicular lesions; later, the lesions become pustular and develop a dark necrotic center. A history of recent sexual exposure may be obtained. In the male, genitourinary symptoms such as penile discharge and dysuria are common; in the female, symptoms related to genitourinary gonococcal infection may not be obvious.

A not uncommon cause of acute polyarthritis in males is *Reiter's syndrome*. Clinically this disease state is characterized by a triad of arthritis, urethritis and conjunctivitis. Mucocutaneous lesions that involve the oral cavity and genitalia are common. In the mouth these lesions take the form of an aphthous stomatitis that is often painless. Genital lesions are characterized by superficial ulcerations of the penis that may coalesce to form a circinate balanitis. Cutaneous lesions most commonly occur on the palms and soles but may appear elsewhere. Small papules rapidly develop a pustular keratotic appearance. The lesions may become confluent and develop a thick keratotic crust, the so-called keratodermia blennorrhagica (Fig. 6-2). Skin lesions, although self-limiting, may last several weeks or months. Involvement of fingernails and toenails results in pitting and keratotic changes similar to those seen in psoriasis. Arthritis most frequently involves the large joints but the joints of the fingers and toes may also be swollen. The initial period of acute polyarthritis is usually followed by a more persistent inflammation, which may last from weeks to months. Urethral discharge or evidence of prostatitis is a characteristic finding. Although conjunctivitis is the classic manifestation in the eyes, iritis is frequently present.

Acute polyarthralgia or polyarthritis frequently follows *rubella infection*[1] or *rubella vaccination*.[2] Joint symptoms are usually self-limited but attacks of brief duration may recur over a period of several years. The disease is more likely to affect adolescents or young adults, whether in association

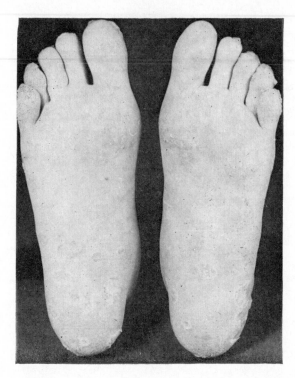

Figure 6-2. Keratodermia blennorrhagica in a patient with Reiter's syndrome. (Courtesy, Dr. A. Mackenzie)

with spontaneously-occurring disease or after vaccination. Small joints of the hands are affected primarily but large joints may also be involved. Articular symptoms usually occur synchronously with the typical maculopapular rash, but may precede or follow it by a few days. Fever and suboccipital lymphadenopathy are common.

Articular symptoms associated with *ulcerative colitis* or *regional enteritis* are variable. The clinical spectrum includes arthralgias, chronic arthritis involving one or a few joints, erythema nodosum with subacute arthritis, and spondylitis. In addition, acute polyarthritis may be observed. Gastrointestinal symptoms usually precede or occur simultaneously with joint symptoms. In certain cases, however, joint symptoms precede bowel symptoms by months or years.

Sarcoid is associated with variable joint manifestations, which include arthralgias or overt arthritis. Acute or chronic monoarthritis or polyarthritis may be seen. Other clinical evidence of sarcoid, such as fever, skin rash, iritis and parotid swelling, is frequently present. Hilar adenopathy and a negative tuberculin skin test support the diagnosis.

Erythema nodosum is a syndrome characterized by acute or subacute polyarthritis, hilar adenopathy, and tender, erythematous, nodular cutaneous swellings. This disorder may occur as a primary disease or secondary to other diseases. Included among the latter are streptococcal infection, coccidioidomycosis, ulcerative colitis or regional enteritis, active tuberculosis and sarcoid. In addition, erythema nodosum is a manifestation of drug sensitivity, particularly to iodides, bromides and sulfonamides. More recently, its occurrence has been noted with the use of oral contraceptives. The nodular skin lesions appear most commonly on the anterior aspect of the lower extremities, especially the tibial areas (Fig. 6-3). Upper extremities are involved occasionally. The lesions are warm, tender and painful, and vary in size from one-half centimeter to several centimeters in diameter. They frequently recur in crops and last for variable periods, from days to weeks. The associated arthritis primarily affects large joints, such as ankles, knees and wrists.

An interesting form of acute polyarthritis occurs in association with *viral hepatitis*.[3] Recent studies suggest that joint symptoms are predominantly or uniquely associated with hepatitis B infection. Joint involvement is often symmetrical and polyarticular. Morning stiffness may occur. Hands, wrists, elbows and knees are involved most often. Urticarial, petechial and macular rashes are common. Tender erythematous subcutaneous nodules have been described. Joint symptoms often resolve as jaundice develops. Serum complement levels are characteristically low. Hepatitis B antigen (HB Ag) is present in the serum. This syndrome may be observed in patients with anicteric hepatitis,[4] in which case the diagnosis is frequently considered

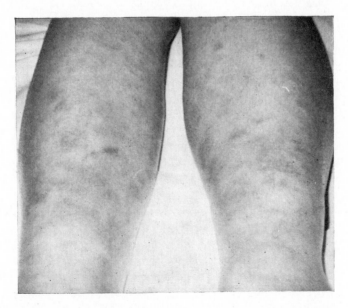

Figure 6-3. Erythema nodosum. Erythematous nodular lesions are seen along both anterior tibial areas. (Courtesy, Dr. B. Michel)

only late or not at all. Infection with hepatitis B virus may also be associated with clinical and pathologic findings of necrotizing vasculitis.[5]

Acute polyarthritis occurs as a manifestation of *serum sickness* or *drug sensitivity* reactions. Low-grade fever, urticaria and lymphadenopathy are associated symptoms. Large and medium-sized joints are usually affected, although any joint may be involved. The arthritis is often migratory and may resemble acute rheumatic fever or gonococcal arthritis.

Severe acute polyarthralgia or polyarthritis is seen in patients with *sickle cell anemia.*[6] Joint symptoms result from local sickling and thrombosis in synovial vessels. Variable degrees of joint swelling occur. Other symptoms of sickle cell disease, such as abdominal crises, are usually present. Diagnostic studies reveal anemia, sickling changes in peripheral red blood cells and the presence of hemoglobin S. Synovial fluid analysis often shows minimal deviations from the normal. Roentgenograms reveal widening of bony medullary cavities, cortical thinning and irregular trabecular markings. Other forms of joint involvement in the hemoglobinopathies include aseptic necrosis, gout, joint hemorrhage, osteomyelitis and septic arthritis.

Palindromic rheumatism is characterized by recurrent attacks of acute arthritis. Articular involvement is usually confined to one or a few joints at a time, but polyarthritis may occur.

Other diseases are associated with acute polyarthritis; these entities are interesting but fortunately relatively uncommon. *Behçet's syndrome,* a disease of unknown cause, is characterized by a clinical triad of oral and genital ulcers and iritis. In many cases, milder eye symptoms, such as conjunctivitis or episcleritis, are observed. Cutaneous lesions, phlebitis, colitis and central nervous system lesions are frequently present. Polyarthritis may be acute or subacute. *Familial Mediterranean fever* is an inherited disorder that primarily affects people in the Eastern Mediterranean area.[7] Recurrent polyserositis is associated with intermittent fever, and pain in the abdomen, chest and joints. Articular symptoms may last for several months; functional recovery is usually complete. *Whipple's disease* is characterized by chronic diarrhea and malabsorption and polyarthritis. The arthritis is usually abrupt in onset and migratory. Knees, ankles and hands are affected most often. Chronic residual articular disease is uncommon. Diagnosis depends on finding PAS-positive inclusion bodies in macrophages of the mucosa of the small bowel on tissue obtained by peroral jejunal biopsy. *Henoch-Schönlein purpura* (anaphylactoid purpura) is characterized by arthralgias or arthritis, cutaneous purpura, abdominal pain, gastrointestinal hemorrhage and renal disease. It occurs mostly in children and young adults. Cutaneous lesions consist of erythematous macules, urticarial papules and purpura (Fig. 6-4). Polyarthritis most frequently affects larger joints. Joint symptoms are transient and unassociated with deformity. Crampy abdominal pain and melena are common. Intussusception may

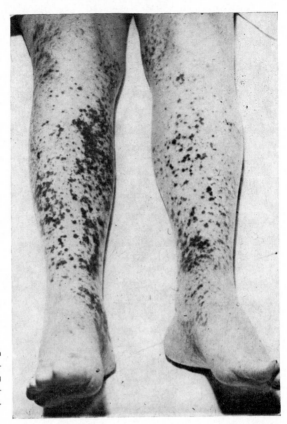

Figure 6-4. Henoch - Schönlein (anaphylactoid) purpura, involving both lower extremities. (Courtesy, Dr. A. Mackenzie)

complicate the clinical picture. Renal involvement is characterized by proteinuria, hematuria and, at times, fatal renal failure. Prognosis is generally good if renal manifestations are mild.

Acute polyarthritis is occasionally seen in other diseases. These latter states do not represent a major problem in differential diagnosis, either because the disease itself or the appearance of joint symptoms as an acute polyarthritis is relatively uncommon. For example, although gout classically initially appears as an acute monoarthritis, patients with acute polyarticular disease as an initial or early manifestation have been described.[8] Two or more joints may be involved. In other gouty patients, acute polyarthritis may occur after a prolonged period of disease when interval therapy has been inadequate. In the latter cases, a careful review of the history usually reveals previous recurrent attacks of acute monoarthritis for many years. Acute polyarthritis also occurs in patients with pseudogout syndrome (chondrocalcinosis). In most cases, however, joint symptoms are limited to one or a few joints at any given time.

Relatively acute polyarthralgia or polyarthritis is seen in patients with leukemia.[9] Joint symptoms and swelling result from leukemic infiltration of synovium, or from leukemic involvement of bone contiguous to the joint. Acute polyarthritis has been described in patients with Type II hyperlipoproteinemia,[10] in which case acute migratory arthritis may simulate rheumatic fever. Attacks last from a few days to one month. Large peripheral joints are usually affected. Episodic tendinitis of the Achilles tendon also occurs in this condition.[11] Associated clinical findings include xanthomatosis, xanthelasma, corneal arcus and early atherosclerosis. Laboratory studies reveal marked elevations of serum cholesterol with normal concentrations of triglycerides. Treatment of acute attacks is symptomatic. Rarely, acute polyarthritis may result from simultaneous involvement of several joints in patients with septic arthritis or hemorrhagic disorders.

DIAGNOSTIC STUDIES

A number of studies are frequently required in the search for the correct diagnosis in patients with acute polyarthritis. Initial studies should usually include a complete blood count, urinalysis, erythrocyte sedimentation rate, throat culture, antistreptolysin-O titer, electrocardiogram, serum protein electrophoresis, serum complement, and tests for rheumatoid factor and antinuclear antibody. A serologic test for syphilis (STS) is valuable because a false positive STS supports a diagnosis of systemic connective tissue disease. Serum glutamic oxaloacetic transaminase and Australia antigen (HAA, HB Ag) determinations should be performed if viral hepatitis is suspected.

Roentgenograms of joints usually have limited diagnostic value, especially early in the course of the various diseases. Articular chondrocalcinosis is seen in pseudogout syndrome. In patients with familial Mediterranean fever, the bones of involved joints reveal a coarse trabecular osteoporosis. A typical "egg shell line" often appears on both sides of the radiolucent osteoporotic zone. Chest x-rays are helpful in the diagnosis of sarcoid or erythema nodosum. More specific diagnostic studies, such as sigmoidoscopy and roentgenograms of the large and small bowel, are indicated if one of the enteropathic arthritides such as regional enteritis or ulcerative colitis is suspected. Blood cultures are often positive in the presence of infectious polyarthritis. Joint fluid studies are especially helpful in delineating the presence of gonococcal or septic arthritis; they have lesser value in the differential diagnosis of other forms of acute polyarthritis because the findings are often similar and nonspecific. If gonococcal arthritis is suspected, a carefully performed culture from the uterine cervix should be obtained in women; in men, cultures of penile discharge or of penile secretions following prostatic massage are indicated. Gram-stain smear and cultures from cutaneous gonococcal lesions may be diagnostically helpful. Rectal swab and pharyngeal cultures are indicated, especially if homosexual contact is suspected.

Despite a carefully performed history and physical examination and detailed diagnostic studies, a specific diagnosis may remain elusive. In these cases, successful diagnosis usually depends on repeated and prolonged clinical observation and followup diagnostic studies.

THERAPY

As noted earlier, patients with acute polyarthritis usually require hospitalization in order to perform detailed extensive diagnostic studies and to institute nonspecific or specific therapeutic measures directed toward relief of symptoms. Bed rest and the appropriate use of splints for immobilization provide pain relief. High doses of aspirin reduce inflammation; in addition, its use may provide valuable clues to differential diagnosis. Rapid and complete resolution of fever and acute joint symptoms in response to high doses of aspirin supports a diagnosis of acute rheumatic fever. Doses of 100 mg/kg/day in small children and 960 mg every four hours in adults are utilized as a diagnostic test. Although aspirin induces some relief from symptoms and fever in other forms of acute polyarthritis, the response is considerably less complete and dramatic than that which occurs in acute rheumatic fever. Physical therapy should be limited to gentle range-of-motion exercises as tolerated. Local applications of superficial heat are usually beneficial, although some patients respond better to cold. Mild analgesic agents such as acetaminophen, propoxyphene HCl (Darvon), or ethoheptazine citrate (Zactane) are helpful; at times, short courses of mild narcotics such as codeine may be necessary. Overly aggressive nonspecific multiple therapeutic regimens should be avoided; symptoms may be temporarily relieved but often at the price of obscuring the diagnosis.

Indomethacin may be given when relief with aspirin is inadequate. Phenylbutazone is similarly beneficial; it should be utilized for relatively short periods of time to avoid side reactions such as bone marrow depression, peptic ulceration, edema and skin rash. The indiscriminate use of corticosteroids to treat acute polyarthritis should be avoided. They are hazardous if given in the presence of undetected infection; in addition, they may suppress symptoms and laboratory findings vital to diagnosis.

Definitive therapy directed to the various disorders is instituted when a specific diagnosis has been confirmed (see Chapter 18). In those cases in which the diagnosis remains uncertain, more aggressive therapeutic measures can be begun when infection has been excluded and a reasonable probable diagnosis has been made.

CASE HISTORIES

History 6-1. Acute Rheumatic Fever

S.F., a 15-year-old white male, was hospitalized on December 27, 1972, for evaluation of the chief complaints of fever and joint pain. He had been apparently well until the first week in December, at which time he developed a mild upper respiratory infection with nonproductive cough. Symptoms resolved in a few days and the patient was well until approximately one week prior to admission. At that time his mother noted that he limped on his right leg and had swelling of the right knee. Two days later, the left ankle and right tarsal areas became warm, swollen and tender and the patient developed a high fever. He was evaluated by his pediatrician, who began penicillin therapy when a throat culture revealed the presence of beta-hemolytic streptococci, group A. That same day, a transient nonspecific rash was noted over the area of both wrists. The patient was admitted to hospital for further study when fever and joint symptoms continued. There was no prior history of symptoms suggestive of acute rheumatic fever and there was no known heart murmur. System review was negative for Raynaud's phenomenon, iritis, conjunctivitis, urethritis, pleurisy, hair loss, sun sensitivity, dry mouth or eyes, alopecia or drug allergy. There were no specific complaints of low back or neck pain. Past medical history was noncontributory.

On physical examination, blood pressure was 130/82 mm Hg. Pulse rate was 120/minute, respiratory rate, 22/minute, and temperature, 39° C. No skin rash was seen. Cardiac examination revealed a Grade I/VI soft systolic murmur, heard best at the cardiac apex. Liver and spleen were not palpably enlarged. The right knee and left ankle were swollen, erythematous, warm and slightly limited in function. The hematocrit was 38%, the white blood cell count, 26,000/mm^3 with a slight shift to the left, and the erythrocyte sedimentation rate, 51 mm/hour (Wintrobe). Urinalysis, serum glutamic oxaloacetic transaminase, and serum bilirubin were normal. Routine serologic test for syphilis was nonreactive. Blood and urine cultures were negative. Throat culture revealed normal flora. Serum studies for febrile and cold agglutinins were negative. Antistreptolysin-O titer was 500 Todd units. C-reactive protein was 4+. Serum studies for rheumatoid factor and antinuclear antibody were negative, as was study for LE cells. Electrocardiograms taken daily for three days were within normal limits. X-rays of the chest, paranasal sinuses, knees, ankles and feet were unremarkable. Serum protein electrophoresis revealed a slight increase in gamma globulin. Ophthalmologic examination showed no evidence of iritis or other abnormalities. During the period of study, the patient continued to have an intermittent fever with daily elevations to approximately 39° C.

A diagnosis of acute rheumatic fever was made, although juvenile rheumatoid arthritis was also a diagnostic consideration. The patient was given aspirin, 960 mg every four hours. The clinical response was striking. Within 36 hours the temperature had become normal and joint symptoms improved considerably. The pulse rate dropped to 82/minute and no cardiac murmur was heard. Repeat erythrocyte sedimentation rate was 34 mm/hour. White blood cell count was 10,000/mm^3 with a normal differential. The patient was discharged on therapy with aspirin, 1280 mg QID, and plans for penicillin prophylaxis.

Discussion: A diagnosis of acute rheumatic fever was made on the basis of acute polyarthritis, fever, evidence of infection with beta-hemolytic streptococci on culture and serologic study, and a dramatic response to aspirin. Although juvenile rheumatoid arthritis was a diagnostic consideration when the patient was first seen, clinical and diagnostic studies supported a diagnosis of rheumatic fever. Juvenile rheumatoid arthritis and acute rheumatic fever may be extremely difficult to differentiate when a limited number of major manifestations of rheumatic fever are present. In cases in which the evidence for diagnosis of rheumatic fever is strong but incomplete, it is safest to treat the patient for acute rheumatic fever. Penicillin prophylaxis should be instituted. If an error in diagnosis has been made and the clinical syndrome is really juvenile rheumatoid arthritis, observation over the ensuing months should clarify the diagnosis.

History 6-2. Rheumatoid Arthritis

P.S., a 40-year-old white male, was in good health until December 2, 1972. At that time he noted sudden onset of chills and fever, followed over a period of several days by acute swelling of the left knee, left ankle, right elbow and several proximal interphalangeal (PIP) joints of both hands. Anorexia and malaise were noted. He was admitted to hospital elsewhere by his physician for study. The white blood cell count was 11,000/mm^3 with 78% polymorphonuclear cells. Erythrocyte sedimentation rate was 55 mm/hour (Westergren). Serum latex fixation study for rheumatoid factor was positive in a titer of 1:40. Serum antinuclear antibody titer and LE cell determinations were negative. Chest x-ray, electrocardiogram, serologic test for syphilis, protein electrophoresis and serum antistreptolysin-O titer were negative or normal. Fluid aspirated from the left knee revealed 8000 WBC/mm^3 with 52% polymorphonuclear cells. Synovial fluid, blood and urine cultures were negative. On system review the patient gave a negative history for urethritis, conjunctivitis, skin rash, pleurisy, Raynaud's phenomenon, hair loss or sun sensitivity. He denied extramarital sexual exposure. The patient was given aspirin, 960 mg QID, with only limited relief of joint symptoms. Low-grade temperature elevation persisted. Symptoms of acute polyarthritis, fever and malaise remained disabling despite an intensive program of conservative therapy using aspirin, 1280 mg QID, indomethacin, 25 mg QID, local heat, bed rest and physical therapy. Prednisone, 7.5 mg per day, was added, and several intra-articular injections of steroid were placed in the left knee, the site of greatest disability. He was discharged on this program of management only to be re-admitted to hospital three weeks later when he had increased inflammatory swelling of the left knee and both ankles. Repeat evaluation showed persistently positive serum rheumatoid factor, weakly positive serum antinuclear antibody titer and negative LE cell preparations. No symptoms or signs of other connective tissue or systemic disease states were noted on full reinvestigation. A course of gold sodium thiomalate (Myochrysine) therapy was begun. Additional medications included aspirin, 1280 mg QID, and prednisone, 2.5 mg BID.

He was first seen in referral January 27, 1973, at which time he was afebrile and joint manifestations were limited to swelling of the left wrist and left knee. He had received a total of 200 mg of Myochrysine. Gold therapy was continued until proteinuria was noted at a total dose of 400 mg, at which time his joint symptoms had greatly improved. Gold was discontinued and the patient was placed on hydroxychloroquine (Plaquenil), 200 mg BID. Aspirin, 1280 mg QID, and prednisone, 2.5 mg BID, were continued in addition to a full physical therapy program. Hydroxychloroquine was reduced to 200 mg once daily after three months when the patient showed continued clinical improvement. When last seen in December, 1973, the patient was doing measurably better. Therapy consisted of aspirin, 1280 mg QID, prednisone, 2.5 mg once daily, and hydroxychloroquine, 200 mg per day. The left wrist and left knee were minimally swollen.

Discussion: This patient appeared initially with an acute onset of polyarthritis associated with systemic manifestations that included fever and chills, anorexia and malaise. Several diagnoses, such as acute rheumatic fever, acute gonococcal arthritis, and systemic lupus erythematosus, had to be considered.

The clinical findings and laboratory studies were consistent with a diagnosis of rheumatoid arthritis of acute onset. The patient responded to a therapeutic regimen for rheumatoid arthritis with a great reduction of symptoms.

History 6-3. Gonococcal Arthritis

G.M., a 24-year-old black female, was first seen in consultation in hospital in August, 1973. She had been in good health until three days prior to admission when she developed migratory polyarthralgia associated with chills and temperature elevations to 39° C. Twenty-four hours later she noted swelling and tenderness in the left first metatarsophalangeal joint, both knees and both ankles. There was no past history of arthritis, sore throat, sun sensitivity, morning stiffness, skin rash, alopecia, Raynaud's phenomenon or pleurisy. She denied recent extramarital sexual intercourse. Menstrual periods were regular and there was no history of increased vaginal discharge. System review was otherwise negative and family history was unremarkable.

On physical examination, the patient's temperature was 37.5° C. There was no lymphadenopathy. Examination of the heart, lungs and abdomen was normal. Pelvic examination revealed a vaginal discharge but no tenderness and no palpable masses. Erythema, tenderness and swelling of both knees and ankles were noted. The right hip was painful on motion and the right shoulder was tender to palpation. Examination of the skin revealed several small erythematous papulovesicular lesions on the hands and forearms. Several lesions were slightly pustular in appearance.

The hematocrit was 36%, the white blood cell count was 5,000/mm³ with a normal differential, and the erythrocyte sedimentation rate was 32 mm/hour (Wintrobe). Urinalysis was normal. Serum studies for rheumatoid factor and antinuclear antibody were negative. No LE cells were seen. Liver function studies, routine serum electrolytes, chest x-ray and electrocardiogram studies were normal. Gram-stain study of material obtained from the uterine cervix revealed gram-negative diplococci in an intracellular location. Neisseria gonorrhoeae was identified on culture of the same material and on material obtained by rectal swab. Blood cultures were negative. A diagnosis of acute gonococcal arthritis was made.

The patient was treated with aqueous crystalline penicillin, six million units daily administered intravenously in divided doses. Joint symptoms resolved dramatically within a 48-hour period. Cutaneous lesions showed similar improvement. Penicillin therapy was continued by intramuscular and then oral routes for a total of 14 days, with complete resolution of symptoms.

Discussion: In this patient, gonococcal arthritis appeared as an acute polyarthritis. The presence of typical cutaneous lesions helped significantly in clinical diagnosis. Bacterial studies confirmed the diagnosis and the patient had an excellent response to therapy. Gonococcal arthritis should be strongly considered in young people with acute arthritis, whether monoarticular or polyarticular in type. Associated manifestations of gonococcal arthritis, such as acute tenosynovitis and typical cutaneous lesions, are extremely helpful in diagnosis.

History 6-4. Rubella Arthritis

J.L., a 17-year-old white female, was first seen in consultation in September, 1970. History revealed acute onset of swelling of the proximal interphalangeal (PIP) and metacarpophalangeal (MCP) joints of the hands, both wrists, knees and ankles two weeks following rubella vaccination. Joint symptoms completely resolved after one week. A second attack of similar joint symptoms of lesser severity occurred several weeks later. Symptoms again remitted completely without therapy after approximately five days. The patient was seen when joint symptoms recurred a third time several weeks later. Symptoms were mild and involved primarily the PIP and MCP joints of the hands and the knees. There were no ancillary symptoms of connective tissue disease such as drug allergy, sun sensitivity, pleurisy, colitis, dry mouth or eyes, hair loss, or psoriasis. Past medical history was essentially negative. Joint examination revealed tenderness and slight swelling of PIP and MCP joints of both hands and the knees. General examination was otherwise normal.

The complete blood count and urinalysis were normal. Erythrocyte sedimentation rate was 5 mm/hour (Wintrobe). Serum studies for rheumatoid factor and antinuclear antibody were negative. Serum uric acid was 5.3 mg/100 ml. Serum glutamic oxaloacetic transaminase and routine serologic test for syphilis were negative. Antistreptolysin-O titer was less than 100 Todd units. EKG and chest x-ray were normal. A diagnosis of rubella arthritis was made.

The patient was placed on therapy with aspirin, 960 mg QID. Joint symptoms remitted after approximately one week. Her general health has been excellent and, on followup examination some four years later, the patient remains in perfect health on no therapy.

Discussion: The sequence of events and the benign nature of the arthritis in this patient are consistent with a diagnosis of rubella arthritis following vaccination. In most cases symptoms are relatively mild and short-lived. The intermittent nature of the symptoms is not inconsistent with the diagnosis, because attacks of brief duration may recur for several years following vaccination.

History 6-5. Arthritis Associated with Ulcerative Colitis

K.P., a 25-year-old white female, had a history of ulcerative colitis beginning at age 23. Abdominal-perineal resection with removal of the colon and rectum was performed one year after the onset of her illness, when medical management with prednisone and salicylazosulfapyridine (Azulfidine) was ineffective in controlling symptoms. The patient did satisfactorily until July, 1973, when she appeared with pain, swelling and tenderness of the right wrist, left knee and left elbow. She denied abdominal pain, diarrhea, dysphagia, rash, photosensitivity, alopecia, pleurisy, dry eyes or dry mouth. There was no prior history of joint disease. The patient had been taking no medications except diphenoxylate hydrochloride with atropine sulfate (Lomotil) and antispasmodics. Physical examination showed marked inflammation and swelling of the involved joints.

The hematocrit was 35%, the white blood cell count was 3600/mm³ with a normal differential, and the erythrocyte sedimentation rate was 38 mm/hour (Wintrobe). Serum electrolytes, glutamic oxaloacetic transaminase and creatine phosphokinase were within normal limits. Urinalysis revealed +1 albuminuria. Serum uric acid was 2.5 mg/100 ml. Serum rheumatoid factor and antinuclear antibody studies were negative, and serologic test for syphilis was nonreactive. Roentgenograms of the wrists, knees and elbows were unremarkable. Analysis of synovial fluid from the left knee revealed 12,000 white cells/mm³ with 55% polymorphonuclear cells. Synovial fluid glucose was 70 mg% when fasting blood sugar was 86 mg%. Mucin clot test was grossly abnormal. No crystals were noted. The fluid was negative for bacterial infection on smear and culture. The patient's symptoms responded well to a program of aspirin, 960 mg QID, in addition to bed rest and application of heat to involved joints. Joint swelling and pain responded sufficiently to allow discharge from hospital after ten days, and the patient was continued on salicylates and a physical therapy program.

Discussion: The presumptive diagnosis in this case is arthritis associated with chronic nonspecific ulcerative colitis. Although joint symptoms in such cases are frequently associated with active ulcerative colitis, joint symptoms may continue or sometimes begin when all evidence of colitis appears to have been removed.

History 6-6. Hepatitis-associated Arthritis

M.J., an 18-year-old white female, was admitted to hospital with a one-week history of pruritus of the legs and arms. Two days prior to admission she had noted painful swelling of the wrists and proximal interphalangeal (PIP) joints. Joint symptoms were intermittent and migratory and remained confined to the upper extremities. On physical examination, both wrists were tender and swollen, and the proximal interphalangeal joints were mildly tender to palpation. Urticarial lesions appeared on the arms and back. Malaise, nausea and anorexia were noted on the fifth hospital day. Clinical jaundice was absent.

The white blood cell count and differential, urinalysis, routine serologic test for syphilis, serum uric acid, heterophile antibody titer, and studies for serum rheumatoid factor and antinuclear antibody were normal or negative. Hematocrit was 34%. Initial serum glutamic oxaloacetic transaminase (SGOT) was 255 Henry units (normal, 9 to 25 units), and total serum bilirubin was 1.3 mg/100 ml. Serum alkaline phosphatase was 11 King-Armstrong units (normal, 3 to 13 units). Sulfobromophthalein retention was 10% at 45 minutes. Serum protein electrophoresis was normal. Serum complement was 35 CH^{50} hemolytic units (normal control, 100 units). Antistreptolysin-O titer was 250 Todd units. LE cell studies were negative. X-rays of the chest, hands and wrists were unremarkable. Oral cholescystogram and liver scan were normal. Cultures of the blood, urine and uterine cervix were negative. Hepatitis-associated antigen (HB Ag) was detected in the serum on the fifth hospital day. On the eighth hospital day, joint abnormalities disappeared. SGOT levels reached a maximum of 1200 units on the 18th day of hospitalization. The patient was discharged after 23 days, with no clinical symptoms and with normal liver function. One month later, she was completely asymptomatic and liver function studies remained normal. Hepatitis-associated antigen was no longer detectable.

Discussion: This patient had the characteristic clinical and laboratory findings of hepatitis-associated arthritis. Joint symptoms and an urticarial rash were noted. Abnormal laboratory results included abnormal liver function studies, a low serum complement and the presence of hepatitis-associated antigen in the serum. As noted in this case, hepatitis-associated arthritis may occur in patients with anicteric hepatitis. Accordingly, hepatitis as an etiology of arthritis may be readily overlooked in patients with this syndrome.

History 6-7. Gout

J.A., a 64-year-old black male, was seen in consultation in January, 1972. He gave a history of joint symptoms of 20 years duration, characterized initially by acute attacks of pain, swelling and tenderness involving the first metatarsophalangeal joints. Attacks lasted several weeks and cleared completely without therapy. Early in the course of his disease, attacks occurred at intervals of approximately one year. Later, attacks became more frequent and were often polyarticular with involvement of MTP joints, ankles, knees and wrists. Joint symptoms cleared completely over a period of one to two weeks, even when several joints were simultaneously involved. No joint symptoms or fibrositis were noted between acute episodes. Past treatment had included the use of aspirin and short courses of steroid therapy at the time of acute symptoms. The patient felt in good health otherwise and had no symptoms of Raynaud's phenomenon, pleurisy, hair loss, sun sensitivity, or skin rash. Past medical history was noncontributory.

Physical examination at the time the patient was first seen revealed marked tenderness and swelling of the right tarsal area and the right first MTP joint. No subcutaneous nodules or tophi were seen. A diagnosis of probable acute gouty arthritis was made and the patient was placed on therapy with phenylbutazone, 100 mg QID, and ACTH gel, 80 units IM. Clinical response was excellent.

Laboratory studies revealed normal urinalysis, hematocrit, white blood cell count and differential. Erythrocyte sedimentation rate was 36 mm/hour (Wintrobe). Serum uric acid was 11.2 mg/100 ml and serum latex fixation test for rheumatoid factor was positive at a titer of 1:20. Serum antinuclear factor study was negative. Diagnostic considerations included: (1) gout with associated positive serum rheumatoid factor of uncertain significance, (2) episodic rheumatoid arthritis with coincidental hyperuricemia, and (3) rheumatoid arthritis and gout. The patient was placed on an interval therapy program of probenecid, 0.5 gm daily, with gradual increases to 0.5 gm QID, which was required to maintain the serum uric acid at normal levels. Colchicine, 0.6 mg BID, was added. The patient had several episodes of acute arthritis involving the MTP joints, ankles, tarsal areas and knees over the subsequent six months. Analysis of synovial fluid removed from the right knee during one of these episodes revealed numerous needle-shaped crystals that were strongly birefringent in a negative direction. Attacks of joint pain gradually subsided and the patient has been essentially asymptomatic over a two-year period of observation. Repeat studies for serum rheumatoid factor have been consistently negative.

Discussion: Gout characteristically appears initially as an acute monoarthritis. However, polyarthritis is not uncommon in later stages when inadequate or no treatment is given. The presence of polyarthritis and a positive test for serum rheumatoid factor when this patient was first seen made diagnosis more complex. The relationship of his symptoms to gout was confirmed later by the finding of crystals consistent with monosodium urate in synovial fluid and the clinical response to an interval therapy program for gout.

REFERENCES

1. Yanez, J. E. et al.: Rubella arthritis. Ann Int Med 64:772, 1966.
2. Thompson, G. R., Ferreyon, A. and Brackett, R. G.: Acute arthritis complicating rubella vaccination. Arth Rheum 14:19, 1971.
3. McCarthy, D. J. and Ormiste, V.: Arthritis and HB Ag-positive hepatitis. Arch Int Med 132:264, 1973.
4. Stevens, D. P. et al.: Anicteric hepatitis presenting as polyarthritis. JAMA 220:687, 1972.
5. Gocke, D. J. et al.: Association between polyarteritis and Australian antigen. Lancet 2:1149, 1970.
6. Schumacher, R. H., Andrews, R., and McLaughlin, G.: Arthropathy in sickle-cell disease. Ann Int Med 78:203, 1973.
7. Sohar, E. et al.: Familial Mediterranean fever. A survey of 470 cases and review of literature. Am J Med 43:227, 1967.
8. Hadler, N. M. et al.: Acute polyarticular gout. Am J Med 56:715, 1974.
9. Silverstein, M. N. and Kelly, P. J.: Leukemia with osteoarticular symptoms and signs. Ann Int Med 59:637, 1963.
10. Khachadurian, A. K.: Migratory polyarthritis in familial hyperlipoproteinemia (type II hyperlipoproteinemia). Arth Rheum 11:385, 1968.
11. Glueck, C. J., Levy, R. I. and Fredrickson, D. S.: Acute tendonitis and arthritis: a presenting symptom of familial type II hyperlipoproteinemia. JAMA 206:2895, 1968.

Chapter 7

SUBACUTE AND CHRONIC POLYARTHRITIS

Rheumatic diseases often occur initially as a subacute or chronic polyarthritis. In other cases subacute or chronic polyarthritis follows monoarthritis or acute polyarthritis as the articular involvement spreads or becomes more persistent.

DIFFERENTIAL DIAGNOSIS

Most likely causes to be considered:

Rheumatoid arthritis
Systemic lupus erythematosus
Other connective tissue diseases (dermatomyositis, scleroderma, periarteritis nodosa, Sjögren's syndrome, mixed connective tissue disease)
Degenerative joint disease (osteoarthritis)
Psoriatic arthritis
Reiter's syndrome
Arthritis of ulcerative colitis and regional enteritis
Sarcoid arthritis
Arthritis associated with malignant neoplasms
Hypertrophic osteoarthropathy
Chronic tophaceous gout; pseudogout

The most common cause of severe chronic polyarthritis is *rheumatoid arthritis*. Classically the proximal interphalangeal and metacarpophalangeal joints of the hands are affected, but all peripheral joints of the body may be involved at one time or another. Although joint involvement is frequently bilateral and symmetric, asymmetric involvement is not uncommon. In addition to the peripheral joints, such as the wrists, elbows, knees and ankles, the temporomandibular, sternoclavicular and cricoarytenoid joints may be affected. Weakness and atrophy of muscles contiguous to involved joints is common.

100

Systemic and extra-articular manifestations are frequent and diagnostically valuable. Generalized fibrositis characterized by stiffness and gelling of joints is most severe on awakening or after a period of inactivity during the day. Low-grade fever is common. Other extra-articular manifestations have prognostic as well as diagnostic importance in that they usually signify more severe disease. Subcutaneous nodules most often occur at the subolecranon areas of the elbows. They may be seen elsewhere, however, and are most apt to involve pressure areas such as the scapulae, buttocks and Achilles tendons. Lymphadenopathy may be striking. Splenomegaly is not uncommon; when associated with leukopenia the combination of symptoms is classified as Felty's syndrome.[1] Anemia may result from any of several causes, including chronic bone marrow depression, impairment of iron absorption, plasma dilution effect, hypersplenism, and drug-induced gastrointestinal blood loss. Eye manifestations may be severe. Band keratopathy is characterized by an equatorial corneal opacity caused by fibrosis of the cornea. Episcleritis involves the anterior cornea and may be localized or diffuse. Intense hyperemia of deep vessels is present. Iritis may occur. Scleritis may be acute, with widespread necrotizing sclerosis. In some cases, scleral involvement with nodular destruction is slow. The wall of the eye softens, and uveal tissue may herniate through the defect. This pernicious

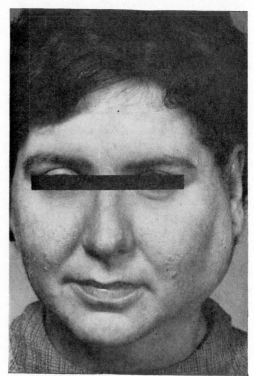

Figure 7-1. Sjögren's syndrome. Note swelling of left parotid gland. (Courtesy, Dr. A. Mackenzie)

form of eye involvement is called scleromalacia perforans. Sicca syndrome with symptoms of dryness of the eyes and a sensation of scratchiness is common. Secondary glaucoma and cataracts are late sequelae of rheumatoid eye disease. Systemic necrotizing vasculitis, which fortunately occurs in only a small percentage of cases, is heralded by skin ulceration, subungual and paronychial infarcts, and neuropathy.

Chronic polyarthritis often identical to that seen in rheumatoid arthritis is common in *systemic lupus erythematosus.* In certain patients, however, joint symptoms are limited to polyarthralgia of varying severity without significant objective changes. Chronic polyarthritis in *other connective tissue diseases* such as dermatomyositis, scleroderma and polyarteritis nodosa is usually much more limited in extent and severity as compared to rheumatoid arthritis.

Sjögren's syndrome, which is a chronic inflammatory disease process characterized by diminished lacrimal and salivary gland secretion,[2] is usually classified with the connective tissue disorders. Joint symptoms consistent with those of classic rheumatoid arthritis occur in many patients. Clinical findings consistent with other connective tissue diseases, such as systemic lupus erythematosus, scleroderma, polymyositis or vasculitis, may also be noted. Chronic inflammatory changes are observed in the salivary and lacrimal glands, and in glandular components of the respiratory tract, gastrointestinal tract and vagina. Classic clinical features include dry eyes, dry mouth and parotid gland swelling (Fig. 7-1). Arthralgia and arthritis are common. Raynaud's phenomenon is seen in 20% of patients.

Several supporting diagnostic studies are available.[3] Parotid salivary flow rates, measured following a stimulus such as lemon juice on the tongue, are diminished. Involvement of the lacrimal glands can be measured by the simple Schirmer test, in which a strip of filter paper is folded and placed

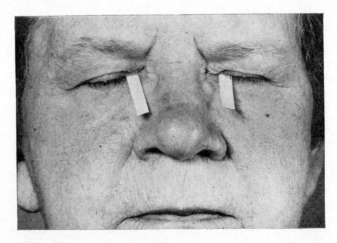

Figure 7-2. Schirmer test, filter paper strips in place. (Courtesy, Dr. A. Mackenzie)

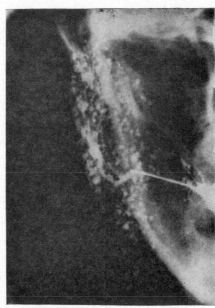

Figure 7-3. Sialogram, Sjögren's syndrome, showing globular and cavitary sialectasis. (Courtesy, Dr. A. Mackenzie)

in the lower conjunctival sac (Fig. 7-2). Normally, after five minutes, the moistened portion of the paper measures 15 mm or greater. In Sjögren's syndrome, the moistened area usually measures 5 mm or less. Secretory sialography, performed by introducing a radiopaque contrast medium into the parotid duct orifice, reveals punctate, glandular or cavitary sialectasis (Fig. 7-3). Salivary scintograms using technetium pertechnetate show decreased uptake, which correlates with impaired glandular function.[4] Biopsy study of mucosal tissue obtained from inside the lower lip demonstrates lymphoid infiltration of the minor salivary glands.

Immunologic abnormalities, such as hypergammaglobulinemia, positive tests for serum rheumatoid and antinuclear factors, and positive studies for LE cells, are common. Lymphoproliferative changes in Sjögren's syndrome lead to pseudolymphomatous hyperplasia. An increased association with reticulum cell sarcoma and Waldenström's macroglobulinemia has been noted.

Artificial tears are useful in relieving eye dryness. Management of joint symptoms should remain conservative whenever possible. Corticosteroid therapy may be helpful when disease manifestations are severe. The use of immunosuppressive agents remains investigative but may be indicated at times, particularly in the treatment of pseudolymphoma.

Chronic polyarthritis may occur in patients whose clinical and laboratory findings represent a composite of several connective tissue disorders. For example, definitive evidence of systemic lupus erythematosus, polymyositis

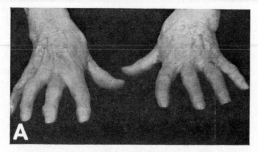

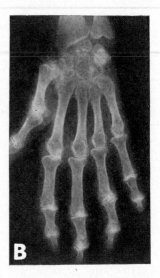

Figure 7-4. Osteoarthritis of hands. (A) Clinical appearance. Knobby swelling of the distal and proximal interphalangeal joints is associated with horizontal joint deviation. Osteoarthritic changes of the first carpometacarpal joints cause a squared appearance in this area. (B) Radiographic appearance. Joint space narrowing and spur formation in involved joints.

and scleroderma may be present in various combinations in the same patient. This overlapping has been given the name *mixed connective tissue disease.*[5] Antibody to a specific extractable nuclear antigen (ENA) is frequently present in the sera of patients with these clinical features.

Degenerative joint disease (osteoarthritis) is usually limited to involvement of one or a few joints. However, manifestations may sometimes be more widespread. Knobby involvement of the distal interphalangeal (DIP) joints of the hands (Fig. 7-4) (Heberden's nodes) is classic and common. This form of osteoarthritis occurs primarily in middle and older years, and affects women ten times more frequently than men. The lesions are usually insidious in development and associated with few or no symptoms. In other cases, however, onset is abrupt and inflammation relatively extensive. Osteoarthritic changes in the distal interphalangeal (DIP) joints are often followed by a similar involvement of proximal interphalangeal (PIP) joints (Fig. 7-4) (Bouchard's nodes). Involvement of metacarpophalangeal joints is relatively uncommon, an important differentiating point from rheumatoid arthritis. Other peripheral joints may be affected by osteoarthritis, often independently of DIP and PIP joint involvement. Particularly susceptible peripheral joints include the first carpometacarpal joint of the hands (Fig. 7-4), hips (Fig. 7-5), knees and first metatarsophalangeal joints. The cervical and lumbar spine are frequently affected. Osteoarthritis rarely affects the wrists, elbows, shoulders and ankles unless secondary to some other disorder such as chronic trauma or injury.

Although osteoarthritis may cause chronic polyarticular disease, evidence of inflammation is usually lacking. Joint swelling is caused mainly by bone and cartilage proliferation. Synovitis is frequently present to mild or mod-

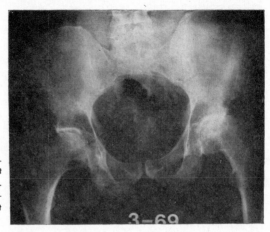

Figure 7-5. Osteoarthritis of hips. Changes are most marked in the left hip. Note joint space narrowing and bony cyst formation.

erate degree on pathologic study but is usually a minimal finding on clinical examination. Morning stiffness, if present, is limited to the specifically involved joints, in contrast to the generalized morning stiffness characteristic of rheumatoid arthritis.

The arthritis associated with *psoriasis* takes several forms[6] and may be difficult to differentiate from rheumatoid arthritis. The most typical form involves the distal interphalangeal (DIP) joints of the hands, usually in association with psoriatic changes in the fingernails. This has some diagnostic significance, because rheumatoid involvement of DIP joints early is uncommon. Of similar significance is involvement of the interphalangeal joints of the toes, which is also rare in patients with rheumatoid arthritis. A second form of psoriatic arthritis is characterized by extensive erosive changes in articulating bone. In the hand, these mutilating changes lead to the "main en lorgnette" or opera-glass hand, in which the fingers are highly mobile and are readily telescoped to shorter size. In the third form of psoriatic arthritis, joint changes are identical to those seen in rheumatoid arthritis; differentiation is essentially impossible. However, the swelling of the small joints involved in psoriatic arthritis often appears sausage-shaped, which aids differential diagnosis (Fig. 7-6). Separation of the two disorders often depends on the results of serum testing for rheumatoid factor —a positive result indicating rheumatoid arthritis. Moreover, spondylitis is common in psoriatic arthritis. Skin changes are usually characteristic and prominent but cases of psoriatic arthritis with minimal skin findings are not uncommon. Although skin and nail changes usually precede or occur simultaneously with articular disease, joint manifestations occasionally precede them by months or years.

Subacute or chronic polyarthritis is a major component of the triad of arthritis, urethritis and conjunctivitis seen in *Reiter's syndrome*.[7] Mucocu-

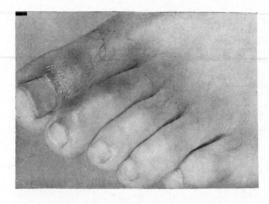

Figure 7-6. Psoriatic arthritis. Sausage-shaped swellings of the interphalangeal joints of the toes.

taneous lesions that involve the skin, oral cavity and genitalia are a common fourth component of the syndrome. More frequent in males, this syndrome is occasionally associated with extra-articular manifestations such as conduction abnormalities of the heart and neuropathy. Spondylitis is a common sequel; it often occurs late in the disease when peripheral joint symptoms are minimal or absent. Histocompatibility antigen, HLA-W27, is present in up to 96% of patients with this disorder.[8]

Polyarthritis is a common associated symptom in patients with *ulcerative colitis* and *regional enteritis*. As in psoriatic arthritis and Reiter's syndrome, spondylitis is an important component of the joint manifestations. Joint symptoms usually occur simultaneously with or following gastrointestinal symptoms. Less frequently, arthritis precedes bowel manifestations. HLA-W27 histocompatibility antigen appears in approximately 75% of patients with ulcerative colitis or regional enteritis when spondylitis is present.[9]

Articular changes occurring in *sarcoid* are variable in type. Chronic polyarthralgia is common; in addition, acute, subacute or chronic monoarthritis or polyarthritis is seen. Joint symptoms may be difficult to differentiate from those of rheumatoid arthritis. Tuberculin skin reaction is usually negative.

Malignant neoplasms may be associated with chronic polyarthritis.[10,11] The clinical features of the joint involvement are similar to those seen in rheumatoid arthritis. This entity should be strongly considered in the differential diagnosis of chronic polyarthritis in older age groups. Although neoplasms in any organ can produce this syndrome, tumors of the genitourinary tract and lungs are particularly frequent. In many cases the offending neoplasm is occult when the patient is first seen. Rheumatoid factor study is usually negative but occasionally positive. Treatment of the neoplasm by surgical, radiologic or chemotherapeutic means may be associated with partial or complete resolution of joint symptoms. Anti-inflammatory agents such as aspirin, indomethacin or phenylbutazone provide symptomatic relief. Steroid therapy is sometimes indicated.

Hypertrophic osteoarthropathy is characterized by clubbing of the fingers, periosteal proliferation and synovitis. Large joints are involved most commonly. In some cases the syndrome is idiopathic or familial. More commonly, it occurs secondary to any of several other disorders, such as neoplasms, suppurative pulmonary disease, cyanotic congenital heart disease, subacute bacterial endocarditis, cirrhosis, chronic diarrheal states and following thryroidectomy for Grave's disease. Aspirin, indomethacin or phenylbutazone therapy provides symptomatic relief in many cases. Steroid therapy may benefit patients with severe joint manifestations. Treatment of underlying disorders such as empyema or bronchiectasis or resection of primary tumors may be associated with resolution of symptoms.

Chronic polyarthritis may be a manifestation of untreated or inadequately treated *gout* when large deposits of urate result in persistent synovitis and joint swelling (Fig. 7-7). Usually, a careful history reveals prior episodes of acute arthritis typical of the gouty diathesis. The other common form of crystal-induced synovitis, *pseudogout syndrome* (chondrocalcinosis), may also produce chronic polyarthritis.[12] In most cases of pseudogout, joint manifestations are characterized by chronic polyarthralgia or by acute or subacute arthritis limited to one or a few joints. Chronic synovitis represents a chronic inflammatory response to synovial deposits of calcium pyrophosphate dihydrate crystals.

The foregoing entities will account for most diagnoses of patients with chronic polyarthritis. However, other disease states must be considered when the diagnosis remains elusive. These latter diseases occur less frequently or less commonly produce chronic polyarthritis as their major articular manifestation. For example, *Behçet's syndrome* is a relatively rare disease in which chronic arthritis may occur in association with the more

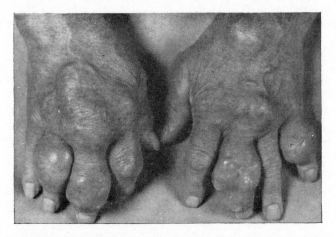

Figure 7-7. Monosodium urate deposits causing chronic polyarthritis in patient with tophaceous gout. (Courtesy, Dr. A. Mackenzie)

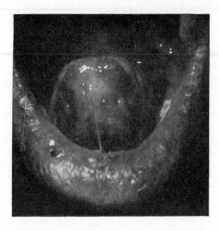

Figure 7-8. Behçet's syndrome. Mucosal ulcerations involve the tongue and
lower lip. (Courtesy, Dr. C. Denko)

classic symptoms of orogenital ulcerations (Fig. 7-8) and recurrent iritis.[13] Additional symptoms include phlebitis, colitis, inflammatory nodular skin lesions (which resemble erythema nodosum), pyoderma gangrenosum and central nervous system manifestations. Another rare cause of chronic poly-arthritis is that associated with *shunting operations of the gastrointestinal tract*. This syndrome has been described following jejunocolostomy per-formed for weight reduction.[14] Articular symptoms frequently remit with correction of the shunt.

Chronic polyarthritis has been described in patients with *hemochromato-sis*.[15] Although large peripheral joints such as the hips and knees may be involved, chronic arthritis affecting the second and third metacarpophalan-geal and proximal interphalangeal joints of the fingers is characteristic. Irregular joint space narrowing, osteoporosis and subchondral cyst forma-tion appear on x-ray. Chronic polyarthralgia and symptoms resembling degenerative joint disease are common. This arthropathy frequently is as-sociated with the radiologic findings of chondrocalcinosis and associated acute symptoms of pseudogout syndrome. Diagnosis is suggested by the typical clinical picture. Confirmation of the syndrome requires demonstra-tion of elevations in serum iron and percent iron saturation of transferrin, and biopsy evidence of tissue deposits of hemosiderin. Articular symptoms of hemochromatosis may precede overt clinical presentation of other mani-festations of the disease, such as skin pigmentation, diabetes mellitus and hepatic cirrhosis.[16]

Chronic polyarthritis may be observed in a small number of patients with *myxedema*.[17] Signs and symptoms of myxedema are usually present when rheumatic symptoms appear. Generalized stiffness is common. The most characteristic objective joint changes are marked synovial thickening and effusions in the knee and small joints of the hands and feet. Signs of inflammation are usually absent. Radiologic findings are not specific. Musculoskeletal manifestations are completely reversible with thyroid replacement therapy.

Chronic polyarticular symptoms occur in patients with familial *type IV hyperlipoproteinemia*.[18] Symptoms consist mainly of recurrent arthralgia; joint swelling is uncommon. Lipoprotein electrophoresis reveals changes mainly in the pre-beta lipoprotein band (type IV).

Although *tuberculous and fungal infections* may result in chronic polyarthritis, joint involvement is most commonly monoarticular or limited to two or three joints. Occasionally, more than three joints are involved and these diagnoses should be considered in the differential diagnosis of perplexing cases. Arthritis attacks in *Whipple's disease* are usually acute and relatively short-lived. Subacute or chronic joint manifestations occasionally appear.

DIAGNOSTIC STUDIES

In most cases of chronic polyarthritis, a well-performed history and physical examination will usually narrow the diagnostic field to a limited number of fairly common entities. In some cases, however, diagnosis is particularly difficult and less common diseases must be considered. Initial laboratory studies should include a complete blood count, erythrocyte sedimentation rate, urinalysis, serologic test for syphilis (to note false positive reactors), serum uric acid, serum latex fixation test for rheumatoid factor, serum antinuclear factor and serum protein electrophoresis.

Roentgenograms of the most severely involved joints should be obtained. They aid in differential diagnosis and, in addition, are valuable in delineating the degree of joint damage. Although radiologic findings are often nonspecific, they may be particularly valuable in certain diseases. Joint space narrowing, erosions and ankylosis of the distal interphalangeal joints are characteristic of psoriatic arthritis. Resorption of the terminal phalanges is common. A characteristic "pencil and cupping" deformity may be seen, in which the sharply tapered end of the proximal bone of the joint fits into the flared end of the distal bony surface. Roentgenograms of affected joints show periosteal elevation and new bone growth in patients with hypertrophic osteoarthropathy. Calcification of fibrocartilages, particularly the menisci of the knees and the triangular cartilage of the wrist, is typical of pseudogout syndrome. Joint space narrowing, osteophyte formation, subchondral bony sclerosis and cyst formation are the classic changes of osteoarthritis. Chest x-ray may demonstrate pulmonary lesions characteristic of several connective tissue diseases, pulmonary sarcoidosis or neoplasms (see Chapter 12).

Additional diagnostic studies such as sigmoidoscopy and gastrointestinal x-rays, serum protein bound iodine and serum lipid studies should be performed when clinical suspicion suggests the presence of less common causes of chronic polyarthritis. Synovial fluid analysis is less helpful diagnostically in this form of articular disease because the findings are often similar and nonspecific for the various disorders. Similarly, synovial biopsy is often nonspecific but may be diagnostically valuable in cases of arthritis due to sarcoid, chronic granulomatous infections, gout or pseudogout. Diagnostic studies should be repeated periodically because they might be negative when the patient is first seen but become positive over the ensuing months or years.

THERAPY

Management should remain conservative until the diagnosis has been established as definitely as possible. Rest and physical therapy relieve joint pain and maintain range of motion and muscle strength. Various forms of heat therapy help to relieve pain and muscle spasm. Canes and crutches should be utilized when lower extremities are severely involved. Aspirin given to maximal tolerance will usually relieve symptoms to some degree in most cases, whatever the etiology. Symptoms are further aided by the use of mild analgesic agents. Other nonspecific anti-inflammatory agents such as indomethacin and phenylbutazone can be considered for use in the more symptomatic cases; they usually will not obscure the diagnosis. Corticosteroid therapy should be considered only when diagnostic studies and observation have led to a reasonable probable diagnosis and to the exclusion of diseases in which their use would be contraindicated. The use of other agents and modes of therapy varies with the final diagnosis (see Chapter 18).

CASE HISTORIES

History 7-1. Rheumatoid Arthritis

M.F., a 52-year-old white female, was well until May, 1963, at which time she noted aching in the posterior cervical area and both shoulders. Shortly afterward she developed swelling and pain of both wrists, proximal interphalangeal (PIP) joints of the second and third fingers bilaterally, and both ankles and knees. Aspirin, 640 mg QID, provided mild relief. There was no past history of arthritis or rheumatic fever. System review was negative for Raynaud's phenomenon, pleurisy, sun sensitivity, psoriasis, diarrhea or alopecia. Additional symptoms included weight loss of ten pounds, prolonged morning stiffness, and easy fatigability. On physical examination, the palms were cool and moist. Swelling and tenderness of the second and third PIP and metacarpophalangeal (MCP) joints of the hands, both wrists, knees and ankles were noted. Pelvic and rectal examinations were normal.

Laboratory studies revealed normal urinalysis, hematocrit of 36%, white blood cell count of 7300/mm³, normal differential white cell count, erythrocyte sedimentation rate of 42 mm/hour (Wintrobe), negative serologic test for syphilis, slightly elevated serum gamma globulin, normal serum uric acid, and normal liver function studies. Chest x-ray was normal. Roentgenograms of the hands, wrists, knees and ankles showed periarticular bone demineraliz-ation. Serum latex fixation test for rheumatoid factor was positive in a titer of 1:1280. Serum antinuclear factor was weakly positive, but LE cell studies were negative.

Discussion: This patient represents a classic case of onset of rheumatoid arthritis. Several other connective tissue diseases that can simulate rheumatoid arthritis had to be excluded by appropriate clinical and laboratory evaluation. The patient was followed regularly over an 11-year period and unfortunately showed progressive changes of rheumatoid arthritis despite a full therapeutic program of aspirin, indomethacin, hydroxychloroquine, gold salt therapy and maintenance low-dose steroids. Bilateral total hip prostheses were required for therapy of severe hip involvement. However, the patient remained indepen-dent in activities of daily living despite persistent progression of her disease.

History 7-2. Systemic Lupus Erythematosus

D.K., a 60-year-old white female, was first seen in consultation in August, 1969. She was well until two years prior, at which time she noted swelling and pain in both wrists. Symptoms resolved completely after a period of one month with no specific therapy. In the fall of 1968 she noted fatigue associ-ated with swelling of both wrists, proximal interphalangeal (PIP) joints of the hands, and both knees. Swelling persisted and other joints were subsequently involved. There was no history of hair loss, pleurisy, drug allergy, skin rash, dry eyes or dry mouth. She had a recent history of sensitivity to sun exposure, characterized by easy burning of the skin, and Raynaud's phenomenon. System review and past medical history were otherwise negative. On physical exam-ination at the time of evaluation, no abnormalities were noted except for musculoskeletal findings. PIP and metacarpophalangeal (MCP) joints of the hands were mildly swollen and tender. The right elbow was swollen, with 15° limitation of extension. Both shoulders were limited to 50° abduction and both knees revealed mild swelling. Initial diagnosis was connective tissue dis-ease, with a note to specifically exclude systemic lupus erythematosus on the basis of sun sensitivity and Raynaud's phenomenon.

Urinalysis, hematocrit, white blood cell count and differential, and routine serologic test for syphilis were normal or negative. Serum rheumatoid factor study was negative but serum antinucelar antibody was present in a titer of 1:1000. Anti-DNA titer in the serum was 1:80. LE cell study showed rosettes and several LE cells. In the absence of any overt major visceral manifesta-tions of systemic lupus erythematosus, a conservative program of aspirin, 960 mg four times a day, mild analgesics and rest was instituted. Indome-thacin, 25 mg TID with food, was added when joint symptoms remained mildly active. The patient did reasonably well on this conservative program of management, but in July, 1973, symptoms became more severe with increased swelling, pain and tenderness of numerous joints. Laboratory studies remained essentially unchanged. Due to the severe exacerbation of her joint symptoms and the economic necessity to remain active in her occupation, therapy with hydroxychloroquine (Plaquenil), 200 mg BID, and prednisone, 2.5 mg BID, was added. A baseline ophthalmologic evaluation was obtained for use in following hydroxychloroquine therapy, which was reduced to 200 mg daily after a period of four months. The patient did extremely well on her re-vised program. When last seen in January, 1974, joint symptoms were under good control and no evidence of intolerance to medications was noted.

Discussion: Arthritis was the major initial clinical manifestation of sys-temic lupus erythematosus in this patient. In the absence of evident involve-ment of critical visceral structures such as the kidneys, it was deemed reason-able to treat the patient with a conservative program of salicylates and indomethacin for a prolonged period of time following diagnosis. Increased joint symptoms prompted the addition of hydroxychloroquine and prednisone. Joint manifestations were identical to those seen in rheumatoid arthritis, and laboratory studies were required to substantiate the diagnosis of systemic lupus erythematosus.

History 7-3. Primary Generalized Osteoarthritis

J.B., a 42-year-old white female, first noted joint symptoms at age 40, at which time she developed pain in both hips with prolonged activity. Increased pain and limitation of motion of both hips was noted over the ensuing two years. One year prior to evaluation she developed pain and swelling of the distal and proximal interphalangeal joints of both hands and both first carpo-metacarpal joints. More recently, both knees had become painful with use, and locking of the left knee had occurred on several occasions. Treatment with aspirin, 640 mg QID, and indomethacin, 75 mg per day in divided doses, afforded some relief early in the course of her symptoms. More recently, this therapy was ineffective in controlling her distress. Mild morning stiffness lasting 15 to 30 minutes involved the knees, hips, and hands. There was no history of Raynaud's phenomenon, hair loss, dry eyes or mouth, dysphagia, sun sensitivity, psoriasis, colitis, or drug allergy. The patient considered herself to be in good health otherwise, and past medical history was noncontributory. Family history of documented severe degenerative joint disease in her father, a paternal uncle, and two paternal cousins was significant. Physical examination at time of consultation revealed bony swelling of the distal and proximal interphalangeal joints of the hands. First carpometacarpal joints bilaterally were tender and limited in motion. Hips were severely limited in range of motion in all directions, and movement was associated with severe pain. Knee swelling was absent but limitation of flexion to 90° bilaterally was evident.

The hematocrit was 43%, the white blood cell count was 8,000/mm³ with a normal differential, and the erythrocyte sedimentation rate was 22 mm/hour (Wintrobe). Serum electrolytes, calcium, phosphorus and alkaline phosphatase, and serum protein electrophoresis studies were within normal limits. Serum uric acid was 2.5 mg/100 ml. Fasting blood sugar was 90 mg/100 ml. Urinalysis was normal and serologic test for syphilis was negative. Urine study for homogentisic acid was negative. Serum studies for rheumatoid factor and antinuclear antibody were negative. X-ray study of the chest was normal. X-rays of the hips revealed significant degenerative changes bilaterally with narrowing of joint spaces, eburnation, and osteophytic spurring. Subchondral cyst formation was present in the femoral heads. Roentgenographic examination of the knees showed extensive degenerative changes bilaterally with narrowing of the joint spaces and spur formation. Multiple loose bodies appeared in the left knee. X-rays of the hands and wrists revealed joint space narrowing and spur formation in numerous distal and proximal interphalangeal joints. A diagnosis of primary generalized osteoarthritis was made. Aspirin and indomethacin therapy was continued with inadequate relief of pain and disability. Multiple surgical procedures were indicated for management of the severe joint symptoms. Loose bodies were removed from the left knee and, at separate intervals, bilateral total hip replacements were performed.

Discussion: This patient had symptoms of severe generalized osteoarthritis at a relatively early age. A history of severe osteoarthritis occurring at an early age in other members of her family suggested a possible hereditary component to her disorder. Underlying disease states such as rheumatoid arthritis, hemophilia, and ochronosis, which are frequently associated with secondary osteoarthritis, were not evident.

History 7-4. Psoriatic Arthritis

R.P., a 34-year-old white male, was well until June, 1973, when he noted a pruritic dry scaly rash over the right temporal area. Shortly thereafter, similar lesions appeared on the scalp, the right ear and the lateral aspect of the right thigh. The lesions healed and itching decreased following therapy with local steroid cream. Approximately two months after onset of the rash, he developed insidious swelling and pain of the distal interphalangeal (DIP) joint of the left index finger and the interphalangeal joint of the third toe of the left foot. Morning stiffness lasted for 10 to 15 minutes. No ancillary symptoms of connective tissue disease were elicited.

Physical examination revealed dry scaly cutaneous lesions involving the scalp, right ear, and right thigh. Fingernails were slightly pitted. Fusiform sausage-like swellings of the DIP joint of the left index finger and the interphalangeal joint of the left third toe were noted. Both joints were warm and tender. Some tenderness of the second and fourth metatarsophalangeal (MTP) joints of the left foot was also observed.

Laboratory studies revealed normal complete blood count and urinalysis. Erythrocyte sedimentation rate was 23 mm/hour (Wintrobe). Serum uric acid was 5.9 mg/100 ml. Serum glutamic oxaloacetic transaminase, serologic test for syphilis, serum protein electrophoresis, electrocardiogram and chest x-ray were normal or negative. Roentgenograms of the involved joints were negative except for evidence of soft tissue swelling. A diagnosis of psoriasis with psoriatic arthritis was made.

The patient was placed on therapy with aspirin, 960 mg QID, with little relief of symptoms. Indomethacin, 25 mg QID, was helpful, but continued involvement of MTP joints caused moderate difficulty in walking. Local injections of steroid into the involved joints of the left hand and left foot provided considerable improvement. The patient remained on therapy with aspirin, 960 mg QID, and indomethacin, 25 mg QID, with only mild joint distress. Cutaneous lesions were kept under control with local applications of steroid cream.

Discussion: The clinical findings in this patient were consistent with the diagnosis of psoriatic arthritis. Fusiform sausage-like swellings of the joints, involvement of the distal interphalangeal joints of the hands and interphalangeal joints of the toes were characteristic. Although joint symptoms usually occur concomitant with or following the onset of psoriasis, arthritis may antedate psoriatic skin changes by months or years.

History 7-5. Overlap Syndrome

S.S., a 51-year-old white female, was well until May, 1968. At that time she noted nonspecific aching in the arms upon rising in the morning. Symptoms were relatively mild and lasted two to three hours daily. Motion aggravated the pain. She was treated symptomatically by her physician with aspirin and phenylbutazone, with little relief. She was admitted to hospital elsewhere in January, 1970, for diagnostic studies when symptoms became more severe and persistent. Pain was located mainly in the muscles of the upper arms and posterior cervical areas. Morning stiffness was a major associated complaint. Routine blood counts, urinalysis, erythrocyte sedimentation rate, serum rheumatoid factor, and serum antinuclear antibody studies and LE cell determination were normal or negative. A diagnosis of primary fibrositis was made. The patient was treated with cervical traction, heat and injections of local steroid into trigger points of tenderness. She was first seen in consultation in August, 1970, with persistent similar complaints. She now complained also of occasional arthralgias that involved the proximal interphalangeal (PIP) and metacarpophalangeal (MCP) joints of the hands and weakness of grip strength. There was no history of Raynaud's phenomenon, pleurisy, hair loss, sun sensitivity, dysphagia, psoriasis or other skin rash, or colitis. No eye or mouth dryness nor frequent canker sores were noted. System review was otherwise negative and past medical history unremarkable. Medications included aspirin, 640 mg QID, and diazepam (Valium), 5 mg TID.

On physical examination the hands were slightly moist and warm. No tremor was noted. Temporal arteries were normal to palpation. Examination of the musculoskeletal system revealed mild but definite weakness of shoulder and hip girdle muscles. Joint examination was unremarkable. Hematocrit was 39%, white blood cell count was 4600/mm³ with a normal differential, and erythrocyte sedimentation rate was 35 mm/hour (Wintrobe). Urinalysis, fasting blood sugar, serum glutamic oxaloacetic transaminase, protein bound iodine, calcium, phosphorus and alkaline phosphatase determinations and serologic test for syphilis were normal or negative. Serum uric acid was 5.5 mg/100 ml. Serum rheumatoid factor test was negative. Serum antinuclear antibody test was strongly positive in a titer of 1:1000, and serum anti-DNA antibody titer was 1:10. Numerous LE cells were present on peripheral blood specimens. Creatine phosphokinase in serum was normal, and daily urinary creatine-creatinine ratio determinations were 18% and 24%. Creatinine clearance was normal. Electromyographic study was normal. Study of biopsy material obtained from the right deltoid muscle revealed variation in muscle fiber size, central migration of sarcolemmal nuclei, and mild infiltration of mononuclear cells. A diagnosis of overlap syndrome with components consistent with systemic lupus erythematosus and polymyositis was made. The patient was placed on prednisone, 5 mg QID, with complete remission of symptoms and good response of muscle weakness.

Discussion: For several years this patient had nonspecific symptoms that were originally diagnosed as primary fibrositis. Although the symptoms were similar to those seen in primary fibrositis, they represented premonitory manifestations of underlying connective tissue disease in this patient. The diagnosis was an overlap syndrome consisting of findings suggestive of systemic lupus erythematosus with polymyositis.

REFERENCES

1. Barnes, C. G., Trumbull, A. L. and Vernon-Roberts, B.: Felty's syndrome. Ann Rheum Dis 30:359, 1971.
2. Mason, A. M. S., Gumpel, J. M. and Golding, P. L.: Sjögren's syndrome—a clinical view. Semin Arthritis Rheum 2:301, 1973.
3. Cummings, N. A. et al.: Sjögren's syndrome. Newer aspects of research, diagnosis and therapy. Ann Int Med 75:937, 1971.
4. Alarcon-Segovia, D. et al.: Salivary gland involvement in diseases associated with Sjögren's syndrome. 1. Radionuclide and roentgenographic studies. J Rheumatology 1:159, 1974.
5. Sharp, G. C. et al.: Mixed connective tissue disease—an apparently distinct rheumatic disease syndrome associated with specific antibody to an extractable nuclear antigen (ENA). Am J Med 52:148, 1972.
6. Moll, J. M. H. and Wright, V.: Psoriatic arthritis. Semin Arthritis Rheum 3:55, 1973.
7. Ford, D. K.: Reiter's syndrome. Bull Rheum Dis 20:588, 1970.
8. Morris, R. et al.: HLA-W27—a clue to the diagnosis and pathogenesis of Reiter's syndrome. N Eng J Med 290:554, 1974.
9. _____.: HLA-W27—a useful discriminator in the arthropathies of inflammatory bowel disease. N Eng J Med 290:1117, 1974.
10. Lansbury, J.: Collagen disease complicating malignancy. Ann Rheum Dis 12:301, 1953.

11. Mackenzie, A. H. and Scherbel, A. L.: Connective tissue syndromes associated with carcinoma. Geriatrics 18:745, 1963.
12. Moskowitz, R. W. et al.: Chronic synovitis as a manifestation of calcium crystal deposition disease. Arth Rheum 14:109, 1971.
13. O'Duffy, J. D., Carney, J. A. and Deodhar, S.: Behçet's disease: A report of ten cases, three with new manifestations. Ann Int Med 75:561, 1971.
14. Shagrin, J. W., Frame, B. and Duncan, V.: Polyarthritis in obese patients with intestinal bypass. Ann Int Med 75:377, 1971.
15. Dymock, I. W. et al.: Arthropathy of haemochromatosis. Ann Rheum Dis 29:469, 1970.
16. Gordon, D. A. and Little, H. A.: The arthropathy of hemochromatosis without hemochromatosis. Arth Rheum 16:305, 1973.
17. Bland, J. and Frymoyer, J.: Rheumatic syndromes in myxedema. N Eng J Med 282:1171, 1970.
18. Goldman, J. A. et al.: Musculoskeletal disorders associated with type IV hyper-lipoproteinemia. Arth Rheum 14:384, 1971.

Chapter 8

INTERMITTENT ARTHRITIS SYNDROMES

In some patients, joint symptoms are characterized by acute attacks that are frequent, recurrent, and intermittent with variable periods of complete remission. Sometimes the recurrences have a periodic character. A limited number of rheumatic diseases produce such a clinical picture, in contrast to numerous arthritic diseases in which articular symptoms are cyclic but exacerbations are usually long in duration and remissions, unfortunately, are limited and incomplete. For example, rheumatoid arthritis, systemic lupus erythematosus and rheumatic fever frequently demonstrate remissions and exacerbations but usually would not be classified as "intermittent arthritis syndromes."

Diseases characterized as intermittent arthritis syndromes include:

Gout
Pseudogout
Episodic rheumatoid arthritis
Palindromic rheumatism
Intermittent hydrarthrosis
Familial Mediterranean fever
Whipple's disease

DIFFERENTIAL DIAGNOSIS

Gout is classically characterized by attacks of acute arthritis abrupt in onset. The usual attack lasts three to seven days followed by variable periods of complete remission during which the joint is normal. Early in the disease, remissions may be prolonged, lasting for months or years. Later, as the disease progresses, acute attacks become more frequent until they recur as often as several times a month. The first metatarsophalangeal joint is most frequently involved (podagra) (Fig. 4-3), but other joints such as the tarsal area, ankle and knee are commonly involved. At times, peripheral joints of the upper extremities are affected. Acute attacks occur spontaneously or may be precipitated by such factors as trauma, surgery,

116

overindulgence in alcohol, intake of high purine foods or diuretic therapy. Acute inflammation results from precipitation of monosodium urate crystals in synovial fluid with subsequent release of various inflammatory mediators. Finding urate crystals in synovial fluid removed from the joint is specific for the diagnosis.

Pseudogout syndrome (chondrocalcinosis) is similarly characterized by acute attacks of joint inflammation that are abrupt in onset. Attacks tend to be less frequent than those seen in true gout. Clinically, the joint most frequently involved is the knee. Other large joints may be involved; podagra occurs but is relatively uncommon. As in true gout, surgery or diuretic therapy may precipitate attacks. Often, there is a background symptomatology of low-grade chronic arthralgia upon which acute attacks are superimposed. Acute symptoms are related to the activation of inflammatory mediators by calcium pyrophosphate dihydrate crystals in synovial fluid. Roentgenograms reveal typical calcifications of articular hyaline and fibrocartilage (Figs. 4-4, 4-5).

Rheumatoid arthritis may occur as an episodic disease, so-called *episodic rheumatoid arthritis,* which is difficult to differentiate from gout and pseudogout. Abrupt onset of acute attacks over a period of several hours is characteristic. Attacks last 36 hours to several days and are followed by complete remission. As the disease progresses, acute attacks become more frequent and prolonged, and complete remission no longer ensues. A similar clinical picture is characteristic of *palindromic rheumatism.*[1] This interesting entity of unknown etiology is also characterized by acute, abrupt attacks of joint inflammation. Symptoms often develop within a period of hours. Severe pain occurs early, followed by joint redness, tenderness and swelling. Any peripheral joint may be affected. Interestingly, joint pain may decrease when swelling is maximal. Duration of attacks varies from a few hours to as long as a week; attacks lasting only several days are most common. One or a limited number of joints are involved at a time. The interval between attacks varies from several days to months. The pattern of attacks with respect to area and frequency of joint involvement may be characteristic in a given patient. Para-articular inflammation characterized by variably-sized painful erythematous swellings in soft tissues adjacent to joints is common. Transient intracutaneous and subcutaneous nodules may be seen. Prognosis is excellent with respect to crippling because, by definition, chronic joint changes do not evolve. On the other hand, control of disease symptoms may be difficult with considerable distress and limitation occurring during the periodic recurrent attacks.

The similarities between palindromic rheumatism and episodic rheumatoid arthritis may cause appreciable diagnostic confusion. It has been suggested that palindromic rheumatism is a prodromal or atypical form of rheumatoid arthritis.[2] Many cases originally diagnosed as possible palindromic rheumatism eventually manifest themselves as rheumatoid arthritis

5

as attacks become more frequent and remissions less complete. The presence of rheumatoid factor in high titer in the serum supports a diagnosis of rheumatoid arthritis. Low titers of rheumatoid factor are less helpful; such findings have been reported in palindromic rheumatism.[2]

Intermittent hydrarthrosis is characterized by acute recurrent attacks of joint swelling of predictable periodicity.[3] Joint effusions are notable for their lack of local inflammatory change and relatively little pain. Systemic signs and symptoms are absent. Usually, symptoms completely resolve and attacks abate in two to four days. Knees are involved most commonly. Although attacks are usually monoarticular, polyarticular involvement does occur. The interval between attacks varies from one week to one month, with intervals of one to two weeks being most common. Attacks at monthly intervals are likely to be related to menstruation in women. In some patients, effusions cease after many years; other patients, unfortunately, will have the syndrome as a life-long condition. There are no characteristic laboratory findings.

Familial Mediterranean fever is an inherited disorder of people from the Eastern Mediterranean area, chiefly Sephardic Jews, Levantine Arabs, Turks and Armenians.[4] The disease is characterized by recurrent acute or subacute attacks of arthritis, frequently associated with fever and with abdominal and chest pain due to polyserositis. Symptoms are usually short-lived, lasting several days to one or two weeks. In some cases, however, arthritis persists for months. Knees, ankles and hips are involved most frequently. Fortunately, functional joint recovery between attacks is usually complete. Many patients develop an erysipelas-like erythema and tenderness around the ankles. Amyloidosis, a dreaded manifestation of the disease, is a common cause of death.

Whipple's disease[5] is characterized by fever, abdominal pain, diarrhea, cutaneous hyperpigmentation, adenopathy and arthritis. Joint symptoms are frequently acute in onset, episodic and transient, lasting only for several hours or days. Residual joint changes are uncommon. In many cases, articular manifestations precede abdominal symptoms by years. Large joints, such as the knee and the ankle, are involved most often, but smaller joints are also affected.

Other diseases, such as Behçet's syndrome, ulcerative colitis, and Henoch-Schönlein purpura, may be associated with intermittent joint manifestations. Articular symptoms are usually overshadowed by serious abnormalities related to other organ systems.

DIAGNOSTIC STUDIES

Clinical similarities may make it extremely difficult to differentiate the foregoing diseases not only from one another but from other forms of rheumatic disease. Close attention to subtle details of the history and physical examination is vital. Diagnosis often depends on carefully considered laboratory investigation. Initial laboratory studies should include a complete blood count, erythrocyte sedimentation rate, urinalysis, serologic test for syphilis, serum latex fixation test for rheumatoid factor, serum antinuclear factor, serum protein electrophoresis, synovial fluid analysis and x-ray of involved joints. Synovial fluid analysis is particularly helpful in the diagnosis of gout or pseudogout, because the finding of intracellular and extracellular crystals of monosodium urate or calcium pyrophosphate dihydrate respectively is diagnostic. Joint fluid examination should be performed early in the acute attack if possible, because crystals are often few or absent during remissions. Although serum uric acid determinations are helpful in corroborating a diagnosis of gout, some studies suggest an increased frequency of coincidental hyperuricemia in pseudogout patients. Serum calcium, phosphorus and alkaline phosphatase and serum iron, iron-binding capacity, and iron saturation studies should be performed in patients with pseudogout to exclude the presence of hyperparathyroidism and hemochromatosis.

A high-titer positive test for serum rheumatoid factor supports a diagnosis of episodic rheumatoid arthritis. Low or negative titers are consistent with rheumatoid arthritis or palindromic rheumatism. Increases in erythrocyte sedimentation rate are common during acute attacks in both diseases. Final differentiation depends on the development of more prolonged attacks and incomplete remissions in patients with episodic rheumatoid arthritis.

There are no specific diagnostic laboratory studies for intermittent hydrarthrosis. The clinical finding of periodic attacks of acute swelling of the knees associated with little or no pain is fairly characteristic, however, and differentiation from the other syndromes described previously usually is not difficult.

Familial Mediterranean fever should be strongly considered in the differential diagnosis of acute intermittent arthritis in patients of Mediterranean origin. Although several abnormal laboratory findings are frequently noted, they are unfortunately nonspecific. The erythrocyte sedimentation rate and the plasma fibrinogen level are elevated during attacks and may even remain slightly elevated during intercritical periods. Massive proteinuria often develops if amyloidosis intervenes. Serum gamma globulin elevations are common. The serum latex fixation test for rheumatoid factor is usually negative. Synovial fluid analysis reveals nonspecific evidence of mild inflammatory disease.

The diagnosis of Whipple's disease depends on demonstrating PAS-positive inclusion bodies in macrophages of the small intestinal mucosa or mesenteric nodes. Jejunal biopsy is performed by peroral approach. Rod-shaped organisms infiltrating the lamina propria of the intestinal mucosa appear on electron microscopic study.

Radiologic studies are helpful in the diagnosis of pseudogout and familial Mediterranean fever. In the former, characteristic calcifications of articular hyaline and fibrocartilage are seen. In familial Mediterranean fever, joints involved for a long period of time show coarse trabecular osteoporosis and pseudocyst formation. Swelling of the knee is associated with enlargement of the femoral condyles. In a few patients, a characteristic "eggshell line" may be found on both sides of the radiolucent osteoporotic zone at the distal femur. This double contoured line may persist after osteoporosis resolves as the attack abates.

THERAPY

Acute attacks of gout or pseudogout may be treated effectively with various therapeutic agents (see Chapter 18). Acute attacks of episodic rheumatoid arthritis of mild severity may respond to high-dose salicylate therapy. In more severe cases, indomethacin, 25 mg QID with meals, or phenylbutazone, 100 mg QID, may be required. In patients who fail to respond to these programs, prednisone in a dose of 5 mg QID is often effective. Acute attacks can often be aborted or lessened in severity by instituting anti-inflammatory therapy at the first sign of pain, before the attack reaches a significant degree of intensity. Continuous prophylaxis with indomethacin, 25 mg QID, may afford long-term suppression when recurrent attacks are frequent. More frequently beneficial for this purpose is long-term therapy with antimalarial agents, such as hydroxychloroquine (Plaquenil), or gold. Hydroxychloroquine is given in a dose of 200 mg twice a day for three to four months, following which the dose usually can be decreased to 200 mg daily. Periodic eye evaluations should be performed to avoid toxicity occasionally associated with long-term use of this agent. Gold therapy, carried out as in the usual case of rheumatoid arthritis, has equal or greater effect. Treatment and prevention of acute attacks of palindromic rheumatism is similar to that described for episodic rheumatoid arthritis. Continuous prophylaxis with hydroxychloroquine or gold is particularly effective in many patients and should be considered if attacks are frequent and severe.

No satisfactory treatment is presently available for the treatment of intermittent hydrarthrosis. Daily salicylate therapy during attacks may ameliorate the swelling and is attended by little hazard. Fortunately, pain is usually not a problem and more aggressive therapy is not required. In patients with familial Mediterranean fever, aspirin, other analgesic agents and local heat may provide partial relief for acute attacks. Corticosteroid agents are surprisingly ineffective. Colchicine, 0.6 mg TID, administered on a regular daily basis, has been shown to be effective in prophylaxis of recurrent attacks.[6] Other agents reported to have therapeutic value include conjugated estrogens[7] and indomethacin.[8]

The response of Whipple's disease to antibiotics is highly successful. A program that includes procaine penicillin G, 1.2 million units, and streptomycin, 1 gm daily for two weeks, followed by tetracycline, 250 mg QID for 10 to 12 months, is currently recommended.

CASE HISTORIES

History 8-1. Gout

N.V., a 42-year-old white male, first noted joint symptoms at age 32, at which time he developed sudden onset of acute pain and swelling of the first metatarsophalangeal (MTP) joint of the right foot. Symptoms resolved after five or six days without specific treatment and the patient was essentially asymptomatic. Recurrent acute attacks of monoarthritis were noted at intervals of approximately six months. Symptoms were acute in onset, extremely painful, and lasted for four to seven days. Right and left first MTP joints and the tarsal areas of the feet were involved. Complete remission occurred after each attack. After approximately six acute episodes, a diagnosis of gout was made on the basis of the clinical picture, the presence of a serum uric acid level of 9.2 mg/100 ml, and a family history of gout in his brother and paternal grandfather. Treatment with probenecid, 0.5 gm daily, was instituted. The patient continued to have similar attacks at intervals of six to nine months. Acute symptoms were treated with short courses of phenylbutazone, but no changes were made in his interval therapy program.

The patient was first seen in consultation in December, 1973, after he had been admitted to the urology service with a history of acute right flank and right lower abdominal pain. Intravenous pyelogram was normal but the patient passed a uric acid stone after two days in the hospital. Serum uric acid on admission, while the patient was still on probenecid, 0.5 gm daily, was 8.6 mg/100 ml. Probenecid therapy was discontinued to study baseline uric acid metabolism. Colchicine, 0.6 mg BID, was given as prophylaxis against acute gouty attacks until studies were completed on an outpatient basis. Laboratory studies performed two weeks after discharge from hospital revealed serum uric acid levels of 9.8 and 10.6 mg/100 ml, and daily urinary uric acid excretions of 1120 mg and 1360 mg on a normal diet. Hematocrit, white blood cell count and differential, urinalysis, and creatinine clearance studies were normal. Colchicine, 0.6 mg BID, was continued, and allopurinol (Zyloprim) was begun in a dose of 100 mg TID. Plans were made to recheck his serum uric acid level in approximately three to four weeks so that appropriate changes in allopurinol therapy necessary to attain a normal serum uric acid could be made.

Discussion: The clinical history in this patient was characteristic of gouty arthritis. Attacks of monoarthritis were acute in onset, lasted four to seven days in duration, and were followed by complete remission. Involvement of first MTP joints was prominent. Inadequate therapy with probenecid was associated with continued symptomatology. The presence of hyperuricosuria and uric acid stone formation prompted use of allopurinol rather than probenecid for treatment of his articular and renal manifestations.

History 8-2. Episodic Rheumatoid Arthritis

H.R., a 56-year-old white male, was first seen in consultation in March, 1971. Joint symptoms had begun approximately one year prior, at which time he developed recurrent acute attacks of pain and swelling that separately involved the left and right knees. Attacks began over a period of hours and resolved in 24 to 36 hours without specific therapy. Acute episodes recurred at intervals of two to six weeks. Especially severe attacks of pain were treated with short courses of phenylbutazone or intramuscular injections of steroids. In January, 1971, he noted similar intermittent acute attacks of pain that involved, at various times, the ankles, proximal interphalangeal (PIP) and metacarpophalangeal (MCP) joints of the hands, and the tarsal areas. Attacks became somewhat more frequent. Remission of symptoms was less complete and attacks were more prolonged. System review was negative for skin rash, sun sensitivity, colitis, iritis, renal stones or hair loss. There was no family history of gout. Past medical history was significant in that the patient had severe urticaria and headaches with use of coal tar products. Therapy consisted of prednisone, 2.5 mg QID.

On physical examination there was acute swelling of the right wrist and the right second MCP joint. Serum rheumatoid factor and antinuclear antibody studies were negative. Serum uric acid was 5.4 mg/100 ml. Hematocrit, white blood cell count and differential, and urinalysis were normal. Serum protein electrophoresis was within normal limits. Roentgenograms of the chest, both knees, and both hands and wrists were negative except for evidence of soft tissue swelling about the right wrist joint. A diagnosis of probable episodic rheumatoid arthritis was made. The patient was maintained on therapy with prednisone, 2.5 mg QID, with instructions to increase the dose temporarily at the onset of acute attacks in the hope of aborting the symptomatic episodes. Hydroxychloroquine (Plaquenil), 200 mg BID, was added to the program. Symptoms improved only minimally on this regimen and hydroxychloroquine was discontinued after a six-month trial. Gold sodium thiomalate therapy was begun. The patient noted great improvement in symptoms at a total dose of 275 mg of gold salt. Shortly thereafter, on a program of 50 mg of gold salt weekly, the patient developed severe stomatitis and generalized pruritus; gold was discontinued. After one month, gold therapy was reinstituted, beginning with a trial dose of 5 mg of gold salt. The dose was gradually increased and weekly maintenance injections of 20 mg were given. The patient tolerated this dose without complication and continued to do well. The interval of gold administration was gradually increased to once a month.

The patient did satisfactorily until December, 1972, when he had a generalized flare of arthritis with extensive swelling and pain of the PIP and MCP joints, both wrists, both knees and ankles. Subcutaneous nodules were noted over both subolecranon areas. Serum rheumatoid factor study, which had been negative on prior repeated testing, was now positive in a titer of 1:256. An increase in the dose of gold salt to 25 mg weekly was not associated with notable clinical improvement. Prednisone, which had been reduced to 2.5 mg BID, was increased to 2.5 mg QID. Further increase in gold therapy to 30 mg weekly was associated with stomatitis and skin rash. The patient was hospitalized in January, 1973, for therapy of his severe uncontrolled joint symptoms. Gold therapy was discontinued and, with the advised consent of the patient, therapy with chlorambucil (Leukeran), 2 mg BID, was begun because of his lack of response to gold therapy in the maximal tolerated dose. The patient continued to have severe, persistent joint symptoms until April, 1973, when he noted a significant progressive improvement. Prednisone intake was gradually reduced to 2.5 mg BID. When last seen in December, 1973, the patient was taking prednisone, 2.5 mg BID, and chlorambucil, 4 mg alternating with 2 mg daily. He was doing satisfactorily with only mild swelling of both wrists, knees and elbows.

Discussion: This patient had acute episodes of arthritis lasting 24 to 36 hours in duration. Attacks became progressively more frequent and severe with less complete remission. Eventually, joint symptoms were chronic and persistent and characteristic of the joint involvement in rheumatoid arthritis. Subcutaneous rheumatoid nodules and a positive test for serum rheumatoid factor eventually appeared. Good control of symptoms was obtained with gold therapy but toxicity necessitated consideration of other therapeutic measures. The patient subsequently appeared to respond well to the use of chlorambucil. Although immunosuppressive agents have been reported as useful in the treatment of rheumatoid arthritis, their utilization remains investigative at this time.

History 8-3. Intermittent Hydrarthrosis

L.S., a 39-year-old white female, was first seen in consultation in November, 1972. She was well until approximately four years prior when, approximately one month after the birth of her third child, she noted acute onset of relatively painless swelling of the left knee. Symptoms receded spontaneously after two days. Since that time she had been afflicted with recurrent episodes of acute attacks of joint swelling that involved the right knee, the left knee or both knees simultaneously. Swelling was relatively painless, lasted two or three days, and resolved without specific therapy. Attacks initially occurred at intervals of one month, beginning several days before the onset of menses. Later, attacks continued to occur on a regular basis, but at intervals of eight or nine days. There were no other joint symptoms. System review was otherwise completely negative and past medical history was unremarkable. On physical examination, performed several days after the onset of one of her attacks in the right knee, a small amount of fluid was noted on palpation and there was a positive bulge sign. No tenderness or increased warmth was noted.

Urinalysis, white blood cell count and differential, hematocrit, and serologic test for syphilis were normal or negative. Erythrocyte sedimentation rate was 22 mm/hour (Wintrobe). Serum studies for rheumatoid factor and antinuclear antibody were negative. Serum uric acid was 3.1 mg/100 ml. Roentgenograms of both knees showed no calcifications or other abnormalities. Differential diagnostic considerations included benign idiopathic intermittent hydrarthrosis, and intermittent hydrarthrosis secondary to rheumatoid arthritis. The patient was advised to use aspirin, 960 mg QID, for mild acute attacks, and short courses of phenylbutazone for more severe episodes. A trial of hydroxychloroquine (Plaquenil), 200 mg BID, was to be added later in an effort to diminish or eliminate the frequency and severity of attacks. She was asked to return at the time of one of the attacks so that synovial fluid could be obtained for analysis. Shortly thereafter, the patient moved to another area of the country and was lost to followup.

Discussion: The clinical picture of acute episodes of relatively painless knee swelling occurring on an intermittent regular basis and resolving spontaneously are consistent with a diagnosis of benign idiopathic intermittent hydrarthrosis. A diagnosis of rheumatoid arthritis could not be completely excluded, because a similar pattern of joint manifestations may be seen in early cases. The increased frequency of attacks prompted concern in this regard. Synovial fluid analysis would have been helpful to exclude crystal-induced synovitis, a less likely diagnostic consideration. Prolonged observation is generally necessary to substantiate a diagnosis of benign idiopathic intermittent hydrarthrosis.

REFERENCES

1. Mattingly, S.: Palindromic rheumatism. Ann Rheum Dis 25:307, 1966.
2. Williams, M. H. et al.: Palindromic rheumatism. Clinical and immunological studies. Ann Rheum Dis 30:375, 1971.

3. Weiner, A. D. and Ghormley, R. K.: Periodic benign synovitis. Idiopathic intermittent hydrarthrosis. J Bone Joint Surg 38A:1039, 1956.
4. Sohar, E. et al.: Familial Mediterranean fever. A survey of 470 cases and review of literature. Am J Med 43:227, 1967.
5. Kelly, J. J. and Weisiger, B. B.: The arthritis of Whipple's disease. Arth Rheum 6:615, 1963.
6. Dinarello, C. A. et al.: Colchicine therapy for familial Mediterranean fever: a double-blind trial. N Eng J Med 291:934, 1974.
7. Bodel, P. and Dillard, G. M.: Suppression of periodic fever with estrogen. Arch Int Med 131:189, 1973.
8. Kats, B. A.: Indomethacin in familial Mediterranean fever. Lancet 2:1202, 1972.

Chapter 9

SYNDROMES OF MUSCULAR PAIN OR WEAKNESS

Diseases in patients whose chief complaint is directed primarily to muscles can usually be divided into three major clinical categories:

Muscular pain without weakness
Muscular pain with associated weakness
Muscular weakness without pain

MUSCULAR PAIN WITHOUT WEAKNESS

Fibrositis (Myofascitis)

Fibrositis is a clinical syndrome characterized by low-grade aching and stiffness of muscles and the connective tissues with which they are intimately related. Stiffness tends to be maximal in the morning or following periods of physical inactivity during the day. Symptoms are worse in cold damp weather and, conversely, are often relieved by heat. Patients may describe symptoms somewhat vaguely, but the term "gelling" is commonly used. Fibrositis is often associated with muscle tenderness and a feeling that the muscles are "knotted up." It may be generalized or local.

Localized Fibrositis. This extremely common entity is usually benign in origin. It may follow a recent nonspecific infection or occur spontaneously in otherwise healthy people. Symptoms are localized to limited, focal anatomic areas. The patient complains of tightness of muscles associated with pain of variable intensity. Movement accentuates the pain, which may become lancinating. The areas of involvement are described as trigger areas of pain from which more diffuse aching radiates. The posterior cervical region, areas around the scapulae, and mid to lower lumbar areas are most often involved. Palpation of tender areas reveals evidence of severe muscle spasm.

Generalized Fibrositis. Generalized fibrositis may be primary (idiopathic) or may be a secondary manifestation of generalized disease. The fibrositis syndrome may be the first manifestation of any of the connective tissue diseases, such as rheumatoid arthritis, systemic lupus erythematosus, scleroderma and polymyositis. Generalized fibrositis also occurs in other systemic diseases, such as hypothyroidism. Symptoms of secondary fibrositis may precede objective findings of underlying systemic disease by many months or years.

A diagnosis of primary fibrositis should be entertained only when typical symptoms occur in the absence of systemic disease or other demonstrable causes. Emotional factors are often important in the pathogenesis of the primary syndrome. A chronic tension state with associated increase in muscle tone and tension is present in a high percentage of cases. Although emotional factors are readily apparent in many patients, they are often subtle and less overt in others. Disturbed sleep patterns have been described. Primary fibrositis should be diagnosed only after underlying diseases have been excluded by a critically performed history and physical examination, appropriate laboratory studies, and prolonged observation.

Polymyalgia Rheumatica

This syndrome, seen primarily in patients over 50 years of age, is characterized by severe pain and stiffness in the shoulder and pelvic girdle areas.[1] Associated symptoms include weight loss, sweating and sometimes depression. Physical examination frequently reveals limitation of shoulder and hip motion but no real muscle weakness. Laboratory studies usually show an elevated erythrocyte sedimentation rate, with values as high as 90 to 100 mm/hour. A normochromic, normocytic anemia is frequently present. Reversal of the albumin/globulin (A/G) ratio due to elevated serum gamma globulins is typical.

Polymyalgia rheumatica syndrome may be idiopathic or associated with several underlying disorders. Many cases are associated with active temporal arteritis[1] (Chapter 13). Occasionally, cases are associated with carcinoma or lymphoma. In some patients, the syndrome represents an early manifestation of rheumatoid arthritis. In those cases related to temporal arteritis, inflammation of the temporal vessels may be relatively asymptomatic and not obvious; the diagnosis is made only by temporal artery biopsy, with or without preceding arteriograms. A thorough search for underlying associated disorders should be carried out before a diagnosis of idiopathic polymyalgia rheumatica is made. Failure to diagnosis the presence of temporal arteritis may be particularly hazardous to the patient, because sudden blindness as a result of occlusion of the ophthalmic artery or nutrient vessels to the optic nerve is a common complication. On the other hand, early treatment with corticosteroids can usually prevent this unfortunate complication in addition to providing relief of generalized muscle symptoms.

Trichinosis

Infestation of muscles with larvae of Trichinella spiralis causes severe disabling muscle pain. History may reveal mild diarrhea preceding larval deposition in the muscle, but this symptom is often absent or so mild and transient as to be overlooked. Other findings include fever and characteristic periorbital edema. Laboratory studies[2] reveal leukocytosis and significant eosinophilia. Serum complement fixation studies for trichina are valuable. Finding larvae in muscle biopsy specimens is diagnostic.

Necrotizing Vasculitis

Polyarteritis nodosa frequently causes muscle pain without weakness. Associated systemic findings such as fever, night sweats and weight loss are common. Symptoms that reflect vascular involvement of organ systems other than the muscles are present, although only muscles are involved for long periods in some cases. Cutaneous involvement leads to a multiplicity of lesions including purpura, urticaria, maculopapular lesions, vesicles, blebs and bullae. Subungual splinter hemorrhages are common. Ulceration, perforation or hemorrhage of any part of the gastrointestinal system causes a wide spectrum of abdominal symptoms. Renal involvement is associated with hypertension and renal failure. Central nervous system lesions produce hemiparesis, cranial nerve abnormalities and convulsions. Involvement of vessels to peripheral nerves causes various forms of peripheral neuropathy. The most characteristic of these is mononeuritis multiplex, in which impairment of several large nerves, such as the median, radial and peroneal, is prominent. Coronary arteritis results in ischemia with symptoms of angina and infarction. Pulmonary lesions include transient or progressive necrotizing pneumonitis.

Laboratory studies reveal leukocytosis, elevated erythrocyte sedimentation rate and frequently eosinophilia. Abnormal urine findings include albuminuria, red cells, white cells and various casts. Electromyograms may demonstrate myopathic abnormalities due to vascular lesions in muscle. In patients with ischemic neuritis, electromyographic study shows neurogenic patterns and slowed nerve conduction velocities.

Muscle biopsy, performed from involved areas, shows evidence of vasculitis. Histopathologic lesions are characterized by fibrinoid necrosis of the vessel wall and infiltration with polymorphonuclear leukocytes, eosinophils, plasma cells and mononuclear cells (Fig. 9-1). Later, healing and fibrosis are evident. In polyarteritis nodosa, small and medium-sized muscular arteries are involved.

In patients with allergic (hypersensitivity) angiitis, vascular lesions involve small arteries, veins and capillaries.[2] In addition, pulmonary artery involvement and extravascular focal necrosis and granulomas are common. Allergic granulomatous angiitis, as described by Churg and Strauss,[3] is

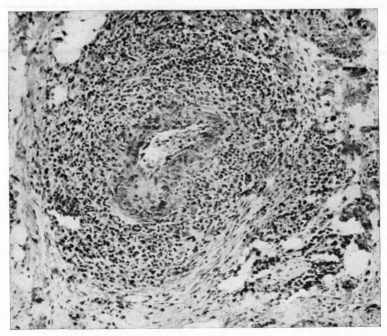

Figure 9-1. Polyarteritis nodosa. Histologic study of involved artery reveals fibrinoid necrosis of vessel wall and diffuse inflammatory infiltrate. (Hematoxylin and eosin) (Courtesy, Dr. A. Mackenzie)

seen in patients with a long history of asthma who develop granulomatous angiitis and diffuse extravascular granulomas. Eosinophilia is characteristic. Wegener's granulomatosis, a variant form of vasculitis, is associated with granulomatous inflammation of the upper respiratory tract, granulomatous disease of the lungs and necrotizing glomerulonephritis.

Athough a specific etiology of polyarteritis nodosa has not been established, recent studies have linked this disease in some patients to infection with hepatitis B virus (HB Ag).[4] In another series of cases, polyarteritis was associated with drug abuse.[5] Methamphetamine was the one drug taken in common by persons so affected.

Arteriograms of renal or mesenteric vessels may be diagnostically helpful in patients with vasculitis because they frequently reveal areas of narrowing and aneurysmal dilation that are pathognomonic.[6]

Polymyositis

The first symptoms of polymyositis may be muscle aching and tenderness, with minimal weakness early in the course of the disease. Later, more profound weakness usually follows (see following section) and allows differentiation of this entity from the preceding syndromes.

Miscellaneous Diseases

Muscle aching may be a major manifestation of metabolic disorders such as hypothyroidism and subacute thyroiditis. In other patients, symptoms simulating diffuse muscle pain may result from involvement of other tissues such as the bones in patients with multiple myeloma or metastatic carcinoma.

MUSCULAR PAIN WITH ASSOCIATED WEAKNESS

Polymyositis (Dermatomyositis)

Polymyositis is often characterized by both muscle aching and weakness. Weakness usually involves the proximal hip and shoulder girdle muscles (Fig. 9-2). Other muscles involved relatively soon in the course of the disease are the cervical and abdominal flexors. As the disease progresses, distal muscles are also involved. The term dermatomyositis is used to define this severe condition when skin manifestations are present. Dusky erythematous lesions appear most frequently on the eyelids (Fig. 9-3) and over extensor surfaces such as the knuckles of the hands, the knees, the malleoli and elbows (see Chapter 10). Cutaneous swelling and induration occur over involved muscles in acute cases. Muscle tenderness may be a prominent finding. Dysphagia results when skeletal muscles in the pharyngeal and upper esophageal regions are involved.

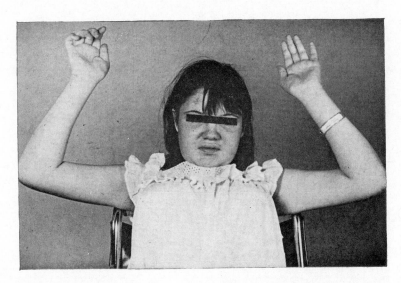

Figure 9-2. Dermatomyositis, illustrating weakness of the shoulder girdles. (Courtesy, Dr. A. Mackenzie)

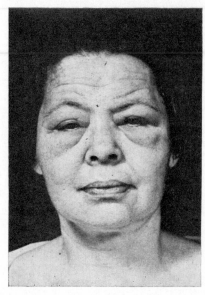

Figure 9-3. Dermatomyositis. Dusky erythematous discoloration of the eyelids is associated with swelling. (Courtesy, the Arthritis Foundation)

Organ systems other than muscle are frequently affected. Raynaud's phenomenon is common and may precede overt evidence of muscle disease. Polyarthralgia or polyarthritis is seen. Although chronic disabling joint changes are uncommon, articular findings sometimes simulate rheumatoid arthritis. Pulmonary fibrosis occurs and can lead to major disturbances in pulmonary function. Chronic polymyositis may be associated with calcinosis

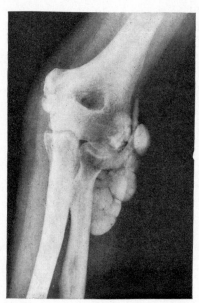

Figure 9-4. Calcinosis universalis. Calcium deposition in subcutaneous soft tissues is extensive. (Courtesy of Dr. A. Mackenzie)

universalis, in which calcium deposits are noted in subcutaneous tissue, deep connective tissue and muscle (Fig. 9-4). Fever, ranging from 101 to 102° F, anorexia, fatigue and weight loss are seen in acute severe cases. Malignant neoplasms are an associated finding in over 50% of patients over age 40. Although more frequently associated with dermatomyositis, neoplasms may be seen in patients with polymyositis as well. For this reason, a thorough physical examination and appropriate diagnostic studies including barium enema, upper gastrointestinal series and intravenous pyelograms are indicated in all patients over age 40 with myositis. The neoplasm may be occult and undetectable when the patient is first seen. Repeat studies may be indicated at one- to two-year intervals for several years following onset of the disease, depending on clinical response. In some patients, polymyositis is associated with other connective tissue diseases, such as systemic lupus erythematosus and scleroderma.

Myoglobinuria

Muscle breakdown with release of myoglobin in the serum and urine results from several diverse causes. In some patients, it follows extreme exercise. Other causes include prolonged muscle ischemia, crush injury and seizure. It may be an associated finding in patients with severe polymyositis. Myoglobinuria is also seen in patients with drug intoxication with phenobarbital, narcotics or alcohol. In these cases, it may result from crush or postural injury to muscle, although a direct toxic effect has also been postulated. A rare cause of myoglobinuria is cobra venom poisoning. Myoglobin release is a frequent concomitant of McArdle's disease (see following).

Clinically, the patient with myoglobinuria complains primarily of severe muscle cramps and pain and passes darkly discolored urine. Serum levels of muscle enzymes such as creatine phosphokinase, aldolase and glutamic oxaloacetic transaminase are elevated. Increased levels of serum potassium result from both muscle breakdown and renal impairment due to pigment casts. Urinalysis reveals proteinuria due to the presence of myoglobin and to tubular dysfunction. A positive urine benzidine test is supportive but not specific of the diagnosis, because hemoglobin gives similar findings. More specific tests for myoglobin include those based on gel electrophoresis, spectrophotometric study, or immunologic methods. Fortunately, most cases are associated with full clinical recovery.

McArdle's Disease

McArdle's disease, an hereditary disorder characterized by deficiency of muscle phosphorylase, is associated with muscle weakness and pain due to inability of muscle to metabolize glycogen for energy. Characteristically, weakness and cramps develop after a period of muscle activity. In severe cases, chronic weakness is seen. Myoglobinuria is common. Samples of venous blood drawn from the arm during muscle use reveal a decreased production of lactic acid as an end-product of glycogen metabolism. Special stains of muscle biopsy specimens reveal excess amounts of glycogen and partial or complete absence of phosphorylase.

Hypothyroidism

Progressively severe hypothyroidism results not only in muscle aching but eventually in muscle weakness. Patients with this combination of findings are frequently overtly myxedematous, and diagnosis is usually not too difficult.

MUSCULAR WEAKNESS WITHOUT PAIN

Muscle weakness without pain may originate in the nerves or muscles. Accordingly, initial diagnostic efforts in these patients should center upon determining whether the etiology is neurologic or myopathic. Neurologic weakness results from involvement of anterior horn cells, nerve roots or peripheral nerves. Involvement of anterior horn cells causes characteristic fasciculations of muscle and loss of deep tendon reflexes in the involved area. Peripheral neuropathy is also associated with loss of deep tendon reflexes, but fasciculations are not seen. In myopathic disorders, deep tendon reflexes are not lost until late when severe atrophy ensues, and fasciculations are not seen.

Neurologic Causes

Primary spinal atrophy, a disease of lower motor neurons, is characterized by severe muscle weakness. Older persons are usually affected. Upper extremity symptoms usually precede involvement of the lower extremities. Muscle atrophy is prominent and fasciculations are pronounced. Weakness usually involves distal muscles early; later, proximal extremity and trunk muscles are affected. Loss of deep tendon reflexes occurs as the disease progresses. Primary spinal atrophy can be considered a variant of *amyotrophic lateral sclerosis,* which affects not only lower motor neurons but lateral corticospinal tracts as well. In this disease, weakness and atrophy of distal muscles of the upper extremity occur first; trunk and lower extremity muscles are affected later. Early in the disease, deep tendon reflexes are overactive; later, these reflexes are lost as anterior horn cell involvement advances. A Babinski sign and ankle clonus are common. In primary spinal atrophy and amyotrophic lateral sclerosis, muscle biopsy shows neurogenic atrophy and electromyography shows denervation changes. Giant potentials and fasciculations are characteristic. Nerve conduction velocities are normal.

One form of spinal atrophy is particularly interesting because it usually begins in early childhood and may simulate muscular dystrophy. This disease, known as *juvenile muscular atrophy* (Kugelberg-Welander disease), affects proximal muscles of the lower extremities first, with resultant weakness of the pelvic girdle. Fasciculations are common but may be absent. Muscle atrophy is prominent. Mildly increased levels of serum creatine phosphokinase may be noted. Muscle biopsy usually shows neurogenic atrophy; electromyography shows denervation changes.

Peripheral neuropathies produce muscle weakness and loss of deep tendon reflexes. Pain is usually defined only vaguely. Frequently, the patient may complain of numbness and paresthesia. The common peripheral neuropathies are diffuse and symmetric, involving both lower and upper extremities. Distal aspects of the limbs are primarily involved. The more common underlying etiologies include diabetes mellitus, alcoholism, nutritional deficiencies, ingestion of various toxins such as lead and arsenic, and carcinoma. Porphyria, though an uncommon disorder, frequently manifests peripheral neuropathy. Involvement of peripheral nerves may be a prominent symptom of various connective tissue diseases, such as systemic lupus erythematosus, necrotizing vasculitis and Sjögren's syndrome.

Certain distinct forms of peripheral neuropathy have been described. *Guillain-Barré syndrome* (infectious polyneuropathy) causes muscle weakness abrupt in onset. Progression of the disease leads to weakness of numerous muscles of the upper and lower extremities. Distal muscles are usually involved first. Muscles of respiration and deglutition, as well as those supplied by cranial nerves, may be affected. Sensory changes occur, but usually are not prominent. Spinal fluid studies characteristically reveal an elevated protein with normal cell count (albuminocytologic dissociation). *Charcot-Marie-Tooth disease* (peroneal muscular atrophy) is an heredofamilial form of peripheral neuropathy. Peripheral nerves demonstrate degeneration of myelin sheaths and axis cylinders, and proliferative changes in Schwann cells. Spinal roots may also be involved. Motor symptoms are prominent and characterized by atrophy and weakness of foot and leg muscles. Peroneal muscles and toe extensors are affected most. Secondary equinovarus is common. Atrophy of the calves and lower thighs leads to an appearance of the lower extremities resembling "inverted champagne bottles." Upper extremities are usually involved late. Sensory disturbances are common; superficial sensation is affected most. A similar disorder, which may be closely related to Charcot-Marie-Tooth disease, is *hypertrophic interstitial neuropathy of Déjérine-Sottas.* Distal atrophy and weakness usually begin in the lower extremities; upper extremities are involved later. Deep tendon reflexes are diminished or absent. Palpable enlargement of involved peripheral nerves is distinctive. Degenerative changes affect the myelin of peripheral nerves; spinal roots may also be involved. In the presence of peripheral neuropathy, nerve conduction velocities are characteristically slowed. Electromyography reveals neurogenic potentials and fibrillation.

Myasthenia gravis often causes distinctive muscle weakness. Early in the disease, weakness is most prominent following activity. Patients with severe progressive disease are chronically weak, with further accentuation of weakness following activity. Involvement of muscles of the eyes, tongue and deglutition leads to symptoms of ptosis, diplopia and difficulty in chewing and swallowing. Improvement in strength with cholinesterase-inhibitors, e.g., neostigmine bromide and edrophonium chloride, confirms the diagnosis. Thymomas are frequent in adults with this disease. Appropriate radiologic studies of the chest and mediastinum should be performed in all cases. A similar syndrome, *myasthenic syndrome of Eaton-Lambert,*[7] is associated with underlying malignancy, most commonly intrathoracic neoplasms. Clinical findings characterized by fatigue, weakness and muscle wasting are related to a defect in neuromuscular transmission. Ptosis, diplopia, dysarthria and dysphagia may occur. Muscle power may temporarily increase after brief exercise.

Myopathic Causes

The differential diagnosis of the primary myopathies requires strict attention to various facets of the clinical history, such as sex, age at disease onset, pattern of muscle involvement and rapidity of disease progression. Physical examination late in the course of these diseases, when muscle involvement is diffuse, no longer reveals characteristic patterns and provides limited diagnostic help.

Polymyositis, as noted earlier, may cause muscle pain with minimal weakness in its early stages, or sometimes both weakness and pain. However, many cases are characterized by progressive weakness with little or no pain. Although this latter symptomatology occurs primarily in cases that are subacute in onset and slowly progressive, weakness without pain is sometimes observed in patients with rapidly advancing disease.

Duchenne's dystrophy (pseudohypertrophic muscular dystrophy) begins in early childhood, usually before age six. It is characterized early by weakness of proximal muscle groups of the hip and shoulder girdles. As the disease progresses, muscle weakness becomes more diffuse and peripheral areas are involved. This disease, the most common of the dystrophies, is inherited by males as a sex-linked recessive. Early symptoms include slowness in walking and difficulty in climbing stairs. There is visible pseudohypertrophy of muscles, especially of the calf and thigh. Myocardial involvement can frequently be identified on electrocardiographic study.

Limb-girdle muscular dystrophy affects both sexes. It tends to begin before the age of five and is characterized initially by weakness in the muscles of the pelvic girdle. Later, weakness involves muscles of the shoulder girdle. Eventually peripheral muscles are affected. *Facioscapulo-humeral dystrophy* occurs in both sexes. Muscle weakness, which may be delayed in onset to any time between the ages five and fifty, is usually mild. Facial and shoulder muscles are involved first; later, as the disease progresses, pelvic muscles are also affected.

Myotonic dystrophy is characterized by dystrophy and by myotonia, an impairment of muscular relaxation. Muscle involvement includes the hands and anterior tibial muscles, the facial muscles, the neck flexors and the muscles of the eyelids. Hip and shoulder girdle muscles are usually spared. Weakness is associated with progressive atrophy. The most common symptom related to myotonia is an inability to rapidly open the clenched fist. Delayed muscle relaxation can be demonstrated by striking involved muscles, such as the thenar eminence, with a reflex hammer; slow muscle relaxation is readily noted. Other manifestations of the disease include cataracts, frontal baldness, testicular atrophy and mental deterioration. The disease is inherited as an autosomal dominant. Mild elevations of serum muscle enzymes may be seen. Electromyography reveals a characteristic continuous firing of muscle fibers, commonly described as a "dive-bomber" pattern.

Muscle weakness may be a major clinical symptom of endocrine disorders. *Thyrotoxicosis* is a primary example of this type of disorder. Weakness is prominent in the proximal musculature, but diffuse weakness develops in severe disease. Serum muscle enzymes, interestingly, are usually normal. Muscle weakness is also noted in patients with *hypothyroidism,* even though gross evidence of myxedema may not be present. Myalgia may be minimal and weakness the predominant manifestation. In contrast to thyrotoxic myopathy, serum muscle enzymes are often elevated. Patients with *hypercortisonism* due to Cushing's syndrome may exhibit variable degrees of muscle weakness in severe cases. Similarly, patients receiving corticosteroid preparations in the therapy of various disorders may develop a toxic *steroid myopathy*. In these patients, proximal muscles of the lower extremities are involved early. Involvement of proximal upper extremity, distal and trunk muscles ensues as the disorder progresses. Urinary excretion of creatine is increased but serum muscle enzyme levels are characteristically normal. Although myalgia may occur, pain is usually minimal. Weakness of involved muscles is the prominent clinical manifestation. Symptoms respond to reduction in steroid dose.

Metabolic disorders may be associated with muscle weakness. Patients with diabetes mellitus may develop a syndrome of muscle weakness termed *diabetic amyotrophy*. Symptoms are usually slow in onset and most pronounced in the proximal aspect of the lower extremities. The pathogenesis of the disorder is uncertain; it may reflect changes primarily of muscle origin, but anterior horn cell degeneration has also been suspected. Symptoms may improve with control of the diabetes, but progressive changes often ensue despite good diabetic management. Several myopathic syndromes have been described in patients with *chronic alcoholism*.[8] One such disorder simulates McArdle's syndrome in that muscle weakness is associated with an inability to metabolize glycogen. Symptoms are usually associated with acute bouts of alcoholism and generally resolve rapidly as alcoholic intake stops. A second syndrome is characterized by chronic muscle weakness that may improve as alcoholic intake ceases, although it may persist despite abstinence from alcohol. The clinical picture simulates polymyositis in that proximal muscles of the extremities are involved most frequently and most severely. *Chronic hypokalemia* is associated with variable degrees of muscle weakness. In other patients, sudden falls in serum potassium are associated with the syndrome *hypokalemic familial periodic paralysis*. Although most often idiopathic, this latter syndrome may be associated with thyrotoxicosis. Symptoms are characterized by acute attacks of diffuse weakness or flaccid paralysis. Weakness may last for hours or days. Lower limbs are usually involved first, followed by involvement of the upper extremities, trunk and face. Speech and swallowing may be affected. Death in an attack is rare. Laboratory studies demonstrate a fall in serum potassium coincident with paralysis. Occasionally, however, familial periodic paralysis is seen in association with normal or high levels of serum potassium.

Muscle weakness may be associated with *amyloidosis*, particularly of the primary type. Weakness progresses slowly as deposition of amyloid in muscle becomes more severe and diffuse. Granulomatous involvement of muscle occurs in many patients with *sarcoidosis*. Despite this finding, clinical symptoms of weakness are uncommon. Nevertheless, some patients develop severe progressive weakness and muscle atrophy. The clinical features resemble chronic polymyositis or one of the dystrophies. Noncaseating granulomas are seen on muscle biopsy.

Muscle weakness may result from a number of rare congenital disorders such as central core disease, myotubular disease, nemaline myopathy, mitochondrial disease[9] and fingerprint body myopathy.[10] These disorders are generally manifest at or shortly after birth. Muscles are hypotonic and walking is delayed. The diseases usually progress slowly, if at all. Diagnosis depends on use of histochemical, light and electron microscopic techniques. These entities should be considered in the differential diagnosis of myopathic disorders not otherwise consistent with the more common entities.

DIAGNOSTIC STUDIES

Obviously, many of the foregoing muscle diseases overlap with respect to clinical symptomatology. Differential diagnosis depends on a clear delineation of subtleties of clinical presentation. A detailed history and physical examination to define age of onset, initial areas of muscle involvement, pattern and pace of disease progression and presence or absence of pain are important clues to diagnosis. Associated systemic findings characteristic of the basic disorder or evidence of associated disease states must also be sought. The following studies are valuable in the diagnosis and management of disorders of muscle.

A detailed manual muscle examination to determine distribution and severity of muscle weakness should be performed as early in the disease as possible; such information is helpful in differential diagnosis. In addition, accurately recorded serial findings can be compared to determine disease progression and response to therapy. Determinations of the ability to rise from a chair with or without the use of hands, the ability to rise from the floor to a standing position, the ability to walk a constant distance and the ability to climb stairs are particularly valuable. These functions should be timed with a stopwatch in order to compare measurements as the patient is observed during the course of disease.

Complete blood count, erythrocyte sedimentation rate, and tests for serum rheumatoid factor and antinuclear antibody are helpful in delineating the presence of associated connective tissue diseases and in differentiating inflammatory from noninflammatory myopathies.

Enzymes released into serum from degenerating muscle cells are important in diagnosis and management. Elevated levels support the presence of a primary myopathic disorder, because they are increased only occasionally and to mild degree in patients with neurogenic atrophy. In addition, these enzyme levels are valuable in following disease progression and response to therapy. The enzyme determinations used most commonly in studies of muscle diseases are serum creatine phosphokinase (CPK), serum glutamic oxaloacetic transaminase (SGOT), and aldolase (see Chapter 2).

As noted, elevated serum enzyme levels support a diagnosis of primary myopathy. However, serum enzyme levels are frequently normal in the presence of significant muscle pathology. Accordingly, normal values for these enzymes do not necessarily exclude primary muscle disease. Elevations of serum enzyme levels are usually proportional to the severity of muscle degeneration or necrosis. High levels are seen in all patients with progressive muscular dystrophy of the Duchenne type until late in the disease. Elevations are common in limb-girdle dystrophy. In facioscapulohumeral dystrophy, enzyme abnormalities are less frequent and only modest in degree. At least one or more of the enzymes are elevated in 50 to 60% of patients with polymyositis. Enzyme levels are frequently elevated in alcoholic and myxedematous myopathies, but are characteristically normal in thyrotoxic and steroid myopathies.

Quantitative determinations of the ratio of creatine to creatinine excreted in the urine are valuable in diagnosis and followup of patients with primary muscle disease (see Chapter 2). Because the degree of creatinuria parallels muscle damage, urinary determinations of creatine-creatinine ratio are valuable not only in diagnosis but also in following disease progression and response to therapy. Elevations in the creatine-creatinine ratio also result from other causes of muscle dysfunction, such as disuse or neurogenic atrophy of muscle.

The electromyogram (EMG) is particularly helpful in distinguishing primary myopathic from neurogenic causes of muscle weakness (see Chapter 2). However, although electromyography and nerve conduction velocity studies will help to differentiate myopathic from neuropathic disorders, they will not differentiate specific disease entities *within* each of these categories.

Muscle biopsy helps to differentiate muscle disorders of neurogenic cause from those of primary myopathic origin; in addition, specific primary myopathies can often be distinguished. Atrophy of groups of muscle fibers innervated by single motor units appears in muscle weakness due to lower motor neuron disease. In polymyositis, several pathologic findings may be noted (Fig. 9-5). Degenerative changes of fibers are common. Central migration of sarcolemmal nuclei occurs. Regeneration is characterized by basophilic staining. Severe cases show fiber necrosis. Variation in muscle fiber size and shape is common. Inflammatory reaction may be prominent and involves interstitial connective tissues, vascular and perivascular structures. Fibrosis occurs as the disease progresses. Similar findings may be noted to various degrees in patients with different forms of muscular dystrophy and, in many cases, biopsy study will not differentiate these entities from polymyositis. However, a striking inflammatory reaction strongly indicates polymyositis. In trichinosis, necrotizing vasculitis, amyloidosis and sarcoid, evidence of Trichinella spiralis larvae, vascular in-

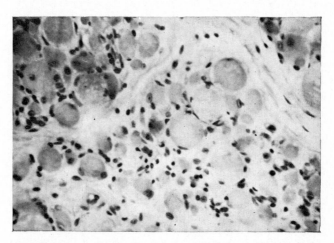

Figure 9-5. Muscle biopsy, polymyositis. Note fiber degeneration, variation in fiber size and shape, and inflammatory cells. (Hematoxylin and eosin) (Courtesy, Dr. A. Mackenzie)

flammation, positive stains for amyloid, and noncaseating granulomas respectively on muscle biopsy provides specific diagnosis.

Special histochemical stains on biopsy material provide additional information. Specific involvement of Type I or Type II fibers, or both, can be determined. Some myopathies are more likely to involve the slowly-contracting Type I fibers, which depend primarily on oxidative mechanisms for energy, while other diseases primarily involve the fast-contracting Type II fibers, which depend on glycogen utilization for energy release. Histochemical studies are required to demonstrate phosphorylase deficiency in McArdle's disease. Histochemical and electron microscopic studies are necessary to diagnose some of the less common myopathies.

To be most informative, muscle biopsy requires the appropriate selection of involved muscles. Prior manual muscle testing or electromyography should be performed in order to determine which muscles are involved. If the disease is acute and recent in onset, biopsy of the weakest muscle is most likely to yield positive findings. In chronic disease, biopsy of a very weak muscle may demonstrate only end-stage, nonspecific characteristics; in these cases, a moderately weak muscle should be selected.

Miscellaneous additional studies are indicated when specific disorders are suspected. Roentgenologic studies of the chest, kidneys and gastrointestinal tract to detect possible neoplasms should be performed in patients over 40 years of age who have polymyositis. Temporal artery biopsy with arteriography should be considered in patients with polymyalgia rheumatica syndrome. Studies for malignancy may be indicated in patients with this syndrome if there is no clinical or biopsy evidence of temporal arteritis.

Additional laboratory studies are helpful in excluding metabolic abnormalities as the cause of the patient's disorder. These should include serum thyroxine determination, glucose tolerance test, and serum potassium. Rectal biopsy for amyloid study is valuable if amyloidosis is suspected.

THERAPY

In most cases of muscle disease, the diagnosis can be pursued with appropriate deliberation with no undue hazard from delay. Symptoms related to inflammation with associated pain are often relieved by a conservative program that utilizes full doses of aspirin, other analgesics, rest and heat. Physical therapy is important, even early in the course of muscle disease, to maintain muscle tone and to retard or prevent deterioration of muscle strength.

Primary fibrositis is benefited by adding anti-inflammatory agents such as indomethacin, 25 mg QID with food, to the therapeutic regimen. Mild tranquilizers may be beneficial in relieving spasm and pain. Injection of local trigger areas of spasm and pain with a combination of long-acting steroids and 1% lidocaine is effective in providing variable periods of symptomatic relief. This therapy is safe in limited administration; several courses may be required. Reassuring the patient regarding the absence of serious underlying disease and the overall benign nature of the syndrome is an important part of the therapeutic program. Paying close attention to chronic tension factors and other psychiatric problems is essential to proper management.

Specific treatment of other diseases varies with the diagnosis. Unfortunately, many patients suffer from disorders for which little specific treatment is available. Adrenocorticosteroids, such as prednisone, are effective in the treatment of polymyositis and polymyalgia rheumatica (see Chapter 18). Corticosteroid therapy may be used as a diagnostic test to differentiate polymyositis from one of the dystrophies, because a positive therapeutic response supports a diagnosis of polymyositis. Steroids are also therapeutically valuable in patients with necrotizing vasculitis and trichinosis. The weakness associated with hyperthyroidism responds to appropriate therapy to diminish overactive thyroid function; the weakness of hypothyroidism responds to thyroid replacement. Diabetic amyotrophy may improve if good control of the diabetes is attainable. Abstinence from alcohol is indicated in the presence of alcoholic myopathy, although unfortunately the disease may persist in some cases despite cessation of alcohol intake. Hypokalemic myopathy usually responds well to potassium replacement. Acute attacks of familial periodic paralysis are precipitated by high sugar intake, which results in rapid utilization of potassium and subsequent lowering of serum potassium levels. A diet high in protein and limited in carbohydrates is often therapeutic. Daily administration of acetazolamide (Diamox) may also be beneficial.

CASE HISTORIES

History 9-1. Primary Fibrositis

B.L., a 38-year-old white female was first seen for evaluation in January, 1972. She had been in apparently good health until approximately six months prior, at which time she noted insidious onset of aching and stiffness involving the posterior cervical, upper dorsal and shoulder girdle regions. Symptoms were aggravated by tension situations. Continuous low-grade aching was punctuated by episodes of pain of increased intensity. Symptoms were worse in cool, damp weather. Musculoskeletal pain was frequently associated with severe blinding headaches similar to migraine headaches from which she had suffered 15 years earlier. There were no complaints of joint swelling, tenderness or limitation. System review was negative for Raynaud's phenomenon, alopecia, sun sensitivity, skin rash, pleurisy, dry eyes or mouth, dysphagia or drug allergy. Past medical history was unremarkable, although family and social history was significant. The patient's mother had died suddenly of myocardial infarction three months prior to onset of the patient's illness; several months later, her mother-in-law died of acute leukemia. In addition to this already severe emotional trauma, the patient was seriously concerned about her daughter when she learned that children of mothers who had received high doses of stilbestrol during pregnancy (as did the patient) had an increased incidence of carcinoma of the cervix.

Physical examination in this pleasant but obviously tense woman was normal except for tenderness and spasm of the upper trapezius and posterior cervical muscles. Deep pressure over areas of maximal spasm and tenderness triggered increased pain, similar in quality to that experienced by the patient during symptomatic flares. No muscle weakness was noted. Temporal arteries were nontender with normal pulsations. Musculoskeletal examination was otherwise negative. Laboratory examinations, which included urinalysis, hematocrit, white blood cell count and differential, erythrocyte sedimentation rate, serologic test for syphilis, serum protein electrophoresis, serum uric acid, protein bound iodine, serum calcium, phosphorus and alkaline phosphatase, serum cholesterol and lipid studies, serum glutamic oxaloacetic transaminase, creatine phosphokinase, serum rheumatoid factor and antinuclear antibody studies were normal or negative, as were x-rays of the chest and cervical spine. A presumptive diagnosis of primary fibrositis was made on the basis of her clinical history and physical examination and negative laboratory findings.

The patient was treated with aspirin, 640 mg QID, diazepam, 5 mg TID, and propoxyphene hydrochloride, 65 mg TID PRN for pain. Periodic injections with steroid and lidocaine were made locally into trigger sites of pain and spasm. Physical therapy, which included hot packs and cervical traction, was extremely helpful in further relieving symptoms. Extensive discussions were carried out regarding the nature of her problem and the important role that emotional factors might play in etiology. With reassurance and better understanding of the illness, the patient was able to tolerate her symptoms with much less distress. No other disease states became apparent over a two-year period of observation. Her symptoms were relatively mild except during periods of extreme emotional stress, at which time exacerbations usually responded to an intensified physical therapy program.

Discussion: At the time this patient was first seen, a diagnosis of primary fibrositis could be made on a presumptive basis only. Similar symptoms are frequently seen in association with systemic disorders, such as one of the connective tissue diseases, temporal (cranial) arteritis, polymyalgia rheumatica, subacute thyroiditis and hypothyroidism. The diagnosis became more secure after observation over a period of time. Appropriate initial and periodic clinical and laboratory evaluations were indicated to exclude more serious disorders. Although many cases of primary fibrositis are associated with emotional factors, psychologic relationships are not always so overt as in this case.

History 9-2. Idiopathic Polymyalgia Rheumatica

J.G., a 75-year-old white male, was seen for evaluation in July, 1973. He was well until November, 1972, at which time he noted pain and stiffness of the shoulders, buttocks and hips. Symptoms were constant, and increased in intensity with activity. Morning stiffness lasted for three or four hours daily. Fever was absent but the patient had noted anorexia and a weight loss of eight pounds during the previous eight months. System review was otherwise negative. In particular, there were no complaints of headaches, dysphagia or joint symptoms. Past medical history was noncontributory. Physical examination revealed slight limitation of motion of the shoulders and severe pain when he attempted to raise his arms above his head. Hip examination was normal except for pain at extreme ranges of motion. Muscle strength was normal and no other abnormalities were noted. Complete physical examination was otherwise unremarkable.

The hematocrit was 36%, the white blood cell count was 8100/mm³ with a normal differential, and the erythrocyte sedimentation rate was 82 mm/hour (Wintrobe). Serum antinuclear antibody and rheumatoid factor studies were negative as were LE cell examinations. Stool examination for occult blood was negative. Serum muscle enzyme determinations were normal. Twenty-four-hour urinary creatine-creatinine ratios were 6% and 8% on two separate evaluations. Serum protein electrophoresis showed 22% gamma globulin with a reversal of the albumin-globulin ratio. Roentgenograms of the chest, upper gastrointestinal tract and colon, and intravenous pyelogram were normal. Sigmoidoscopic examination was unremarkable. Biopsy of the right temporal artery revealed no inflammatory changes. Clinical impression was polymyalgia rheumatica.

The patient was given prednisone, 10 mg TID; significant symptomatic improvement was noted in 48 to 72 hours. The dose of prednisone was gradually decreased as symptoms improved and the erythrocyte sedimentation rate fell to high normal levels. Symptoms were eventually controlled with prednisone, 5 mg daily.

Discussion: The clinical findings were consistent with a diagnosis of idiopathic polymyalgia rheumatica. Symptoms are usually severe in the areas of the shoulder and hip girdle muscles. Although muscle weakness is absent, pain may limit muscle function. Since this syndrome is frequently associated with temporal (cranial) arteritis and, at times with neoplasm, careful studies to exclude both entities should be carried out. Clinical response of symptoms to steroid therapy is usually dramatic and supports the diagnosis.

History 9-3. Temporal (Cranial) Arteritis with Polymyalgia Rheumatica

B.R., an 82-year-old white female, was first seen for evaluation in July, 1973. She was in good general health until six months prior, at which time she noted a flu-like syndrome characterized by anorexia, malaise and low-grade fever. Shortly thereafter, she developed muscle aching that was particularly severe in the shoulder and hip girdle areas. Weight loss of 15 pounds was noted. The patient had no history of eye symptoms and no muscle weakness. She complained of temporal and occipital headaches. System review was otherwise noncontributory and past medical history was unremarkable. On physical examination blood pressure was 120/70 mm Hg, pulse 72 per minute, and temperature 37° C. Both temporal arteries were thickened and tender to palpation. Eye examination was normal. There was full range of motion of all joints with no tenderness or swelling. Muscles were nontender and had normal strength. A clinical diagnosis of temporal (cranial) arteritis with polymyalgia rheumatica was made and the patient hospitalized for further studies.

Hematocrit was 31%, white blood cell count was 6400/mm³ with a normal differential, reticulocyte count was 1.1%, platelet count was 225,000/mm³, erythrocyte sedimentation rate was 55 mm/hour (Wintrobe), and urinalysis was normal. Serum electrolytes, calcium, phosphorus and alkaline phosphatase, fasting blood sugar and liver function studies were normal or negative. Serum protein electrophoresis revealed slight elevation of alpha-2 globulin. Chest x-ray was negative, and electrocardiogram was normal. Sigmoidoscopy and x-rays of the upper and lower gastrointestinal tract were normal. Erythrocytes appeared normal on smear, and red cell indices revealed normochromic, normocytic results. Stools were negative for occult blood. Serum iron content and total iron binding capacity were normal; saturation was 37%. Bone marrow examination was within normal limits. Arteriography and biopsy of the left temporal artery were performed on November 13, 1973. The arteriogram revealed focal areas of vessel narrowing. Histopathologic examination showed extensive infiltration of all layers of the artery with lymphocytes and polymorphonuclear cells. The internal elastic membrane was well preserved and giant cells were not identified. Therapy consisted of prednisone, 20 mg QID, antacids, and a no-salt-added diet. Within 24 hours the patient had notable relief of pain and tenderness in the area of the temporal vessels and loss of muscle stiffness and pain.

Discussion: This patient's history was characteristic of temporal (cranial) arteritis with polymyalgia rheumatica. Response to steroid therapy was dramatic. The patient was discharged to the care of her physician with the recommendation to continue high dose steroid therapy until the erythrocyte sedimentation rate had returned to essentially normal values. At that time, gradual reduction in dose was to be carried out and the patient maintained on the lowest dose possible that would keep her free of symptoms with a normal sedimentation rate. Treatment for a period of one to three years is usually required. Although the temporal arteritis that was clinically apparent in this patient with polymyalgia rheumatica provided a reasonable explanation for her anemia, a neoplasm evaluation was considered necessary for completion of her workup.

History 9-4. Dermatomyositis

D.K., a two-year-old black male, was in good health until age 21 months, at which time his mother noted that the child appeared "lazy." He was less active than usual and refused to walk stairs, complaining that he was too tired. Weakness became more overt and the patient had difficulty walking, rising from a chair, or rising from the floor to a sitting or standing position. He walked with a waddling gait. He had no history of difficulty in chewing or swallowing nor changes in speech or articulation. System review was otherwise completely negative. Past medical history was noncontributory. The patient was hospitalized approximately six weeks after the onset of symptoms. Physical examination revealed moderate erythema over the knuckles of the proximal interphalangeal (PIP) joints of the hands. No muscle fasciculations were noted. The child was unable to lift his neck off the bed and there was moderate weakness of shoulder and hip girdle muscles. Neurologic examination was normal.

Urinalysis, white blood cell count and differential, serologic test for syphilis, and erythrocyte sedimentation rate were normal or negative. Serum electrolytes were normal. Serum glutamic oxaloacetic transaminase was 11 Henry units (normal, 9 to 25 units), and creatine phosphokinase was 1200 IU/ml (normal, less than 150 IU/ml). Twenty-four-hour urinary creatine–creatinine ratio determinations were 54% and 48% on two successive days. Serum protein electrophoresis and protein bound iodine were normal.

Chest x-ray and electrocardiogram were normal. Barium swallow revealed no abnormalities of esophageal function. Electromyographic study showed multiple polyphasic potentials consistent with primary myopathic disease. Spinal fluid studies revealed normal pressure, no cells, protein 10 mg%, and sugar 41 mg%. Biopsy of the right vastus lateralis muscle was performed. Histopathologic examination revealed extensive variability of muscle fiber size, degenerative vacuolation, and regenerative changes. Moderate numbers of inflammatory cells were seen throughout the specimen. An occasional vessel was slightly thickened and hyalinized. No perivascular infiltrates were seen. No changes specific for one of the congenital myopathies were noted on electron microscopic study.

A diagnosis of childhood dermatomyositis was made and the patient was placed on prednisone, 15 mg TID. Antacids were added as a prophylactic measure. Progressive improvement in strength was noted. Serum muscle enzyme determinations returned to normal levels over a period of two months. Urinary creatine–creatinine ratios similarly improved. Prednisone therapy was gradually reduced and symptoms were well controlled on a dose of 5 mg daily. Following this, the patient was successfully converted to an alternate day program in which prednisone, 10 mg, was administered every other day only. This latter schedule was utilized in the hope of lessening growth retardation and other complications of steroid therapy. Attempts to further reduce his steroid dosage were associated with slow onset of increased weakness.

Discussion: This patient had a history consistent with childhood dermatomyositis. Initial diagnostic considerations included infectious polyneuritis and other forms of primary myopathic disease. Laboratory and pathologic studies and the response to steroid therapy were consistent with a diagnosis of dermatomyositis.

History 9-5. Amyotrophic Lateral Sclerosis

W.J., a 70-year-old white male, was in good health until approximately six months prior to consultation. At that time he noted a change in his usual strong voice, which became high-pitched and nasal. In addition, he had difficulty swallowing and regurgitated food through the nose. He developed weakness in climbing stairs and, later, weakness in his upper extremities. There was no history of diplopia nor difficulty in chewing. On physical examination there was notable atrophy of interosseous muscles. Extensor and flexor muscles of the wrists were weak, and diffuse atrophy of the muscles of the shoulder and hip girdles was noted. The patient spoke with a nasal voice. Sensory examination was normal except for a slight decrease in vibratory sensation of both feet. Bilateral positive Babinski reflexes were elicited. Deep tendon reflexes of the left arm were increased. No clonus was present. Eye examination was normal and there was no weakness of extraocular muscles. Diffuse fasciculations were noted in the muscles of the upper extremities, trunk, abdominal wall, and thighs.

Chest x-ray and upper gastrointestinal series were normal. X-rays of the skull and cervical spine were within normal limits. Electrocardiogram was normal. Other laboratory studies revealed normal hematocrit and white blood cell count and differential. Urinalysis revealed slight albuminuria. Serum uric acid was 6.2 mg/100 ml. Serum calcium, phosphorus and alkaline phosphatase studies, serum protein electrophoresis, and serum electrolytes were normal. Protein bound iodine was 6.3 μg%. Fasting blood sugar was normal. Twenty-four-hour urinary creatine–creatinine ratios were 25 and 20% on two different occasions. Serum muscle enzyme determinations were normal. Electromyographic study revealed large spikes consistent with denervation atrophy. A diagnosis of amyotrophic lateral sclerosis was made.

Discussion: The findings of diffuse weakness, muscle atrophy, muscle fasciculations and involvement of the corticospinal tracts were characteristic of the diagnosis of amyotrophic lateral sclerosis. Abnormal sensory changes are not seen. The disease is usually gradual in onset and relentless in progression. Fasciculations are characteristic of neurogenic atrophy and differentiated the symptoms in this patient from those seen in primary myopathy. Abnormal creatinuria occurs in muscle disorders related both to primary myopathy and neurogenic atrophy. The clinical picture as described in this patient should not be readily confused with primary myopathic disease.

History 9-6. Thyrotoxic Myopathy

N.A., a 43-year-old black female, was first seen in consultation in the hospital in January, 1974. She had been in good health until several months prior when she noted onset of fatigue and generalized weakness. She had difficulty climbing stairs, needed help getting up from her bed, and had to use her hands to get up from a chair. Despite increased appetite and food intake, she had lost 13 pounds in the previous two months. System review revealed palpitations of the heart, increased sweating, and heat intolerance. Diarrhea alternated with constipation. She had a choking feeling in the anterior neck area. No aching was noted in the joints or muscles. There was no family history of muscle disease, and the patient gave no history of rash, sun sensitivity, Raynaud's phenomenon, dryness of the eyes or mouth, pleurisy, alopecia or drug allergy. Past medical history was noncontributory.

On physical examination, blood pressure was 120/70 mm Hg, pulse rate was regular at 100 beats per minute, and temperature was 37° C. The skin was smooth and moist and hair texture was fine. A slight tremor of the hands was noted. No lid lag or exophthalmos was seen. The thyroid was diffusely enlarged to approximately three times normal size and a bruit was heard over the gland. Lungs were clear to examination. Cardiac examination revealed a Grade II/VI systolic murmur, best heard at the apex. Deep tendon reflexes were symmetric but generally increased. Neurologic examination was otherwise within normal limits. Muscle evaluation revealed mild to moderate weakness of the muscles of the hip and shoulder girdles and neck flexors.

Hematocrit was 31%, white blood cell count was 4200/mm³ with a normal differential, platelet count was 350,000/mm³, and erythrocyte sedimentation rate was 52 mm/hour (Wintrobe). Urinalysis showed trace albumin. Serum electrolytes, fasting blood sugar, protein electrophoresis and routine serologic test for syphilis were normal or negative. Serum iron content, iron binding capacity and iron saturation were 65 μg/100 ml, 300 μg/100 ml and 22% respectively. Serum studies for rheumatoid factor and antinuclear antibody were negative. Serum creatine phosphokinase was 30 IU/ml (normal, less than 150 IU/ml). Serum glutamic oxaloacetic transaminase was normal. Twenty-four-hour urinary creatine-creatinine ratio determination was 32%. Serum protein bound iodine was 14.4 μg/100 ml. Total serum thyroxine was "over 16 μg/100 ml." T-3 sponge resin uptake and 24-hour I^{131} uptake studies were significantly elevated. Serum calcium was 10.9 mg/100 ml and 12.1 mg/100 ml on two separate occasions. Serum phosphorus was 6 mg/100 ml. Serum creatinine was 0.5 mg/100 ml and creatinine clearance was 92 ml/min. Chest x-ray was normal.

Endocrine consultation was requested. A diagnosis of classic Grave's disease with associated thyrotoxic myopathy was made. The increased calcium was considered a manifestation of thyrotoxicosis. The patient was placed on therapy with propranolol, 10 mg QID, and referred for I^{131} therapy. Although other causes of muscle weakness and hypercalcemia were not completely excluded, it was elected to observe the patient following I^{131} therapy and to perform further diagnostic studies if muscle weakness and laboratory evidence of hypercalcemia did not resolve.

Discussion: This patient had classic clinical findings of hyperthyroidism. Muscle weakness was severe and was a major initial complaint. The distribution of muscle weakness was characteristic of thyrotoxic myopathy but was also consistent with other primary myopathies such as polymyositis. Clinical observation after discharge revealed progressive improvement in muscle strength and a fall in serum calcium to normal values.

REFERENCES

1. Healey, L. A., Parker, F. and Wilske, K. R.: Polymyalgia rheumatica and giant cell arteritis. Arth Rheum 14:138, 1971.
2. Blankenhorn, M. A., Zeek, P. and Knowles, H. C.: Periarteritis nodosa and other forms of necrotizing angiitis: a clinical pathological correlation. Trans Assoc Am Physicians 66:156, 1953.

3. Churg, J. and Strauss, L.: Allergic granulomatosis, allergic angiitis, and periarteritis nodosa. Am J Path 27:277, 1951.
4. Gocke, D. J. et al.: Association between polyarteritis and Australia antigen. Lancet 2:1149, 1970.
5. Citron, B. P. et al.: Necrotizing angiitis associated with drug abuse. N Eng J Med 283:1003, 1970.
6. Bron, K., Stratt, C. and Shapero, A.: The diagnostic value of angiographic observations in polyarteritis nodosa. Arch Int Med 116:450, 1965.
7. Rooke, E. D. et al.: Myasthenia and malignant intrathoracic tumors. Med Clin N Am 44:977, 1960.
8. Perkoff, G. T.: Alcoholic myopathy. Ann Rev Med 22:125, 1971.
9. Pearson, C. M. et al.: Skeletal muscle: basic and clinical aspects and illustrative new diseases. Ann Int Med 67:614, 1967.
10. Engel, E. G., Angelini, C. and Gomez, M. R.: Fingerprint body myopathy. A newly recognized congenital muscle disease. Mayo Clin Proc 47:377, 1972.

Chapter 10

SKIN RASH AND ARTHRITIS

Joint symptoms are the common thread connecting the various rheumatic disorders. Since these joint manifestations frequently resemble one another, close attention to ancillary associated findings such as skin lesions is important in diagnosis. Careful observation and characterization of these cutaneous manifestations can often lead to the correct rheumatologic diagnosis.

DIFFERENTIAL DIAGNOSIS

Diseases to be considered:

Systemic lupus erythematosus | Rheumatic fever
Dermatomyositis | Rheumatoid arthritis
Scleroderma | Juvenile rheumatoid arthritis
Psoriasis | Rubella arthritis
Reiter's syndrome | Gonococcal arthritis
Behçet's syndrome | Ulcerative colitis and regional enteritis
Stevens-Johnson syndrome |
Erythema nodosum | Hepatitis-associated arthritis
Vasculitis | Lipoid dermatoarthritis (multicentric reticulohistiocytosis)

Cutaneous lesions are common in *systemic lupus erythematosus* (SLE) at all stages of the disease. These lesions may be the initial symptoms, with joint symptoms following later. In other cases skin lesions occur concomitantly with or follow other manifestations of the disease. The classic lesion is the macular erythematous butterfly rash of the face in which involvement of malar areas is bridged by a lesion across the skin of the nose (Fig. 6-1). Other areas of frequent involvement are the neck, upper chest, and the extremities. The lesions tend to be symmetric. The rash may be transient, lasting only a few days, or may be chronic. Chronic lesions are characterized by erythematous plaques with scaling and follicular plugging; the skin often becomes atrophic and scarred. Other characteristic compo-

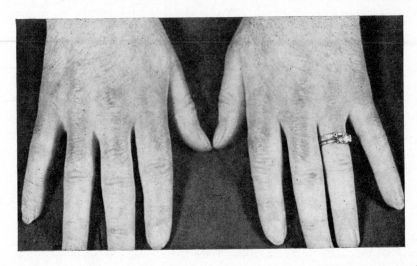

Figure 10-1. Rash, systemic lupus erythematosus. Involvement between knuckles is prominent, although extension over knuckles is also seen.

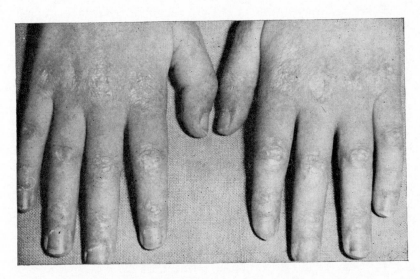

Figure 10-2. Rash, dermatomyositis. Lesions over the extensor surfaces of the knuckles are characteristic. (Courtesy, the Arthritis Foundation)

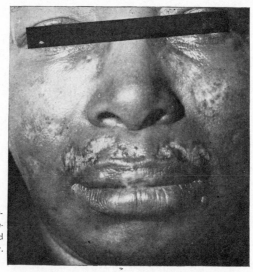

Figure 10-3. Rash, discoid lupus erythematosus. Chronic lesions reveal atrophy and scarring. (Courtesy, Dr. B. Michel)

nents of the rash are erythematous lesions in the paronychial areas of the fingers, and lesions scattered over the palms associated with palmar erythema. Lesions of the hands in SLE characteristically involve the dorsal skin *between* the knuckles (Fig. 10-1) rather than at the knuckles. This differentiates them from the skin lesions of dermatomyositis, which characteristically involve extensor surfaces over the knuckles (Fig. 10-2). The skin lesions of SLE and dermatomyositis may overlap in form and location, however, and be difficult to differentiate.

The rash of chronic discoid lupus is similar to chronic lesions of systemic lupus erythematosus (Fig. 10-3). The dermatitis is usually focal and often confined to the face, neck and scalp. In some patients, discoid lupus is present in disseminated form, with numerous discrete lesions occurring in many locations.

Skin rash is a prominent component of *dermatomyositis.* The characteristic rash consists of a symmetric dusky erythematous lesion in the periorbital region, associated with periorbital edema (Fig 9-3). Their unusual violaceous color has given rise to the term "heliotrope eyelids." The facial rash may be more diffuse, involving a butterfly distribution on the face as in systemic or discoid lupus, and extending to the forehead, neck and upper thorax and back. Lesions on the extremities characteristically affect extensor areas such as elbows and knees, and malleoli at the ankles. These lesions, similar to those seen in the face and neck area, consist of dusky red patches that are slightly elevated and sometimes slightly scaly. Hyperemia occurs about the base of the fingernails. The areas of skin involvement may become somewhat atrophic with time. Less common skin features include cutaneous changes that simulate those of scleroderma, with thickening of the skin of the hands and arms and evidence of hyperpigmentation or vitiligo.

Skin rash is the classic and most characteristic change seen in patients with *scleroderma*. Early, changes are characterized by painless edema of the hands, fingers, feet and legs. This swelling, which lasts for variable periods of time, is gradually replaced by chronic thickening and tightening of the skin. The term acrosclerosis is often used to describe the form of the disease in which lesions are localized to the hands and feet. In other patients, cutaneous lesions are diffuse and involve not only peripheral areas of the extremities but the trunk as well. Following the initial phase of cutaneous edema, the skin becomes less pliant and somewhat shiny (Fig. 10-4). A hardening of the tissues leads to loss of normal skin folds; a characteristic "pinched facies" is noted (Fig. 10-5.) Generalized hyperpigmentation of the skin and areas of patchy vitiligo are common. Telangiectases are frequently noted on the fingers, face (Fig. 10-5), lips and tongue (Fig. 10-6) as the disease becomes chronic. Ulceration (Fig. 10-4) and infection of the fingers and bony eminences and subcutaneous calcification are noted. The clinical combination of calcinosis, Raynaud's phenomenon, esophageal dysfunction, sclerodactyly and telangiectasis in scleroderma has been given the term CREST syndrome, after the initials of the five associated manifestations. These symptoms probably reflect degenerative changes that have been allowed to develop in patients with more benign scleroderma of longer duration rather than a specific disorder.

There is an increased frequency of arthritis of various forms in patients with *psoriasis*[1] (see Chapter 7). In any form of psoriatic arthritis, joint symptoms may be acute or insidious, and few or many joints may be involved. Spondylitis involving the spine and sacroiliac joints is common. In

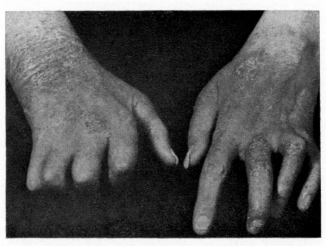

Figure 10-4.   Scleroderma. Cutaneous involvement leads to tightening of the skin. Small healed ulcerations are seen at the proximal interphalangeal joints.

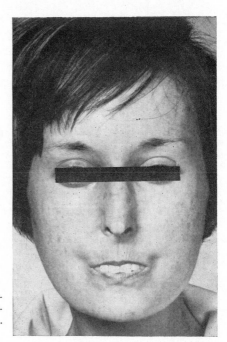

Figure 10-5. Scleroderma. Note the characteristic "pinched facies" and telangiectases. (Courtesy, Dr. A.
Mackenzie)

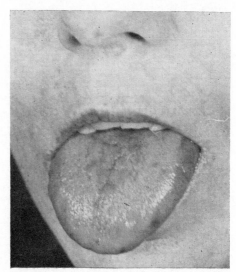

Figure 10-6. Scleroderma. Telangiectases
of the tongue are seen as
dark red areas.

most cases, psoriasis precedes the onset of arthritis; in others, psoriasis and arthritis begin concomitantly. In a few patients, arthritis precedes psoriatic lesions by one or more years. Nail and skin lesions are identical to those seen in psoriatic patients without arthritis; they are often minimal and overlooked. Nail changes in women may be missed if nail polish is worn at the time of examination. Nail lesions are characterized by discoloration, pitting, thickening and onycholysis. Skin lesions are characterized by erythematous scaling plaques, located most frequently on extensor areas such as the elbows and knees. Involvement of the scalp and intergluteal areas is common. In addition, any region of the skin may be affected.

Involvement of the skin and mucous membranes in *Reiter's syndrome* is so frequent that a tetrad of symptoms consisting of arthritis, urethritis, conjunctivitis and mucocutaneous lesions is often used to clinically define the syndrome.[2] Lesions of the penis are especially common. They are characterized by superficial ulcerations, especially around the urethral meatus (Fig. 10-7). Coalescence of lesions on the glans penis gives rise to a characteristic circular lesion called balanitis circinata. Mucous membrane ulcers are seen frequently in the mouth, with involvement of the buccal mucosa, tongue and gums. The lesions are often small and painless but may be irritating and painful in some patients. Papular and pustular lesions are common on the palms of the hands and soles of the feet. They may be small and discrete at onset, but frequently become confluent and covered

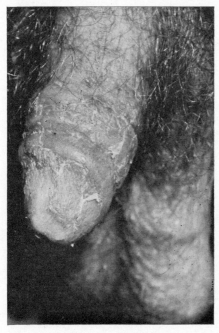

Figure 10-7. Mucocutaneous lesions of the penis in a patient with Reiter's syndrome. (Courtesy, Dr. C. Denko)

by a thick keratotic crust that eventually peels with no evidence of scar formation. The diffuse keratotic lesions of the soles have been termed keratodermia blennorrhagica (Fig. 6-2). Hyperkeratosis may occur around the finger and toe nails. The lesions of Reiter's syndrome may be almost identical in appearance to those seen in pustular psoriasis and, indeed, impossible to differentiate. In some patients, there appears to be an actual overlap between psoriatic arthritis and Reiter's syndrome, with various features of both diseases being present at the same or different times. The skin and joint lesions of Reiter's syndrome are usually self-limiting and resolve after several weeks or months. Of pathogenic and diagnostic interest is the recent observation that histocompatibility antigen, HLA-W27, is present in up to 96% of patients with Reiter's syndrome, whether or not spondylitis is present.[3]

Behçet's syndrome is characterized by a basic triad of lesions that includes mucocutaneous ulcers of the oral and genital tracts and recurrent iritis. Arthritis is common. Oral ulcerative mucous membrane lesions resemble aphthous stomatitis (Fig. 7-8). Ulcerative lesions of the penis are common and usually painful. In women, similar ulcerations may be seen on the vulva and in the vagina. They are characteristically painfree and easily overlooked. Pyoderma gangrenosum and lesions that resemble erythema nodosum are common.

Stevens-Johnson syndrome may be regarded as a variant of erythema multiforme. Characteristically, patients have high fever and severe stomatitis characterized by ulcerative lesions of the oral mucous membranes. Similar lesions may appear on the genitalia. A bullous erythematous skin eruption may occur elsewhere on the body. Symptoms in joints and muscles may be present but are usually a minor manifestation of the disease. Transient arthralgia is the most frequent associated musculoskeletal finding. The presence of bullous vesicular lesions and stomatitis is usually required to make the diagnosis.

The syndrome of *erythema nodosum* is characterized by painful subcutaneous nodules. Hilar adenopathy, fever and arthritis are frequent associated findings (see Chapter 6). The syndrome is more frequent in females. Characteristic skin lesions consist of cutaneous and subcutaneous inflammatory nodules that appear in crops. Lesions are red, tender and painful. Their color may change as the lesion ages, becoming somewhat violaceous in hue. Lesions usually heal completely without scarring. In most cases, lesions are confined to the legs below the knees and involve the anterior tibial areas (Fig. 6-3). In some patients, however, the lesions are more widespread and involve the upper extremities as well. Joint symptoms usually occur concomitantly with skin findings, but they may precede or follow cutaneous manifestations. Joint symptoms may be limited to arthralgia, but swelling and synovial effusion are common. Although knees and ankles are most frequently involved, other joints may be affected. Erythema

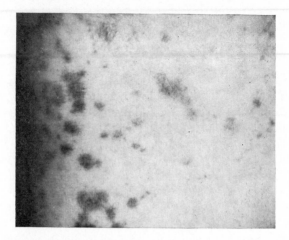

Figure 10-8. Necrotizing vasculitis. Typical purpuric lesions of skin.

nodosum may occur as a primary disease, or secondary to other disorders, which should be diagnostically excluded (see Chapter 6).

Skin lesions are a prominent component of various forms of *vasculitis,* such as polyarteritis nodosa, allergic angiitis and Henoch-Schönlein purpura. The lesions are extremely pleomorphic and many forms may be seen simultaneously. Purpuric eruptions are very common (Fig. 10-8). Other forms include nodular lesions, vesicular or bullous eruptions, urticaria, livedo reticularis and gangrene. Small necrotic lesions that involve the paronychial or subungual areas (Fig. 10-9) are common and are similar to the splinter hemorrhages seen in subacute bacterial endocarditis.

Subcutaneous nodules and erythema marginatum are the characteristic skin lesions of *rheumatic fever.* Subcutaneous nodules vary in size from a few millimeters to one or two centimeters and appear most frequently over bony surfaces such as the olecranon areas and at the wrists and malleoli. Although these nodules are similar in appearance to those seen in patients with rheumatoid arthritis, certain differences are notable: the nodules in rheumatic fever appear more commonly at the point of the olecranon pro-

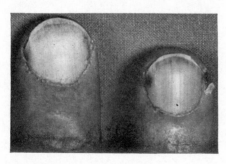

Figure 10-9. Necrotizing vasculitis. Paronychial and subungual lesions secondary to ischemia. (Courtesy, Dr. A. Mackenzie)

cess, rather than in the subolecranon area characteristic of rheumatoid arthritis. In addition, the nodules in rheumatic fever tend to last for a shorter period of time; the duration rarely exceeds more than three or four weeks.

Erythema marginatum is characterized by nonpruritic macular pink lesions that tend to be evanescent. The trunk and limbs are affected most often; the face is never involved. The lesion extends peripherally while the skin in the center gradually returns to normal. Lesions that are continuous and form a ring are called erythema annulare; they probably represent a form of erythema marginatum. Lesions may appear and disappear over a matter of hours. They change shape rapidly and are often more evident following a hot bath or shower. Both the subcutaneous nodules and erythema marginatum lesions are considered major manifestations in diagnosis.

Although joint manifestations are the hallmark of *rheumatoid arthritis,* extra-articular lesions are common and can be helpful in diagnosis. Rheumatoid nodules, characterized by firm subcutaneous nodular lesions, are a significant diagnostic finding. Although located most frequently in subcutaneous areas, they often involve deeper connective tissue structures such as periosteum and tendon sheaths, as well as tendons themselves. They tend to appear in areas subjected to repeated trauma, such as the subolecranon areas of the elbow (Fig. 1-3), the ischial tuberosities, the Achilles tendons, and the scapular areas of the back. Involvement of hands and feet is common in severe cases. These lesions must be differentiated from gouty tophi, sebaceous cysts, xanthoma tuberosum, granuloma annulare, amyloid deposits and the subcutaneous nodules of rheumatic fever.

Other cutaneous manifestations associated with rheumatoid arthritis are seen when necrotizing vasculitis is a complicating manifestation of the disease. The lesions are similar to those described in the preceding section on vasculitis. Particularly frequent are purpuric lesions of the skin and infarctive lesions of the fingernail beds. The purpuric lesions should be distinguished from ecchymotic or purpuric lesions that occur spontaneously or follow mild trauma in rheumatoid arthritis patients on prolonged steroid therapy. Secondary skin ulcers are common.

A characteristic erythematous rash occurs in approximately 30% of patients with *juvenile rheumatoid arthritis* (JRA). The rash consists of macular and maculopapular lesions that are usually discrete but are sometimes confluent (Fig. 10-10). They are distributed mainly on the limbs and trunk, but are also seen on the face, palms and soles. As with erythema marginatum, the rash of juvenile rheumatoid arthritis tends to be evanescent. It frequently appears primarily in the evening or concomitantly with high fever spikes. Heat or irritation intensify the rash. Pruritus occurs but is uncommon. In contrast to the frequent finding of subcutaneous nodules in adult rheumatoid arthritis, subcutaneous nodules are uncommon in children, especially at the youngest age levels.

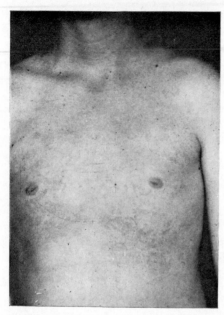

Figure 10-10. Rash, juvenile rheumatoid arthritis. Diffuse macular and maculopapular lesions are seen. (Courtesy, the Arthritis Foundation)

Rubella infection is characterized by a diffuse maculopapular rash, fever, and suboccipital lymphadenopathy. Acute polyarthralgia or polyarthritis commonly occurs in adolescents or young adults.[4] Joint symptoms usually occur in association with the rash, but may precede or follow it. Small joints of the hands are affected most commonly, but large joints may also be involved. Joint manifestations are usually self-limited.

A distinctive skin rash is seen in patients with *gonococcal arthritis*.[5] The lesions represent either septic metastatic foci with infectious angiitis, or a systemic hypersensitivity reaction. Small erythematous macules, vesicles and pustules are common (Fig. 10-11). As the lesions progress, central necrosis occurs. Bullous lesions are occasionally seen. Skin lesions in all stages of development may be present simultaneously.

Skin lesions and arthritis are seen in patients with *ulcerative colitis* and *regional enteritis*. Erythema nodosum is present in approximately 5% of patients with ulcerative colitis and somewhat less often in patients with regional enteritis. Oral ulcerations are common. Pyoderma gangrenosum, associated with ulcerative colitis, is seen most frequently on the lower extremities. Early lesions appear as pustules that later coalesce and ulcerate. The lesions are frequently multiple and may become quite extensive. They are slow to heal and scarring is common. New lesions may appear at sites of trauma.

Skin rash is a common concomitant of the *arthritis associated with hepatitis*.[6] Although urticarial pruritic lesions are seen most frequently, erythe-

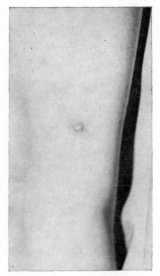

Figure 10-11. Pustular necrotic lesion of leg in patient with acute gonococcal arthritis. (Courtesy, Dr. F. Bishko)

matous maculopapular lesions, petechiae, and tender erythematous nodules have been described. Large joints are involved most commonly in the associated arthritis. Low serum complement levels and a positive test for hepatitis B antigen (HB Ag) are characteristic laboratory findings.

Lipoid dermatoarthritis (multicentric reticulohistiocytosis) is an uncommon disorder characterized by cutaneous nodules and severe, often mutilating, polyarthritis.[7] In most cases arthritis precedes the skin rash, but the two may occur simultaneously. Skin lesions consist of firm brownish-yellow papular nodules, seen most commonly on the face, hands, scalp, neck and chest. Small raised lesions, similar to coral beads in appearance, appear around the nail folds. Lesions tend to vary in size and usually disappear without a trace. Mucosal papules occur on the lips, tongue and buccal mucosa. The associated polyarthritis is usually symmetric and often simulates rheumatoid arthritis. Some patients suffer from severe arthritis mutilans. Roentgenograms of involved joints show extensive destructive changes with loss of cartilage and absorption of subchondral bone. Biopsy study of lesions reveals multinucleated giant cells and histiocytes with a ground-glass appearance.

DIAGNOSTIC STUDIES

Close attention to history and physical examination is important in the initial differential diagnosis of disease characterized by skin rash and arthritis. Appropriate laboratory studies are then directed toward the most highly suspected diagnoses. Skin biopsy can be performed with little hazard and discomfort utilizing a punch biopsy technique under local anesthesia. Pathologic findings on routine histologic study are often sufficiently characteristic to allow accurate diagnosis. Special immunofluorescent studies of biopsy tissue are often helpful when a diagnosis of chronic discoid lupus or systemic lupus erythematosus is being considered (see Chapter 2). Immunofluorescent localization of gamma globulin at the epidermal-dermal junction is seen in 85 to 95% of cases of discoid or systemic lupus erythematosus (SLE) in biopsy specimens from involved skin. Similar findings are noted in normal uninvolved skin in approximately 60% of patients with SLE but are absent in studies of normal skin of patients with chronic discoid lupus.

THERAPY

Treatment of the cutaneous manifestations varies with the specific diagnosis. The lesions of discoid and systemic lupus erythematosus are usually aided by direct application of local steroid creams or by intralesional injections of corticosteroids. Enclosing the areas of treatment with an occlusive covering augments the therapeutic response to local steroid creams. More severe lesions require the use of systemic agents such as hydroxychloroquine (Plaquenil), 200 mg BID, or quinacrine hydrochloride (Atabrine), 100 mg daily, and oral or parenteral steroids. Sun screen lotions diminish aggravation of the rash by sun exposure. The rash of dermatomyositis may respond to systemic steroids utilized in treatment of the muscular component of the disease, in addition to local steroid creams. Management of cutaneous changes in scleroderma requires trial with a variety of agents (see Chapter 18). Psoriasis responds to various regimens including coal tar ointments and ultraviolet light, or local steroid creams or ointments. Intractable cases may require more potent agents, such as methotrexate, 6-mercaptopurine, azathioprine or hydroxyurea. All of these agents except methotrexate are still investigational for use in this disease. The cutaneous lesions of Reiter's syndrome usually respond to local steroid therapy. Oral lesions benefit from applications of triamcinolone (Kenalog) in Orobase. Tetracycline suspension used three or four times a day as a mouthwash is effective in reducing secondary infection. Pain is often lessened by use of Viscous Xylocaine. Genital ulcerations similarly respond to local steroids. Severe diffuse lesions may require systemic steroids. Management of Stevens-Johnson syndrome usually requires high-dose steroids, such as prednisone, 15 mg QID, by mouth. Offending allergenic drugs implicated in etiology should be discontinued. The lesions of Behçet's syndrome that involve the mouth or genitalia are treated similarly to lesions in Reiter's syndrome. Systemic steroids or immunosuppressive agents[8] are worthy of trial in severe cases.

The nodular lesions of erythema nodosum require little specific therapy if the disease is mild. Full doses of aspirin reduce inflammation and relieve pain. Local steroids combined with plastic wrap occlusion may be beneficial. Severe cases may require systemic steroids for relief of joint and cutaneous manifestations. The skin lesions of necrotizing vasculitis require high-dose systemic steroids for management; 60 to 100 mg of prednisone daily are not unusual. Use of topical steroids with occlusion may also be beneficial. The cutaneous lesions of rheumatic fever spontaneously disappear and do not require specific attention. Subcutaneous nodules in patients with rheumatoid arthritis are often asymptomatic, in which case no specific therapy is required. Large lesions in pressure-sensitive areas may benefit from local steroid injection therapy. Large persistent nodules require surgical removal. Recurrences are lessened by avoiding pressure over previously involved areas. No specific therapy is indicated for the rash of juvenile rheumatoid arthritis. Antipruritic lotions or oral antihistamines are helpful if pruritus is bothersome. Gonococcal skin lesions respond readily to penicillin therapy used in management of the basic gonococcal infection. Pyoderma gangrenosum seen in ulcerative colitis may require systemic steroid therapy. Although no specific therapy is available for treatment of the lesions of lipoid dermatoarthritis, immunosuppressive agents have been described as possibly beneficial.[9]

CASE HISTORIES

History 10-1. Dermatomyositis

C.H., a 15-year-old white female, had a history of weakness of the pelvic and shoulder girdle muscles beginning nine months earlier. This symptom was associated with periorbital edema and the presence of slightly scaly violaceous macular lesions over the extensor surface of both elbows and knees and the malleoli of the ankles. Muscle weakness progressed in severity over the ensuing months. Shortly prior to consultation the patient observed pallor and paresthesia of the fingers on exposure to cold. There was no history of dysphagia, sun sensitivity, pleurisy, dry eyes or mouth, frequent canker sores, arthralgia or arthritis. System review was otherwise negative, and past history was unremarkable. Family history for muscle disorders was negative.

On physical examination, the cutaneous lesions were readily visible. No thickening of the skin was observed. Moderate weakness of the hip and shoulder girdle muscles and the cervical and abdominal flexors was demonstrated. Muscles were nontender. The remainder of the examination was normal.

Hematocrit was 38%, white blood cell count was 6200/mm³ with a normal differential, and erythrocyte sedimentation rate was 18 mm/hour (Wintrobe). Routine serologic test for syphilis was negative; serum protein electrophoresis was normal. Urinalysis revealed trace protein. Serum glutamic oxaloacetic transaminase and alkaline phosphatase were normal. Studies for serum rheumatoid factor and antinuclear antibody were negative. Serum creatine phosphokinase (CPK) was 1500 IU/ml (normal, up to 150 IU/ml). Twenty-four-hour urinary creatine-creatinine ratio determinations were 34% and 39% on two successive days. Electromyographic study of involved muscles demonstrated small numbers of polyphasic potentials. Right deltoid muscle biopsy was performed. Examination of the specimen revealed variation in fiber size, increased amounts of connective tissue, and mononuclear inflammatory infiltrates. A diagnosis of dermatomyositis was made and the patient was placed on prednisone, 15 mg QID.

Excellent response with improvement in muscle strength was noted over a period of six weeks. Repeat serum CPK was 70 units. Urinary creatine-creatinine ratios were 16% and 21%. Slow reduction of prednisone dosage was instituted and the patient monitored closely by periodic manual muscle evaluation, serum CPK and urinary creatine-creatinine ratio studies. Muscle symptoms were eventually well-controlled on a maintenance dose of prednisone, 2.5 mg TID. Cutaneous lesions improved but did not disappear despite additional therapy utilizing local steroid creams.

Discussion: The clinical diagnosis related to muscle weakness in this patient was simplified by the presence of cutaneous lesions characteristic of dermatomyositis. Periorbital edema with a violaceous rash of the eyelids (heliotrope eyelids) is a typical finding, as is the presence of the rash over extensor surfaces such as the knuckles, elbows, and knees. Cutaneous lesions improved but did not completely resolve with steroid therapy, despite excellent response of muscle weakness.

History 10-2. Psoriatic Arthritis

S.B., a 42-year-old white male dentist, was first seen in consultation in January, 1972. Approximately one year prior he noted arthralgias of the proximal interphalangeal (PIP) joints of the hands, wrists, elbows, and knees. Six months later he developed persistent swelling of the metatarsophalangeal (MTP) joints of the feet, both knees, and the right wrist. Morning stiffness was minimal. In November, 1971, he had onset of scaly erythematous pruritic patches on the extensor surfaces of both elbows and over the right scalp. There was no history of pleurisy, colitis, back pain, sciatica, iritis, or urethritis. Physical examination revealed scaly erythematous lesions over both olecranon areas and the right scalp. There was swelling of the IP joint of the left thumb, the right second and third PIP and DIP joints, the left knee, and the second, third and fourth MTP joints of the right foot. In addition, the interphalangeal joints of the left third and fourth toes showed a sausage-like fusiform swelling. Several fingernails exhibited pitting and thickening with whitish discoloration.

Urinalysis, white blood cell count and differential, hematocrit and serologic test for syphilis were normal or negative. Erythrocyte sedimentation was 18 mm/hour (Wintrobe). Serum studies for rheumatoid factor and antinuclear antibody were negative. Serum uric acid was 5.4 mg/100 ml. Roentgenograms of the hands showed several small erosions of periarticular bone in the second and third PIP joints of the right hand. A diagnosis of psoriatic arthritis was made.

The patient was treated with aspirin, 640 mg QID, physical therapy, and transverse metatarsal pads for the shoes. Psoriatic cutaneous lesions responded well to local use of steroid creams. Joint symptoms were well controlled for several months on this conservative program. Indomethacin, 25 mg TID, was added when a moderately severe episode of the arthritis did not respond to increased doses of aspirin. Swelling and pain were well controlled, and the patient was able to carry on his dental activities without major difficulty.

Discussion: The involvement of distal interphalangeal joints of the hands and sausage-like fusiform swelling of the interphalangeal joints of the toes were characteristic manifestations of psoriatic arthritis in this patient. As may occasionally occur, joint symptoms preceded onset of psoriatic skin lesions.

History 10-3. Reiter's Syndrome

R.B., a 32-year-old white male, was admitted to hospital on January 19, 1972. His illness began two weeks prior, at which time he noted pain and burning on urination and a white urethral discharge. The right eye appeared red. Pain and swelling of the right knee and left ankle developed one week later. During hospitalization, the right heel became painful and tender, and inflammation of the right eye increased. In addition, several scaly maculopapular lesions were noted on the plantar surfaces of both feet and a scaly erythematous lesion appeared in the area of the penile meatus. There was an erythematous aphthous lesion of the tongue. Further history revealed extramarital sexual contact seven days prior to onset of his acute illness. Physical examination showed acute swelling and inflammation of the right knee and left ankle, and mucocutaneous lesions on the feet, penis and tongue.

The hematocrit was 42%, and the white blood cell count was 5700/mm³ with a normal differential. Erythrocyte sedimentation rate was 33 mm/hour (Wintrobe). Urine contained 1+ albumin with a few white cells per high power field. Smear and culture of the urethra and urine culture were negative. Study of fluid aspirated from the right knee revealed 7000 white cells/mm³, 45% of which were polymorphonuclear cells. Synovial fluid glucose was 80 mg/100 ml when blood glucose was 100 mg/100 ml. No crystals were seen. Synovial fluid culture was negative. Serum studies for rheumatoid factor and antinuclear antibody were negative. Creatinine clearance was normal. Serum protein electrophoresis revealed slight elevation of alpha-2 globulin. Roentgenograms of the chest and involved joints were normal except for soft tissue swelling of the right knee. Ophthalmologic examination revealed conjunctivitis and mild uveitis. A diagnosis of Reiter's syndrome was made.

Tetracycline, 500 mg QID, was begun for his genitourinary symptoms, with resolution of complaints after a period of five to six days. Attempts to control his relatively severe arthritic symptoms with full doses of aspirin, indomethacin and, later, phenylbutazone were unsuccessful. The patient was placed on prednisone, 10 mg QID, for treatment of uveitis and joint symptoms. In addition, steroid eye drops were used locally. Triamcinolone in Orabase was prescribed for his oral lesion. The patient responded well to the above program and prednisone dosage was gradually reduced as joint and eye symptoms improved. Clinical symptoms resolved completely after four months and all therapy was discontinued. The patient did well for approximately one and a half years, at which time he had recurrence of iritis in the right eye. This was treated successfully with oral and local steroids and was not associated with recurrence of joint, genitourinary or mucocutaneous lesions.

Discussion: The patient presented with a classic tetrad of symptoms of Reiter's syndrome, including arthritis, conjunctivitis and iritis, urethritis, and mucocutaneous lesions of the skin, mouth and genitalia. Although all components of the tetrad were present simultaneously in this patient, it is not uncommon for various facets of the syndrome to occur independently of one another at separate times during the clinical course of this disease. Joint symptoms in many patients with this syndrome will respond satisfactorily to conservative therapy with salicylates and indomethacin, but some patients require short courses of steroids to control severe articular manifestations. Steroids used both systemically and locally are valuable for treatment of iritis. Genitourinary symptoms may respond to a short course of tetracycline therapy.

History 10-4. Behçet's Syndrome

A.H., a 15-year-old black male, was first seen for evaluation in December, 1973. He was well until approximately four weeks prior, when he noted onset of fever, malaise, myalgia and polyarthralgia. Several days later he developed swelling, tenderness and limitation of motion of the right ankle. Shortly afterwards, pain was noted in both shoulders and he developed swelling and pain in the right knee. The patient was treated with buffered aspirin, 640 mg QID, with some relief of muscle and joint pain. Three weeks prior to admission he developed painful subcutaneous nodules over the anterior aspect of the right leg and the dorsal aspect of the right forearm. Furuncle-like lesions were noted over the right side of his forehead. Temperature elevations up to 38.5° C daily were recorded. There was no history of eye symptoms, pleurisy, Raynaud's phenomenon, sun sensitivity, dry eyes or dry mouth, dysuria or drug allergy. Several days prior to admission, the patient developed painful oral ulcers and a painless ulcer on the scrotum. He was admitted to hospital by his pediatrician for evaluation and rheumatologic consultation. Further system review was negative, and past medical history was noncontributory.

Physical examination revealed normal blood pressure, pulse and respiration. Intermittent daily temperature elevations to 38.5° C were noted. Furuncle formation was seen over the right side of his forehead. Multiple oral ulcerations were present in the buccal mucosa and at the inferior aspect of the tongue. Small lymph nodes were palpable in each axillary area. Cardiorespiratory examination was normal. Abdominal examination revealed no enlargement of the liver or spleen. Examination of the extremities revealed slight swelling and tenderness of the right knee, and more extensive swelling, tenderness and limitation of motion of the right ankle. Tender, erythematous, warm discrete nodules, measuring 2 × 3 cm, appeared over the anterior aspect of the right leg and the dorsal aspect of the right forearm. A small ulcer of the scrotum was observed. The remainder of the musculoskeletal examination and muscle evaluation was normal.

The hematocrit was 41%, white blood cell count was 10,000/mm^3 with a normal differential, and the platelet count was 342,000 per mm^3. The erythrocyte sedimentation rate was 12 mm/hour (Wintrobe). The serum uric acid was 6 mg/100 ml, serum calcium was 10.7 mg% and serum phosphorus was 4.4 mg%. Serum protein electrophoresis, creatinine, and muscle enzymes were normal. Serologic test for syphilis was negative. Serum studies for rheumatoid factor and antinuclear antibody were negative, as were blood studies for LE cells. Throat culture revealed normal flora. Culture of the furuncle from the right forehead revealed Staphylococcus albus. Blood and urine cultures were negative. Upper gastrointestinal series, barium enema and chest x-rays were normal. Roentgenograms of both knees and ankles were unremarkable. Sigmoidoscopic examination to 25 cm revealed slightly edematous mucosa at 20 cm. No ulcers were seen. Ophthalmologic examination was normal. PPD and fungus skin tests were negative. A diagnosis of probable Behçet's syndrome was made.

Aspirin was increased to 960 mg QID. Oral ulcerations were treated with tetracycline suspension used as a mouthwash, Viscous Xylocaine, and triamcinolone in Orobase. It was advised that prednisone, 20 to 30 mg daily, be started if the patient failed to respond to a conservative program of therapy. Joint symptoms, myalgia, malaise and fever responded after four days of conservative therapy, however, and the patient was discharged to the care of his pediatrician.

Discussion: The symptoms in this patient, which included orogenital ulcerations, pyoderma, erythema nodosum-like lesions, arthritis and fever were consistent with a diagnosis of Behçet's syndrome. Although the classic syndrome includes conjunctivitis or iritis, components of the basic triad of symptoms may occur at separate times. Other diagnostic considerations included Reiter's syndrome and ulcerative colitis. Absence of symptoms involving the eye and genitourinary tract militated against a diagnosis of Reiter's syndrome. No evidence of ulcerative colitis was noted on radiologic or sigmoidoscopic study.

History 10-5. Erythema Nodosum

C.T., a 26-year-old white female, was seen in consultation in March, 1969. She was well until approximately one month prior, when she noted aching in the knees, hips and shoulders associated with mild morning stiffness. Two weeks later, she developed increased aching in numerous peripheral joints and objective swelling of the ankles and knees. Red, painful, tender nodules were noted in both anterior tibial areas. Nodule formation occurred in crops at intervals of several days. Treatment with aspirin, 640 mg QID, provided mild relief. She gave no past history of arthritis or rheumatic fever. Recent history was negative for upper respiratory infection or sore throat. On system review the patient denied pleurisy, Raynaud's phenomenon, sun sensitivity, dry eyes or mouth, iritis, canker sores, diarrhea or drug allergy. There was no known exposure to tuberculosis and the patient had not traveled outside the midwest for several years. The patient gave no history of prior drug ingestion; in particular, no intake of bromides, iodides, sulfonamides or contraceptive pills was noted.

Physical examination revealed blood pressure 100/64 mm Hg. Cutaneous examination showed a number of discrete, warm, erythematous nodules on the anterior aspects of both tibial areas. Individual lesions were characterized by a central area of induration. Lesions varied from 1 to 1½ cm in diameter. Cardiorespiratory examination revealed a Grade I/VI apical systolic murmur. Liver and spleen were not palpably enlarged. Musculoskeletal examination showed swelling of both wrists and both ankles with mild limitation of motion.

Hematocrit was 38%, and white blood cell count was $7700/mm^3$ with 8% eosinophils on differential white count. Erythrocyte sedimentation rate was 27 mm/hour (Wintrobe). Urinalysis was normal. Serum calcium was 9.4 mg%. Routine serologic test for syphilis and C-reactive protein studies were negative. Antistreptolysin-O titer was less than 100 Todd units. Heterophile antibody titer was 1:28. Serum studies for rheumatoid factor and antinuclear antibody were negative, and LE cells were not seen. Throat culture revealed normal flora. PA and lateral roentgenograms of the chest showed bilateral hilar adenopathy. Electrocardiogram was normal. Skin test with intermediate PPD was negative. A diagnosis of erythema nodosum was made.

The patient was continued on aspirin, 960 mg QID. When seen in followup one month later the cutaneous lesions had almost completely resolved. Joint swelling was absent and only mild polyarthralgia remained. Repeat chest x-ray at that time was completely normal. The patient went on to complete clearing of symptoms over a period of several more weeks and had no recurrence of a similar syndrome during a four-year followup.

Discussion: The findings of tender, erythematous nodular skin lesions over the anterior tibial areas, arthritis, and hilar adenopathy were consistent with a diagnosis of erythema nodosum. History, physical examination and laboratory studies did not reveal the presence of any underlying disease with which erythema nodosum is commonly associated. Lesions responded to a conservative program of management.

Prolonged observation for the presence of primary disease states that are associated with erythema nodosum is important, because the underlying disorder may not become evident for some time. A diagnosis of primary idiopathic erythema nodosum can be made safely only after a reasonable period of followup.

History 10-6. Henoch-Schönlein (Anaphylactoid) Purpura

G.G., a 10-year-old white male, was admitted to hospital for evaluation in April, 1973. He was well until one week prior, at which time he noted onset of fatigue, fever, red spots on the skin about the ankles, and pain in both elbows and knees. The night prior to admission he developed nausea and epigastric pain and vomited clear gastric fluid. Physical examination revealed many discrete purpuric cutaneous lesions, 3 mm to 2 cm in size, over the lower extremities and buttocks. Lesions did not blanch with pressure. Cardiorespiratory examination was normal. There was generalized abdominal tenderness and the spleen was palpable 1 cm below the costal margin. Joint examination was normal except for tenderness of the elbows and knees to palpation.

The urine contained 10 to 20 red blood cells per high power field. Hematocrit was 38%, white blood cell count was 11,500/mm^3 and differential white cell count was normal. Erythrocyte sedimentation rate was 26 mm/hour (Wintrobe). Prothrombin time, partial thromboplastin time, platelet count, bleeding time and coagulation time were normal. Throat culture revealed normal throat flora, and antistreptolysin-O titer was negative. Studies for serum rheumatoid factor, antinuclear antibody, complement and serum protein electrophoresis were normal or negative. Serologic test for syphilis was negative. Stool guaiac studies were strongly positive. Creatinine clearance was 104 ml/minute. Electrocardiogram and roentgenograms of the chest and abdomen revealed no abnormal findings.

Re-examination on the second day of hospitalization demonstrated definite swelling of the right wrist and the presence of fresh blood in the stool. Purpuric cutaneous lesions became larger and more widespread and the patient continued to pass grossly bloody stools. Prednisone was begun in a dose of 10 mg BID by mouth. After four days, skin lesions notably diminished, there was no abdominal tenderness or gross gastrointestinal bleeding, and joint examination was normal. Urinalysis revealed no abnormalities. The patient was discharged with plans to slowly decrease steroid therapy while under clinical observation. Clinical manifestations continued to improve and steroids were discontinued after three weeks.

Discussion: The clinical findings of purpura, abdominal pain and gastrointestinal bleeding, hematuria and joint symptoms were typical of those seen in patients with Henoch-Schönlein (anaphylactoid) purpura. Prognosis is generally good unless chronic renal disease intervenes. Other forms of necrotizing vasculitis that might produce similar clinical manifestations must be excluded if symptoms are atypical.

History 10-7. Gonococcal Arthritis

P.D., a 19-year-old black male, was first seen in consultation in December, 1972. He had been in good heatlh until four days prior to admission, at which time he noted pain in the right wrist with use. Pain increased in intensity, with severe symptoms at rest. Pain was followed by swelling of the right wrist and the dorsum of the right hand. Two days prior to admission, the patient developed fever and chills. There was no history of sun sensitivity, Raynaud's phenomenon, morning stiffness, skin rash, diarrhea, urethritis or pleurisy. The patient denied past history of venereal disease and recent sexual intercourse. System review was otherwise normal and past medical history was unremarkable.

Physical examination revealed temperature of 38° C. No lymphadenopathy was present. Examination of the heart and lungs revealed no abnormal findings. The abdomen was soft and the liver and spleen were not palpably enlarged. Several acute papulovesicular lesions with erythematous borders were observed. Joint examination revealed acute inflammation of the right wrist and hand with notable erythema, increased heat and tenderness. Movement of the fingers produced pain in the region of the dorsum of the right hand and the wrist. No other abnormal joint findings were observed.

Hematocrit was 42%, the erythrocyte sedimentation rate was 30 mm/hour (Wintrobe), and white blood cell count was 9000/mm³ with 88% neutrophils. Urinalysis, liver function studies, electrocardiogram and chest x-ray were normal. X-rays of the right wrist and hand revealed only soft tissue swelling. A few drops of purulent-looking material were removed by arthrocentesis from the right wrist. Gram stain revealed a moderate number of polymorphonuclear cells but no bacteria. Culture was positive for Neisseria gonorrhoeae. Blood, urethral, and throat cultures were negative. A diagnosis of acute gonococcal arthritis and tenosynovitis was made.

The patient was treated with aqueous crystalline penicillin, 6 million units daily in divided doses, by intravenous route. Swelling of the right hand and wrist and fever subsided notably over a two-day period. He was discharged five days after admission to continue oral penicillin for a total of 14 days of therapy.

Discussion: Gonococcal arthritis may appear in several different clinical forms. Acute migratory polyarthralgia or polyarthritis may precede localization of infection to one or two joints. Systemic findings such as fever and chills and cutaneous lesions are common associated symptoms. In some patients, preceding polyarticular disease may be absent and the infection appears as an acute monoarthritis. In this patient, joint symptoms were limited to the right wrist and dorsum of the right hand. The right hand symptoms were consistent with acute tenosynovitis, a common manifestation of gonococcal infection. Cutaneous lesions were characteristic of those seen in gonococcal infection and strongly suggested the correct diagnosis even before bacterial confirmation. Although a history of recent sexual exposure can frequently be elicited, the diagnosis cannot be excluded in the absence of such information.

REFERENCES

1. Moll, J. M. H. and Wright, V.: Psoriatic arthritis. Semin Arthritis Rheum 3:55, 1973.
2. Ford, D. K.: Reiter's syndrome. Bull Rheum Dis 20:588, 1970.
3. Morris, R. et al.: HLA-W27—a clue to the diagnosis and pathogenesis of Reiter's syndrome. N Eng J Med 290:554, 1974.
4. Yanez, J. E. et al.: Rubella arthritis. Ann Int Med 64:772, 1966.
5. Keiser, H. L.: et al.: Clinical forms of gonococcal arthritis. N Eng J Med 274:234, 1968.
6. McCarty, D. J. and Ormiste, V.: Arthritis and HB Ag positive hepatitis. Arch Int Med 132:264, 1973.
7. Barrow, M. V. and Holubar, K.: Multicentric reticulohistiocytosis. Medicine 48:287, 1969.
8. Buckley, G. E. III and Gills, J. P. Jr.: Cyclophosphamide therapy of Behçet's disease. J Allerg 43:273, 1969.
9. Hanauer, L. B.: Reticulohistiocytosis. Remission after cyclophosphamide therapy. Arthritis Rheum 15:636, 1972.

Chapter 11

GASTROINTESTINAL SYMPTOMS AND ARTHRITIS

Patients with arthritis may suffer from diseases characterized by gastrointestinal abnormalities. In some patients, the arthritis and gastrointestinal symptoms occur concomitantly, or the arthritis follows gastrointestinal manifestations. In others, the arthritis may occur first, in which case the relationship between the two sites of involvement becomes obvious only with observation over a period of time.

DIFFERENTIAL DIAGNOSIS

Diseases to be considered:

Ulcerative colitis, regional enteritis
Whipple's disease
Reiter's syndrome
Behçet's syndrome
Hypertrophic osteoarthropathy
Scleroderma
Necrotizing vasculitis
Carcinoma of the bowel
Amyloidosis
Tuberculosis
Gastrointestinal shunts
Miscellaneous gastrointestinal disorders

Arthritis often accompanies *chronic ulcerative colitis*[1,2] or *regional enteritis*.[2,3] The arthritic features of these disorders are similar. Different patterns of peripheral joint involvement occur. In classic cases, peripheral joint symptoms parallel gastrointestinal symptoms with respect to remissions and exacerbations. Large and small joints are involved. Arthritis may be limited to one or a few joints or involve numerous articulations. Migratory spread is common. Some patients complain of arthralgia with little or no objective swelling or tenderness. Rheumatoid factor tests are

166

characteristically negative. Prognosis is usually good with regard to permanent joint disability.

In some patients, joint symptoms may more closely simulate rheumatoid arthritis; attacks are prolonged and lack an association with exacerbations and remissions of bowel disease. In other patients with inflammatory bowel disease, joint symptoms may be a reflection of associated disorders, including erythema nodosum and hypertrophic osteoarthropathy. Systemic manifestations of inflammatory bowel disease such as pyoderma gangrenosum, oral ulcerations, uveitis, and hepatic abnormalities are common associated findings.

Spondylitis that resembles ankylosing spondylitis occurs with increased frequency in patients with ulcerative colitis and regional enteritis. Evidence supports the interpretation that the spondylitis seen in these patients is an independent associated finding rather than a systemic manifestation of the bowel disease. For example, spondylitis often antedates bowel symptoms and there is little clinical correlation between the spondylitis and bowel disease. Effective treatment of the bowel is usually unassociated with relief of back symptoms. Interestingly, HLA-W27 histocompatibility antigen has recently been found in approximately 75% of patients with spondylitis and inflammatory bowel disease.[4] This increased frequency parallels the increased association of this antigen in patients with ankylosing spondylitis. No such increase is seen in patients with colitis or enteritis in the absence of spondylitis.

Whipple's disease is characterized by abdominal pain, diarrhea, fever, cutaneous hyperpigmentation, peripheral lymphadenopathy and arthritis[5,6] (see Chapter 8). In addition, there is a tendency to hypotension and pleural reactions. Peripheral joint manifestations are similar to those described for patients with colitis and regional enteritis. Joint complaints often precede symptoms of diarrhea; symptoms of arthritis and diarrhea usually do not occur simultaneously. The arthritis is usually episodic with a migratory pattern. Joint symptoms last for one to several days and long remissions are frequent. Chronic residual arthritis is rare. Large joints such as the knees and ankles are involved most frequently; fingers, wrists, elbows and other joints are also affected. Back symptoms may be present and findings of spondylitis have been described.[5,6] Rheumatoid factor studies are negative.

Diagnosis of Whipple's disease depends on demonstrating PAS-positive inclusion bodies in macrophages of small intestinal mucosa or mesenteric nodes. Biopsy of the jejunum by a peroral approach is utilized to obtain tissue for study. Electron microscopic studies demonstrate rod-shaped organisms infiltrating the lamina propria of the intestinal mucosa. Although these rod-shaped structures are probably related to disease etiology, experimental transmission of disease to animals has not been successfully accomplished. Initial treatment with penicillin and streptomycin for 10 to

14 days, followed by tetracycline for 10 to 12 months, has given favorable results in most cases.

Reiter's syndrome is associated with arthritis, urethritis, conjunctivitis and mucocutaneous ulcerative lesions. In addition, patients occasionally have involvement of the gastrointestinal tract. Diarrhea is usually mild and short in duration; in some cases, however, it is severe, bloody and prolonged. A relationship between Reiter's syndrome and Shigella flexneri infections during episodes of epidemic dysentery has been described.

Arthritis is most frequently seen in large joints, but toes and fingers may be involved. As in patients with ulcerative colitis and regional enteritis, spondylitis with involvement of sacroiliac joints and the spine is a common sequela of the disease. Close evaluation of roentgenographic spinal changes is helpful in differentiating the spondylitis of Reiter's syndrome from that seen in ulcerative colitis and ankylosing spondylitis. In Reiter's syndrome, paravertebral spurs (syndesmophytes) are more rounded and thicker than those seen in ankylosing spondylitis. Unilateral syndesmophytes are common in Reiter's syndrome.

Behçet's syndrome is a multisystem disorder characterized by a triad of recurrent oral and genital ulcerations and relapsing iritis. In addition, lesions occur in the gastrointestinal tract that may be severe and resemble the pathologic changes of ulcerative colitis. In most patients, arthralgia is more frequent than true arthritis. Large joints such as knees, ankles, wrists and elbows are involved most frequently. Fortunately, chronic permanent changes and joint disability rarely develop.

Hypertrophic osteoarthropathy is characterized by clubbing of the fingers and toes, periostitis of the ends of long bones and arthritis. Although usually seen secondary to infectious or neoplastic diseases of the lungs and pleura (see Chapter 12), this syndrome also occurs in association with gastrointestinal disorders such as ulcerative colitis, regional enteritis, intestinal tuberculosis, sprue, and carcinoma of the colon.

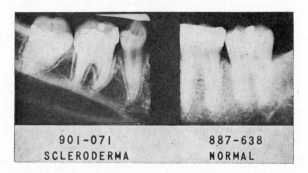

901-071
SCLERODERMA

887-638
NORMAL

Figure 11-1. Dental z-rays, scleroderma. Widening of the periodontal membrane due to collagen deposition is contrasted with normal findings. (Courtesy Dr. A. Mackenzie)

Joint and gastrointestinal symptoms are common concomitant findings in *scleroderma*. In most patients joint symptoms are characterized by pain with little or no swelling; other patients, however, show mild to severe degrees of joint disability. Involvement of skeletal muscle results in weakness which, when severe, simulates polymyositis. Lesions of the gastrointestinal tract may be present from the mouth to the anus. Roentgenograms of the teeth show widening of the periodontal membrane (Fig. 11-1). Esophageal dysfunction with symptoms of dysphagia and esophagitis is common; on x-ray examination, peristaltic activity may be diminished or totally absent (Fig. 11-2). Hiatal hernia is frequent as reflux of gastric juices leads to stricture and secondary herniation. Involvement of the small bowel causes bloating, cramps, vomiting, episodic diarrhea and constipation. Malabsorption syndrome results from severe involvement of the small bowel.[7] Roentgenologic examination reveals dilatation of the second and third portions of the duodenum (Fig. 11-3). X-ray examination of the small intestine demonstrates irregular flocculation of barium, areas of dilatation, hypersegmentation and evidence of hypomotility. Pneumatosis cystoides intestinalis may be seen in the form of radiolucent cysts or streaks of gas within the walls of the small bowel. When rupture of one of these cysts leads to pneumoperitoneum, the symptoms are highly suggestive of a perforated viscus. The disproportion between radiologic findings and benign clinical symptoms is the clue to diagnosis. Atrophy of the muscularis of the large intestine produces characteristic wide-mouthed diverticula (Fig. 11-4).

Gastrointestinal symptoms may be a major clinical feature in patients with various forms of *necrotizing vasculitis*. Abdominal pain is often ac-

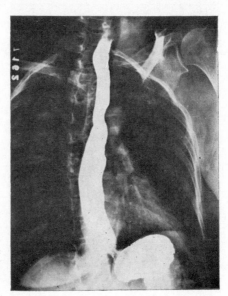

Figure 11-2. Roentgenogram of esophagus, scleroderma, showing generalized dilatation. Fluoroscopic study revealed loss of peristaltic activity. (Courtesy, Dr. A. Mackenzie)

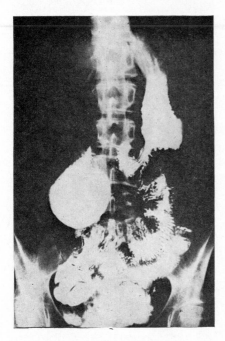

Figure 11-3. Roentgenogram of stomach and small bowel, scleroderma. Note widely dilated duodenum. (Courtesy, Dr. A. Mackenzie)

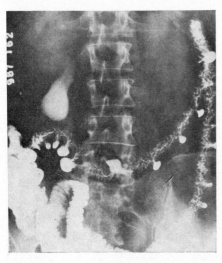

Figure 11-4. Roentgenogram of large intestine, scleroderma. Note numerous wide-mouthed diverticula. (Courtesy, Dr. A. Mackenzie)

companied by nausea, vomiting, diarrhea or bloody stools. The latter result from ischemic involvement of the bowel. Acute inflammation of various abdominal viscera, such as the appendix, intestine, stomach, gallbladder or pancreas, causes acute abdominal pain and sometimes rupture of the involved viscus. Mesenteric arteritis leads to thrombosis and bowel infarction; the clinical picture may superficially resemble ulcerative colitis. Henoch-Schönlein purpura is a specific vasculitic syndrome characterized by arthralgia or arthritis, cutaneous macules, papules and purpura, renal disease and gastrointestinal symptoms. Crampy abdominal pain and gastrointestinal hemorrhage are common. Intussusception may be a complicating factor.

Carcinoma of the bowel, as with carcinomas elsewhere, may be associated with peripheral arthritis that simulates rheumatoid arthritis.[8] Joint symptoms may appear when the neoplasm is occult and the true diagnosis becomes evident only after prolonged observation. The association of arthritis and malignancy should always be considered as a diagnostic possibility when arthritis begins in older persons. Large joints are characteristically involved but small joints may also be affected. Joint symptoms may recede following resection or other forms of treatment of the carcinoma. Recurrence of joint symptoms should suggest the possibility of recurrence of the neoplasm.

Arthritis may be a manifestation of either primary or secondary *amyloidosis.* Actual joint swelling may be noted. Cutaneous deposits of amyloid form subcutaneous nodules that simulate those seen in rheumatoid arthritis. Amyloidosis is frequently accompanied by gastrointestinal symptoms, including gastrointestinal bleeding. Infiltration of the esophagus or small bowel may lead to obstruction. Malabsorption syndrome results from infiltration of the small bowel. The diagnosis of amyloid may be made safely by study of tissue obtained by biopsy of the rectum, gingiva, or subcutaneous abdominal fat.[9]

An uncommon cause of arthritis and gastrointestinal symptoms is *tuberculosis.* These patients are usually severely ill and other findings to support the diagnosis are usually obvious.

An unusual form of arthritis is that seen in association with *gastrointestinal shunts.* This syndrome has recently been noted in patients subjected to jejunocolostomy for weight reduction.[10] Large joints are involved most commonly. Symptoms usually regress when normal bowel anatomy is restored. The etiology of joint manifestations in this syndrome is unknown.

Peptic or gastric ulceration is common in patients with various diseases of connective tissue. Their frequency is increased by use of various therapeutic agents that are highly irritating to the gastrointestinal tract. Indomethacin, commonly used in the treatment of inflammatory arthritides, may cause ulcerative lesions of the bowel. It is contraindicated in the presence of ulcerative colitis, regional enteritis and diverticulitis.

DIAGNOSTIC STUDIES

In addition to general diagnostic studies, specific examinations directed to the bowel are required. Sigmoidoscopic examination and barium enema are indicated if ulcerative colitis is suspected. Small bowel roentgenograms are utilized in patients with symptoms consistent with regional enteritis. The diagnosis of Whipple's disease is based on demonstration of specific pathologic findings in small bowel specimens obtained by peroral biopsy as previously described. Roentgenologic findings in patients with gastrointestinal symptoms due to Reiter's syndrome may be nonspecific or absent. The diagnosis usually rests on the overall clinical presentation. Ulcerative bowel lesions on radiologic study of patients with Behçet's syndrome are usually difficult to differentiate from ulcerative colitis. Indeed, the two diseases may be clinically indistinguishable. Sigmoidoscopic and vaginal examination to demonstrate ulcerative lesions characteristic of Behçet's syndrome are diagnostically helpful.

Studies in patients with hypertrophic osteoarthropathy should be directed toward diseases to which it is a secondary manifestation; chest x-rays are mandatory. Tuberculin skin testing, chest x-ray and cultures of sputum and urine are indicated in patients with symptoms suggestive of intestinal tuberculosis.

Scleroderma is usually obvious on clinical examination, but visceral changes may occur with minimal or no skin changes. Roentgenograms often reveal characteristic changes at various levels of the bowel, as previously described. Radiologic changes in vasculitis of the bowel are nonspecific and resemble changes seen in other types of bowel ischemia. Dilatation and irritability of the bowel may be seen in association with edema and thickening of the bowel wall. Muscle biopsy is usually indicated for diagnosis. Arteriography of mesenteric, hepatic or renal vessels may demonstrate characteristic areas of thrombosis and aneurysm formation.

Carcinoma requires careful radiologic and sigmoidoscopic evaluation for diagnosis. Amyloidosis can be diagnosed in many cases by specific amyloid stains of tissue obtained at biopsy. A long history of inflammatory bowel disease should suggest the possible presence of a jejunocolic shunt, which is readily demonstrable on radiologic study.

THERAPY

The management of arthritis associated with the foregoing disorders includes nonspecific measures directed toward symptomatic relief and specific measures directed to the underlying disorders. Nonspecific therapeutic programs such as rest, heat, exercise and mild anti-inflammatory and analgesic agents can often be instituted safely prior to completion of studies without obscuring the diagnosis. Full doses of aspirin, such as 640 to 960 mg four times daily, are effective in relieving painful joint manifestations to some degree. Aspirin should be used with caution, if at all, in patients whose underlying disease state may be aggravated by its use, such as patients with peptic ulcer disease. Special forms of salicylates, such as enteric-coated aspirin, can be utilized more safely in such cases. Analgesic agents including acetominophen, 320 to 640 mg QID, propoxyphene hydrochloride, 65 mg QID, or ethoheptazine citrate (Zactane), 75 mg QID, may be substituted or added without fear of causing significant gastric irritation. Indomethacin is a useful anti-inflammatory agent, but is contraindicated in the presence of peptic ulcer disease or ulcerative disease of the small or large bowel. Phenylbutazone or oxyphenbutazone (Tandearil), 100 mg three to four times daily, can be safely used for short periods to treat acute attacks of joint pain; use is contraindicated in patients with a history of significant peptic ulcer disease. Systemic corticosteroid therapy should not be instituted for symptomatic relief, but should be limited to those specifically diagnosed conditions in which it has a definite and safe therapeutic effect. However, local steroid injections into the joint can be safely considered a nonspecific approach to overall management.

The arthritis of ulcerative colitis or regional enteritis often responds to measures directed at control of the disease. Therapeutic agents include salicylazosulfapyridine (Azulfidine), systemic corticosteroids and, at times, immunosuppressive agents such as azathioprine. Colectomy or small bowel resection should be considered only for treatment of bowel disease unresponsive to conservative measures, and not as a therapeutic approach for the arthritis per se. The symptoms of Whipple's disease, including the arthritis, usually respond favorably to antibiotic therapy. Initially, procaine penicillin G, 1.2 million units, and streptomycin, 1 gm daily, are given for a period of 10 to 14 days. This is followed by tetracycline, 250 mg QID, which is continued for at least 10 to 12 months.

The arthritis of Reiter's syndrome, if mild, often responds to high doses of salicylates. More severe cases require additional anti-inflammatory agents such as indomethacin, phenylbutazone or corticosteroids. Patients with Behçet's syndrome are handled in similar fashion with respect to joint manifestations. Severe cases with diffuse systemic symptoms warrant consideration of high-dose steroids or immunosuppressive agents[11] for control.

Treatment of the arthritis of hypertrophic osteoarthropathy involves nonspecific anti-inflammatory agents for symptomatic relief. Prolonged or complete relief depends on the ability to effectively treat and remove those factors to which the syndrome is often secondary. Therapy of musculoskeletal symptoms in scleroderma is usually a minor part of overall management. Although joint symptoms may be severe, they are more often mild and respond to the simpler anti-inflammatory agents. Various forms of therapy are effective for gastrointestinal symptoms, depending upon the area of bowel involved. Dysphagia is improved by use of bethanechol (Urecholine), 5 to 10 mg TID, chewed 30 minutes before meals. Antacids are helpful in relief of esophagitis. Malabsorption symptoms sometimes respond to periodic or continuous administration of tetracycline. A diet utilizing short-chain fatty acids may also provide some symptomatic relief. Bowel softeners or mild laxatives, such as dioctyl sodium sulfosuccinate (Colace) or bisacodyl (Dulcolax), relieve severe constipation.

Bowel manifestations of vasculitis reflect the basic underlying vascular pathology seen elsewhere and may respond to corticosteroid therapy. Unfortunately, steroid therapy may represent a two-edged sword, in that rapid healing may result in ischemic occlusion of mesenteric and other vessels. Nevertheless, steroid therapy is usually indicated because uncontrolled vasculitis will usually lead to even more serious pathologic manifestations.

Joint symptoms related to carcinoma of the bowel are relieved to variable extent by nonspecific anti-inflammatory agents. Successful removal of the neoplasm is sometimes associated with rapid and complete relief of articular symptoms. Incomplete relief or recurrence of joint symptoms suggests incomplete removal or recurrence of the tumor. Tuberculosis of the joints and bowel is managed by the usual antitubercular regimens. Multiple drug therapy using various combinations of isoniazid, ethambutol and rifampin are usually indicated. Treatment should be continued for a minimum of one year to 18 months, and in certain cases even longer, before the patient is considered permanently cured.

Amyloid disease is difficult to treat. No consistently effective specific therapy has been found. Arthritic manifestations associated with jejunocolic shunts are aided by various anti-inflammatory agents such as high-dose salicylates; corticosteroid therapy is necessary in severe cases. Symptoms often resolve when normal bowel anatomy is restored.

CASE HISTORIES

History 11-1. Chronic Ulcerative Colitis with Arthritis

J.B., a 49-year-old white female, was first seen in January, 1974. She gave a history of having been well until approximately two years prior, when she noted onset of fever, abdominal cramps and bloody diarrhea. Gastrointestinal studies revealed changes consistent with chronic nonspecific ulcerative colitis. At that time, the patient was placed on therapy with prednisone and salicylazosulfapyridine (Azulfidine). Remission of symptoms occurred after approximately one month. All medications were discontinued several months later when the patient continued to be completely asymptomatic. She did well until September, 1973, when symptoms of colitis recurred; this was controlled with prednisone, 5 mg BID. A mild exacerbation of symptoms was noted in December, 1973. At that time the patient developed acute onset of pain and swelling in both ankles. Symptoms were worse in the morning and did not respond to aspirin, 960 mg QID, added to her usual dose of prednisone. There were no ancillary symptoms of connective tissue disease such as pleurisy, alopecia, sun sensitivity, drug allergy, Raynaud's phenomenon, dry eyes or mouth, or frequent canker sores in the mouth. On physical examination no abnormal findings were noted except for moderate swelling, increased heat and tenderness of both ankles.

Laboratory studies revealed negative serum rheumatoid factor and antinuclear antibody studies and a normal serum uric acid. Hematocrit, white blood cell count and differential were normal. Erythrocyte sedimentation rate was 29 mm/hour (Wintrobe). Roentgenograms of both ankles were normal. Studies of synovial fluid aspirated from the left ankle revealed a white cell count of 8300/mm³ with 42% mononuclear cells. No crystals were seen. Smears and cultures for routine organisms, tuberculosis and fungi were negative. A presumptive diagnosis of arthritis related to ulcerative colitis was made. The patient responded well to local injections of steroid with lidocaine into both ankles. She was maintained in a relatively comfortable state on a program of aspirin, 960 mg QID, added to her daily dose of prednisone, 5 mg BID.

Discussion: Although a diagnosis of arthritis associated with ulcerative colitis was only presumptive in this patient with joint symptoms of recent origin, the clinical findings were consistent with the diagnosis. No evidence of articular disease of other etiology was present on clinical or laboratory study. Onset of joint symptoms at a time of exacerbation of her colitis was supportive of the diagnosis. Further observation should substantiate the initial clinical impression.

History 11-2. Regional Enteritis with Arthritis

G.W., a 15-year-old white male, was in good health until age 13, at which time he developed anorexia, vomiting, weight loss and fever. Diagnostic studies were consistent with regional enteritis and the patient was begun on prednisone therapy, 15 mg daily. Six months later, he had a severe episode of gastrointestinal symptoms associated with a painless effusion of the left knee. Swelling improved following joint aspiration and injection of intra-articular steroids. Prednisone was increased to 10 mg BID for a short period of time, and reduced later to a maintenance dose of 5 mg BID. Subsequently, the patient had intermittent swelling of the left knee which was treated with periodic injections of local steroids. The patient was referred for rheumatologic evaluation when swelling of the right knee was noted. There was no history of morning stiffness, pleurisy, Raynaud's phenomenon, dysphagia, sun sensitivity, iritis, urethritis, psoriasis or other skin rash. Bowel symptoms were quiescent and other aspects of the system review were negative.

Physical examination revealed a slightly pallid, well-developed young man. Abdominal examination was within normal limits. Musculoskeletal examination revealed moderate swelling and increased warmth of the right knee and minimal swelling of the left knee. No limitation of knee motion was noted. Examination of other joints was negative.

Hematocrit was 40%, white blood cell count was 9700/mm³ with a normal differential, erythrocyte sedimentation rate was 10 mm/hour (Wintrobe) and urinalysis was normal. Serum glutamic oxaloacetic transaminase, serologic test for syphilis, serum studies for antinuclear antibody and rheumatoid factor, and LE cell studies were normal or negative. Slight elevation of gamma globulin was seen on serum protein electrophoresis study. Analysis of synovial fluid removed from the right knee revealed a mildly inflammatory fluid that was negative on culture for routine organisms, tuberculosis and fungi. Chest x-ray was normal. X-rays of the knees showed a small suprapatellar effusion in the right knee. Barium enema revealed a normal mucosal pattern of the colon. Small bowel x-rays showed narrowing and mucosal irregularities consistent with regional enteritis. The right knee was treated with an intra-articular injection of steroid and lidocaine. The patient was continued on prednisone, 10 mg daily, in addition to aspirin, 640 mg QID. A physical therapy program was instituted.

Discussion: The clinical and laboratory findings in this case are consistent with a diagnosis of arthritis related to regional enteritis. No evidence of other forms of arthritis was noted. The patient did satisfactorily on a program of rest, physical therapy, and salicylates added to his maintenance prednisone. Joint symptoms were relatively mild and not disabling.

History 11-3. Arthritis Associated with Gastrointestinal Shunt

I.H., a 46-year-old black female, was in good health until 1945 when, at age 26, she underwent uterine myomectomy, right salpingo-oophorectomy and coincidental appendectomy for treatment of chronic pelvic inflammatory disease. Six years later, she had surgical lysis of adhesions for treatment of intestinal obstruction. Panhysterectomy was performed later that same year for management of menometrorrhagia. Over the ensuing 11 years, abdominal surgery was performed on four more occasions for treatment of recurrent intestinal obstruction due to adhesions. Surgical management included lysis of adhesions, multiple small bowel resections and, in 1962, performance of a jejunocolostomy.

In 1963 the patient developed severe diarrhea, with 10 to 25 bowel movements a day. Stools were characterized as frothy and foul-smelling and were noted to float in the toilet bowl. Diagnostic studies revealed marked malabsorption with associated metabolic changes. The patient's clinical problems were later complicated by the development of hypercalcemia in 1969. Diagnostic studies suggested a diagnosis of hyperparathyroidism. Exploration of the parathyroid glands revealed a large parathyroid adenoma. Parathyroidectomy was performed.

The patient was first evaluated by the rheumatology service in February, 1972, when she was admitted to hospital with complaints of pain and swelling of the right knee and right ankle since May, 1971. Persistent swelling had been treated with intermittent injections of intra-articular steroids, aspirin, and analgesic medications. System review revealed diarrhea, with five to six stools daily. There was no history of Raynaud's phenomenon, hair loss, pleurisy, skin rash, psoriasis, dry mouth or eyes, sun sensitivity or drug allergy. On physical examination blood pressure was 150/90 mm Hg. Moderate swelling of the right knee and right ankle were noted. The patient had been on no medications other than buffered aspirin, 960 mg four times a day, and diphenoxylate hydrochloride with atropine sulfate (Lomotil) as needed for diarrhea.

Hematocrit was 37%, white blood cell count was 4200/mm^3 with a normal differential count, and erythrocyte sedimentation rate was 25 mm/hour (Wintrobe). Urinalysis, serum electrolytes, serum calcium, phosphorus and alkaline phosphatase, serum muscle enzymes and uric acid determinations were normal. Routine serologic test for syphilis was negative. Serum studies for rheumatoid factor and antinuclear antibody were negative, as were LE cell determinations. Serum protein electrophoresis was normal. Chest x-ray was unremarkable. Roentgenographic examination of the knees revealed bilateral calcification of menisci consistent with pseudogout. No calcifications of the ankles were noted. During hospitalization, the patient developed swelling of the right wrist. X-rays of both wrists were normal; no calcium deposits were seen. Synovial fluid was aspirated from the right knee for study. The fluid was mildly inflammatory; no crystals were observed. Histopathologic study of synovial tissue removed at closed biopsy of the right knee revealed inflammatory granulation tissue and mild infiltration of mononuclear cells. No granulomas or calcium deposits were present. A diagnosis of arthritis secondary to jejunocolostomy was made.

The patient was placed on prednisone, 2.5 mg TID, in addition to buffered aspirin, 640 mg QID. Psyllium hydrophilic mucilloid (Metamucil) 4 cc TID, and dicyclomine hydrochloride (Bentyl), 20 mg TID, were used in treatment of diarrhea. The patient was followed regularly after discharge. Joint symptoms were limited to chronic swelling of the right ankle, right knee and right wrist with periodic acute exacerbations. No evidence to suggest a different diagnosis as a cause of her symptoms was seen. Repeated studies of synovial fluid were consistently negative for the presence of crystals. Symptoms were only poorly controlled with prednisone, 2.5 mg QID, aspirin 960 to 1280 mg QID, and periodic injections of intra-articular steroids. Chlorambucil therapy, 2 mg BID, was initiated when persistent symptoms became disabling. Subsequently, the patient had fewer acute exacerbations and moderately good reduction in chronic synovial swelling. Improvement persisted and prednisone dosage was reduced to 2.5 mg BID.

Discussion: This patient presented an interesting diagnostic challenge with respect to her rheumatologic symptoms. No evidence to support a diagnosis of one of the more common causes of chronic arthritis was seen. Although chondrocalcinosis (pseudogout syndrome) may cause chronic polyarthritis, absence of crystals in the synovial fluid and the absence of calcium deposits on synovial biopsy suggest that her symptoms were due to some other disorder. The association of hyperparathyroidism and chondrocalcinosis was of interest. The patient's joint findings were consistent with arthritis described in patients with jejunocolostomy and malabsorption syndrome. This clinical syndrome has been described in a number of patients in whom jejunocolostomy was performed as a short-circuiting procedure for control of obesity.

REFERENCES

1. Wright, V. and Watkinson, G.: The arthritis of ulcerative colitis. Brit Med J 2:670, 1965.
2. Palumbo, P. J. et al.: Musculoskeletal manifestations of inflammatory bowel disease. Mayo Clin Proc 48:411, 1973.
3. Soren, A.: Joint affections in regional ileitis. Arch Int Med 117:78, 1966.
4. Morris, R. I. et al.: HL-A-W27—a useful discriminator in the arthropathies of inflammatory bowel disease. N Eng J Med 290:1117, 1974.
5. Kelly, J. J. and Weisiger, B. B.: The arthritis of Whipple's disease. Arth Rheum 6:615, 1963.
6. LeVine, M. E. and Dobbins, W. O.: Joint changes in Whipple's disease. Semin Arthritis Rheum 3:79, 1973.
7. Kahn, I. J., Jeffries, G. H. and Sleisinger, M. H.: Malabsorption in intestinal scleroderma. Correction by antibiotics. N Eng J Med 274:1339, 1966.
8. Calabro, J. J.: Cancer and arthritis. Arth Rheum 10:553, 1967.
9. Westermark, P. and Stenkvist, B.: A new method for the diagnosis of systemic amyloidosis. Arch Int Med 132:522, 1973.
10. Shagrin, J. W., Frame, B. and Duncan, H.: Polyarthritis in obese patients with intestinal bypass. Ann Int Med 75:377, 1971.
11. Buckley, G. E. III and Gills, J. P. Jr.: Cyclophosphamide therapy of Behçet's disease. J Allerg 43:273, 1969.

Chapter 12

PULMONARY-ARTICULAR SYNDROMES

Pulmonary disease is commonly seen in association with various forms of arthritis. In some patients, the pulmonary lesions represent systemic extra-articular manifestations of the primary rheumatologic disorder. In others, the pulmonary lesions are primary and articular manifestations secondary.

DIFFERENTIAL DIAGNOSIS

Diseases to be considered:

Rheumatoid arthritis
Systemic lupus erythematosus
Polymyositis-dermatomyositis
Necrotizing vasculitis
Rheumatic fever
Scleroderma

Sarcoidosis
Erythema nodosum
Hypertrophic osteoarthropathy
Tuberculosis; fungal infection
Lung carcinoma

Pulmonary manifestations are common in association with many of the systemic connective tissue diseases. Although the lung changes in these disorders may be similar, they are frequently specific enough to be useful clues in differential diagnosis.

Lesions involving the lung and pleura are common in patients with *rheumatoid arthritis*.[1] They occur more frequently in males and sometimes precede the actual onset of arthritis. The form of involvement varies. Rheumatoid nodules, similar to those seen in subcutaneous areas of the skin, develop within the pleura or within the lung parenchyma (Fig. 12-1). They are more likely to be seen when serum rheumatoid factor is present in high titer. The nodules may persist for some time without change or they may disappear spontaneously. Other nodules slowly enlarge, with considerable progression in size. Nodules may be single or multiple; differentiation of these discrete shadows from primary or metastatic carcinoma on x-ray may be impossible. Cavitation occurs but is not common. In addi-

178

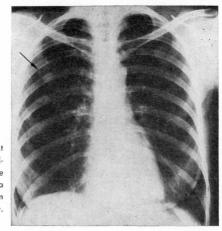

Figure 12-1. Chest roentgenogram in patient with rheumatoid arthritis. A solitary nodule (arrow) had the pathologic characteristics of a typical rheumatoid nodule when studied following thoracotomy. (Courtesy, Dr. M. Pazirandeh)

tion to discrete nodules, rheumatoid lung disease is characterized by diffuse interstitial fibrosis. Progression is associated with dyspnea, cough, sputum and occasionally clubbing of the fingers. Early, roentgenologic examination reveals soft fluffy patches of fine reticular mottling, most prominent at the lung bases. With disease progression, the fibrosis becomes more dramatic: a honeycombing picture, with cyst formation and fibrosis characterizes the end-stage disease (Fig. 12-2). Pleural disease is also common in the form of asymptomatic pleural effusion or pleural thickening on x-ray.[2] The fluid is exudative with increased protein and cells. Characteristically, the glucose content of the pleural fluid is reduced[3]; this finding, however, is variable. Examination of the fluid for rheumatoid factor frequently yields positive results and helps to confirm the diagnosis. Pleural fluid complement levels may be reduced.[4]

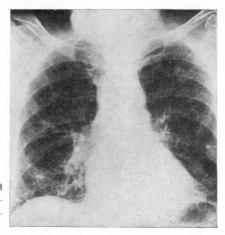

Figure 12-2. Chest roentgenogram, rheumatoid arthritis. Diffuse interstitial fibrosis with honeycomb appearance. (Courtesy, Dr. M. Pazirandeh)

An interesting type of rheumatoid lung disease is that associated with pneumoconiosis, the so-called *Caplan's syndrome*. Pulmonary lesions result from the interplay of silicosis and rheumatoid arthritis, both of which are present in these patients. Radiologic examination of the lung reveals well-defined nodular lesions usually greater than 1 cm in diameter. Cavitation is common and nodules are usually diffuse. Characteristic fibrotic and nodular changes of pneumoconiosis appear in the background. A similar syndrome has been described for rheumatoid arthritis and lung disease associated with agents other than silica, such as asbestos and abrasives.

Pulmonary symptoms are extremely common in patients with *systemic lupus erythematosus* (SLE)[5] as a result of pleural involvement, pneumonitis or congestive heart failure. Pleuritic pain and associated pleural effusions are frequent. Basilar plate-like atelectasis is a notable finding. Pleural effusions associated with congestive heart failure may be difficult to differentiate from similar changes induced by inflammatory pleuritis. A low pleural fluid complement indicates an inflammatory origin.[4] The combination of pleural disease and plate-like atelectasis on x-ray is a common finding in patients with SLE. Because secondary infection is not uncommon in patients with SLE, infectious pneumonitis due to bacteria or fungi should always be considered in the differential diagnosis of pulmonary lesions.

Diffuse pulmonary fibrosis may develop in patients with *dermatomyositis* or *polymyositis* (Fig. 12-3). The symptoms may be difficult or impossible to differentiate from those seen in rheumatoid arthritis or other entities causing pulmonary fibrosis. Pulmonary neoplasms should be routinely excluded, because 50% or more of cases of dermatomyositis occurring in persons over age 40 may be associated with malignancy.

Necrotizing vasculitis is associated with pulmonary manifestations. Roentgenologic study reveals a patchy nonspecific pneumonitis that resembles that seen in a number of diverse infectious or inflammatory pulmonary disorders. Involvement is often progressive. In some cases, new areas of the

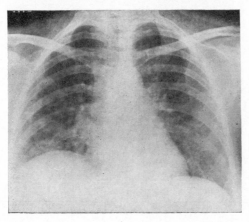

Figure 12-3. Diffuse pulmonary fibrosis in a patient with dermatomyositis. Similar lesions are seen in rheumatoid arthritis and scleroderma. (Courtesy, Dr. M. Pazirandeh)

lung become involved while lesions in formerly involved areas spontaneously regress.

Pulmonary artery involvement is rare in periarteritis nodosa but is commonly seen in allergic angiitis, in which case thrombosis with infarction may develop. Wegener's granulomatosis is characterized by systemic necrotizing vasculitis, granulomatous inflammation of the upper respiratory tract, vasculitic and granulomatous disease of the lungs, and necrotizing glomerulonephritis. Pulmonary involvement is characterized by discrete nodules or diffuse widespread pneumonitis.[6] Cavitation is not uncommon. In some patients with a forme-fruste of the disease, pulmonary lesions alone may be seen for variably long periods of time.

The syndrome of *"rheumatic fever pneumonitis"* is open to question. Patients with rheumatic fever and rheumatic heart disease frequently develop congestive heart failure; the associated pulmonary and pleural changes may simulate nonspecific inflammation or infection.

Pulmonary involvement occurs in many patients with *scleroderma*. The most common lesion is interstitial pulmonary fibrosis. This may be accompanied clinically by dyspnea on exertion, chronic cough with little or no sputum, and bouts of pleuritic chest pain. Many patients, however, are asymptomatic for prolonged periods of time. Roentgenologic evaluation reveals a reticular pattern of linear and nodular densities, usually most pronounced in the lower two-thirds of the lung fields. Honeycombing, the result of cystic lesions, is common in advanced cases and is similar to that seen in rheumatoid arthritis.

Laboratory studies reveal low pulmonary diffusion capacity and a restrictive ventilatory deficit. Bronchograms of the lungs show a characteristic bronchiectatic pattern. Electron microscopic examination of lung tissue occasionally reveals a notable thickening of the basement membrane of alveolar lining cells. Alveolar or bronchiolar cell carcinoma occurs with some increased frequency in patients with scleroderma. These lesions may result from the chronic intense stimulation of bronchiolar epithelial cells that accompanies the fibrosis.

A diagnosis of *sarcoidosis* should be strongly considered when joint symptoms occur in association with pulmonary symptoms. Sarcoid arthropathy is characterized by diffuse poylarthralgia, monoarthritis or polyarthritis. Chronic joint inflammation simulates that seen in rheumatoid arthritis. Pulmonary lesions include hilar adenopathy, diffuse parenchymal nodular granulomatous lesions, restrictive lung disease with fibrosis, and secondary cor pulmonale.

Erythema nodosum (see Chapter 6) is characterized by tender painful subcutaneous nodules occurring most commonly on the anterior aspects of the legs. Hilar adenopathy is common on roentgenologic examination. Cutaneous lesions are often associated with an acute or subacute polyarthritis that lasts for weeks or several months.

7

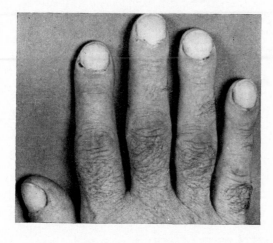

Figure 12-4. Clubbing of fingers in a patient with hypertrophic osteoarthroppathy. (Courtesy, Dr. A. Mackenzie)

The syndrome of *hypertrophic osteoarthropathy* is characterized by clubbing of the fingers (Fig. 12-4) and toes, periostitis of the ends of long bones, synovial swelling of joints, and sometimes gynecomastia. Large joints, such as the wrists, knees and ankles, are involved most frequently. The syndrome may be idiopathic but frequently occurs secondary to some other disorder, such as neoplasm, subacute bacterial endocarditis, cirrhosis, and chronic diarrheal disorders. An association with bronchogenic carcinoma and pleural mesotheliomas is particularly common. Although in the past this syndrome was commonly seen secondary to pulmonary infections such as empyema, lung abscess and bronchiectasis, this relationship is now infrequent due to the availability of more successful antibiotic therapy for the underlying infections. Rarely, osteoarthropathy may be associated with pulmonary tuberculosis or pneumoconiosis.

Chronic infectious arthritis may be associated with pulmonary infection with *tuberculosis, atypical mycobacteria, or fungal organisms.* Articular lesions are usually limited to one or a few joints.

Chronic joint findings characterized by pain, swelling, and objective evidence of synovitis may be associated with *carcinoma.* Although seen with neoplasms originating in almost any site, tumors of the lungs and the genitourinary and gastrointestinal tracts are frequent associated lesions. Joint manifestations often simulate rheumatoid arthritis, but subcutaneous nodules are not characteristically seen. Studies for serum rheumatoid factor are usually negative; when present, rheumatoid factor may diminish or disappear when the tumor is effectively removed. This diagnosis should always be entertained when joint disease has its onset in older persons.

Pulmonary lesions and joint symptoms may rarely be associated with other disorders, such as Reiter's syndrome, Behçet's syndrome and ulcerative colitis. These causes should be considered when the more common disorders affecting the two systems have been excluded.

DIAGNOSTIC STUDIES

Detailed history and physical examination will usually limit the diagnostic entities to be considered to a reasonable number. The Routine laboratory studies should include a complete blood count, erythrocyte sedimentation rate, urinalysis, studies for rheumatoid and antinuclear factors, and serum protein electrophoresis. Serial roentgenologic examinations of the chest may prove invaluable in defining the problem at hand. Pleural fluid, when present, should be removed for analysis and studied for total and differential white cell count, protein, glucose, complement, cytology, and culture for routine organisms, tuberculosis and fungi. A low pleural fluid glucose strongly suggests a diagnosis of rheumatoid arthritis. Low pleural complement is seen in rheumatoid arthritis and systemic lupus erythematosus. Rheumatoid factor may be present in fluid from rheumatoid patients. Fluid from patients with systemic lupus erythematosus may reveal LE cells on appropriate cytologic study.

Skin tests for tuberculosis and fungi should be performed when these diseases are suspected. Fungus skin tests should be delayed, however, until sera have been drawn for complement-fixation studies. In some cases, open or closed biopsy of the lung or pleura is necessary for diagnosis.

THERAPY

Management of the arthritis associated with pulmonary disease can be divided into nonspecific symptomatic measures and specific measures directed at the basic disease process. Symptomatic measures include rest, heat and mild anti-inflammatory and analgesic agents. In patients with one of the systemic connective tissue diseases, specific measures of value can be added when the diagnosis has been confirmed (see Chapter 18). Acute sarcoid arthritis may respond to full therapeutic doses of colchicine as used in attacks of acute gout.[7] The chronic polyarthralgia or polyarthritis of sarcoid may benefit from daily use of salicylates, indomethacin or phenylbutazone. Corticosteroid therapy may be indicated in severe cases. Antimalarial agents, such a hydroxychloroquine (Plaquenil), 200 mg BID, are helpful in selected instances. The dose can be reduced to once daily after three or four months if a response has been obtained. Baseline and periodic eye examinations for antimalarial toxicity are essential.

Oral salicylates or indomethacin benefit patients with arthritis related to erythema nodosum if symptoms are mild; severe cases require steroid therapy. Underlying causes of erythema nodosum should be removed or treated if possible. Articular symptoms of hypertrophic osteoarthropathy respond to anti-inflammatory agents such as aspirin, indomethacin or phenylbutazone; steroid therapy may be necessary if joint symptoms are severe. Removal of any underlying causes is usually essential for complete remission of symptoms. Tuberculous or fungal infections of the joints are treated with the same agents used in treatment of these diseases in other locations. Long-term therapy is indicated. Joint symptoms associated with carcinoma may benefit to some degree from nonspecific anti-inflammatory agents. Complete or significant remission depends on the ability to adequately treat the tumor.

Therapy of the pulmonary manifestations of these disorders varies with the diagnosis. The treatment of the pulmonary lesions of rheumatoid arthritis is often difficult. Lung manifestations may respond to antimalarial agents, gold or steroids used in management of the basic rheumatoid process. In many cases, however, lung changes persist despite improvement in joints. Pleural effusions may clear spontaneously. Persistent effusions should be aspirated in order to prevent pleural thickening and loss of lung volume. Treatment with intrapleural administration of nitrogen mustard or radioactive colloidal gold is sometimes successful. Surgical decortication may be indicated if ventilatory restriction is severe. Moderate to high doses of steroids may prevent progression of pulmonary fibrosis; this therapy should be considered in patients with deteriorating pulmonary function. The pulmonary manifestations of systemic lupus erythematosus usually respond to systemic steroid therapy; the lesions are usually short-lived and reasonably well-controlled with this agent. The progressive pulmonary fibrosis seen in dermatomyositis does not lend itself to any specific therapeutic agent. Treatment with steroids is worth a try when progressive deterioration in pulmonary function ensues.

CASE HISTORIES

History 12-1. Rheumatoid Arthritis with Pulmonary Manifestations

I.K., a 64-year-old white male, was first seen in September, 1970, with a history of rheumatoid arthritis of ten years' duration. Physical examination revealed classic joint deformities of rheumatoid arthritis and subcutaneous rheumatoid nodules. Serum latex fixation test for rheumatoid factor was positive in a titer of 1:1280; antinuclear antibody was absent. The patient was continued on his prior therapeutic program of aspirin, 960 mg QID, hydroxychloroquine, 200 mg daily, and prednisone, 2.5 mg TID. Symptoms improved only slightly and Myochrysine therapy was substituted for hydroxychloroquine. In March, 1971, the patient complained of sticking pains in the left lower chest unassociated with cough, expectoration of sputum, or hemoptysis. Chest x-ray revealed a left pleural effusion and the patient was admitted for study. Repeat chest x-ray after aspiration of pleural fluid showed no parenchymal lung disease. Pleural fluid cell count, differential and protein studies were consistent with a mild exudate. Blood sugar and pleural fluid sugar determinations done simultaneously with the patient in a fasting state were 96 mg% and 16 mg% respectively. Serum CH^{50} complement was 90 units; pleural fluid complement was 42 units. Pleural fluid cultures for tuberculosis and fungi were negative, and cytologic examination revealed no abnormalities. Intermediate PPD, histoplasmin and coccidioidin skin tests were negative. Pulmonary consultation was requested.

Clinical findings were considered consistent with a diagnosis of rheumatoid pleural effusion and further studies such as pleural biopsy were deemed unnecessary. The patient's medical regimen was continued unchanged and he was discharged to be followed with periodic chest x-rays and clinical observation. Periodic followup chest roentgenograms showed no recurrence of pleural effusion nor other pulmonary abnormalities. Joint symptoms slowly improved.

Discussion: The development of pleural effusion in a patient with rheumatoid arthritis requires exclusion of other causes such as tuberculous or fungal infection or neoplasm. The presence of a reduced pleural fluid glucose, characteristically seen in rheumatoid pleural effusion, was strong evidence that the pulmonary symptoms in this patient were related to his basic rheumatologic disorder. A fall in pleural fluid complement levels has been reported in pleural effusion secondary to rheumatoid arthritis or systemic lupus erythematosus. No special management other than aspiration of the pleural fluid and maintenance of his primary treatment program for rheumatoid arthritis was necessary in this patient. Pulmonary manifestations of rheumatoid arthritis are not uncommon, particularly in patients with high serum rheumatoid factor and subcutaneous nodules, both of which were noted in this patient.

History 12-2. Necrotizing Vasculitis with Vasculitic Pneumonitis

J.B., a 60-year-old white male, was first seen in April, 1972, when he was referred to hospital for evaluation of fever and arthritis. The patient gave a history of rheumatoid arthritis of five years' duration for which he had been treated with aspirin, 960 mg QID, and prednisone, 5 mg BID. Ten days prior to admission he noted increased stiffness in his joints, high fever and shaking chills. Physical examination in hospital revealed multiple rheumatoid arthritis deformities with active synovitis. Numerous small purpuric lesions were diffusely scattered over both lower extremities. Neurologic examination showed decreased sensory response to pinprick in the distal aspects of both lower extremities. Initial diagnostic considerations included acute exacerbation of rheumatoid arthritis, pyogenic or granulomatous infection, and vasculitis.

Hematocrit was 48%, white blood cell count was 16,500/mm³ with a normal differential, and blood urea nitrogen was 27 mg%. Erythrocyte sedimentation rate was 42 mm/hour (Wintrobe). Urinalysis demonstrated trace albumin and occasional white cells, red cells and hyaline casts. Serum rheumatoid factor was positive in a titer of 1:1280. Serum study for antinuclear antibody was negative. No LE cells were seen. Creatinine clearance was 89 ml/min. Cultures of the pharynx, blood and urine were negative. Chest x-ray was within normal limits.

On the third day of hospitalization, the patient developed sudden onset of numbness and weakness of dorsiflexion of the right foot. Peripheral pulses were normal. Biopsy of the right gastrocnemius muscle was performed the following morning. Histopathologic examination revealed diffuse inflammatory infiltrates of lymphocytes and polymorphonuclear cells throughout all coats of numerous small and medium-sized arteries. Fibrinoid necrosis of some vessel walls was evident. Prednisone was increased to 15 mg QID with excellent response of clinical symptoms over a period of 48 hours. Intermittent high fever receded and the patient had notable improvement in muscle aching. The right foot-drop improved over a period of several weeks, during which good position was maintained with physical therapy exercises and a foot-drop splint. The patient was discharged on prednisone, 15 mg BID, one month after admission. Isoniazid, 300 mg daily and pyridoxine, 50 mg daily, were added while awaiting culture results. Symptoms of vasculitis and rheumatoid arthritis were in good control.

The patient was readmitted to hospital ten days after discharge for evaluation of acute right sided chest pain and fever. He gave no history of cough, dyspnea or hemoptysis. His therapeutic program had not been altered. Physical examination revealed dry rales at the right lung base. Chest x-ray showed patchy infiltrates in the right first and second interspace. Chest films taken at intervals of one to two days revealed enlargement and consolidation of the right lung lesions; infiltrates were seen in the left lower lobe as well. Pertinent laboratory studies revealed negative blood cultures, normal throat culture, and absence of acid-fast and fungus organisms on examination of sputum smears. Serum cold agglutination study was positive in a titer of 1:128. Pulmonary consultation was requested.

Differential diagnosis lay chiefly between rapidly progressive necrotizing vasculitis of the lungs versus pneumonia due to a pyogenic organism. Pulmonary mycosis, tuberculosis, atypical pneumonia or Pneumocystis carinii infection seemed less likely causes of the pulmonary findings. Repeat sputum culture showed small numbers of gram-positive diplococci. Intravenous oxacillin and gentamicin were added to his therapeutic program. Despite several days of high dose antibiotic therapy, the lung lesions progressed rapidly. Prednisone was increased to 20 mg QID, and tetracycline, 2 gm daily, was added. The patient had an excellent response to this program over 48 hours. Antibiotic therapy was discontinued after several days, and prednisone therapy alone was maintained. Progressive clinical improvement was associated with clearing of pulmonary infiltrates on x-ray. The patient was discharged on a program of gradually decreasing doses of prednisone. He did well over a two-year period of observation, but required a maintenance dose of prednisone, 5 mg BID, to control vasculitis symptoms.

Discussion: This patient with biopsy evidence of necrotizing vasculitis developed a severe progressive pneumonitis. Numerous diagnostic possibilities had to be considered and excluded. The clinical course and response to steroid therapy were consistent with pulmonary lesions due to necrotizing vasculitis.

History 12-3. Hypertrophic Osteoarthropathy

J.H., a 56-year-old white male, was first seen for evaluation in December, 1972. He had been in good health until two months prior when he developed pain and swelling of both knees and wrists. Swelling and disability were relieved only slightly by aspirin, 640 mg QID. The patient had no other complaints except for a seven-pound weight loss over the preceding two months. System review was completely negative and past medical history was noncontributory. On physical examination both knees and wrists were tender, warm and swollen. In addition, moderate clubbing of the fingers and toes was present.

Hematocrit was 35%, white blood cell count was 7200/mm³ with a normal differential, urinalysis was normal, and erythrocyte sedimentation rate was 38 mm/hour (Wintrobe). Serum rheumatoid factor and antinuclear antibody tests were negative. Chest x-ray revealed a mass lesion in the right middle lobe. Tuberculin and fungus skin tests were negative. Cytologic examination of induced sputum samples was normal. Roentgenograms of the wrists and knees revealed periosteal new bone formation at the distal aspects of the radial and femoral bones. A clinical diagnosis of bronchogenic carcinoma with pulmonary hypertrophic osteoarthropathy was made.

Exploratory thoracotomy was performed. Pathologic studies revealed bronchogenic carcinoma and a right pneumonectomy was performed. The patient had mild remission of musculoskeletal symptoms postoperatively. Residual joint symptoms were controlled with aspirin, 640 mg QID, and indomethacin, 25 mg TID. The patient returned to his referring physician for followup.

Discussion: This patient appeared with arthritis consistent with that seen in many of the connective tissue diseases. The presence of clubbing suggested a clinical diagnosis of hypertrophic osteoarthropathy. Roentgenographic studies of involved joints revealed abnormalities characteristic of this syndrome. Variable degrees of symptomatic remissions may be seen following tumor resection.

REFERENCES

1. Walker, W. C. and Wright, V.: Pulmonary lesions and rheumatoid arthritis. Medicine 47:501, 1968.
2. Lillington, G. A., Carr, D. T. and Mayne, J. G.: Rheumatoid pleurisy with effusion. Arch Int Med 128:764, 1971.
3. Carr, D. T. and Mayne, J. G.: Pleurisy with effusion in rheumatoid arthritis, with reference to the low concentration of glucose in pleural fluid. Am Rev Resp Dis 85:345, 1962.
4. Hunder, G. G., McDuffie, F. C. and Hepper, N. G. G.: Pleural fluid complement in systemic lupus erythematosus and rheumatoid arthritis. Ann Int Med 76:357, 1972.
5. Eisenberg, H. et al.: Diffuse interstitial lung disease in systemic lupus erythematosus. Ann Int Med 79:37, 1973.
6. Israel, H. L. and Patchefsky, A. S.: Wegener's granulomatosis of lungs: diagnosis and treatment. Ann Int Med 74:881, 1971.
7. Kaplan, H.: Further experience with colchicine in the treatment of sarcoid arthritis. N Eng J Med 268:761, 1963.

Chapter 13

VASCULAR ABNORMALITIES AND CONNECTIVE TISSUE DISEASE

Vascular symptoms may be the initial complaint in patients with systemic connective tissue disease. In some patients, the vascular manifestations precede articular symptoms by several or many years. In others, the vascular changes occur concomitant with or subsequent to articular symptoms. An awareness of the important inter-relationship of vascular changes and connective tissue disease is helpful in diagnosis.

RAYNAUD'S PHENOMENON AND RAYNAUD'S DISEASE

Clinical Features

Although several vascular diseases are associated with systemic connective tissue disorders, the most common abnormality is *Raynaud's phenomenon.*[1] This entity is characterized by color changes in the skin that occur either spontaneously or in response to certain precipitating factors such as cold. Color changes occur most frequently in the hands, but the toes, nose and ears may sometimes be involved. In the typical sequence, the skin first becomes white because of arteriolar spasm and subsequent diminished blood supply. Cyanosis follows, caused by stagnation of blood in capillaries and venules. As warming and reactive vasodilation ensue, the skin becomes red. Thus, the classic color sequence is white to blue to red. In many patients, this sequence is not present, and various combinations of color change are seen. Tingling and paresthesia are common accompanying symptoms and may occur in the absence of definitive color changes. Severe recurrent Raynaud's phenomenon may produce chronic vasomotor instability with a persistent blue mottling of the skin on which the typical color changes are intermittently superimposed. Among the connective tissue diseases, Raynaud's phenomenon occurs most frequently in patients with systemic lupus erythematosus, and scleroderma. Rheumatoid arthritis, dermatomyositis and necrotizing vasculitis are less common causes.

188

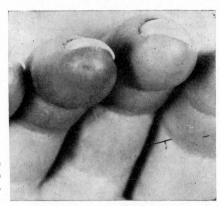

Figure 13-1. Cyanosis and trophic ulceration
of the fingertip in a patient with
long-standing Raynaud's disease.
(Courtesy, Dr. A. Mackenzie)

Raynaud's phenomenon should be differentiated from *Raynaud's disease.* The latter is an idiopathic primary disorder with color changes identical to those seen in patients with Raynaud's phenomenon; however, evidence of an underlying disorder is persistently absent. Over a period of time, vascular insufficiency may produce trophic changes such as ulceration of the fingertips (Fig. 13-1). A diagnosis of Raynaud's disease should be made with caution when symptoms are recent in onset, because secondary Raynaud's phenomenon may be present for long periods of time prior to the appearance of other symptoms of connective tissue disease. The presence of Raynaud's changes for over two years in the absence of any underlying disorder supports a diagnosis of idiopathic Raynaud's disease. Unfortunately, some patients manifest Raynaud's changes for years before connective tissue disease becomes apparent. Constant reappraisal of the significance of the patient's vascular symptoms is usually indicated.

Differential Diagnosis

Besides occurring in association with connective tissue diseases, Raynaud's phenomenon may occur secondary to other disorders. The following are non-connective tissue diseases that must be considered as possible underlying disorders in the differential diagnosis of Raynaud's phenomenon.

Patients with *disorders of the cervical spine, such as cervical disk herniation or thoracic outlet compression syndromes,* may develop Raynaud's phenomenon secondary to vascular instability induced in the involved extremity. *Carpal tunnel compression* may produce similar vascular abnormalities.

Patients may develop Raynaud's phenomenon as a result of *chronic trauma,* as occurs in pneumatic hammer workers or in industrial occupations that require repetitive pounding motions of the hands. Raynaud's phenomenon is associated with diseases of large vessels, such as *atheroscle-*

rosis obliterans and *Buerger's disease* (*thromboangiitis obliterans*). Peripheral pulses are usually diminished.

Raynaud's phenomenon is seen in patients with various *hematologic disorders* such as polycythemia vera. Patients with multiple myeloma, hypergammaglobulinemia of Waldenström, lymphoma, chronic leukemia or idiopathic cryoglobulinemia may have Raynaud's phenomenon. The vascular changes may result from the presence of blood cryoglobulins, cryofibrinogens or cold agglutinins or from hyperviscosity changes.

Intoxication with heavy metals, such as arsenic, or poisoning with ergot derivatives may produce Raynaud's phenomenon. A careful history and studies for suspected toxic agents are essential in diagnosis.

Laboratory Diagnosis

A full laboratory evaluation should include a complete blood count, erythrocyte sedimentation rate, serologic test for syphilis (for false-positive serology), serum studies for rheumatoid and antinuclear factors, serum cold agglutinins and cryoglobulins, plasma cryofibrinogen, and serum protein electrophoresis. Chest x-rays may demonstrate an associated underlying disorder. Cervical spine roentgenograms including PA, lateral and oblique views are helpful in excluding etiologic factors emanating from this area. Barium swallow often demonstrates abnormal function in patients with scleroderma. This finding is not diagnostic, however, because similar dysfunction may be noted in patients with idiopathic Raynaud's disease. Other laboratory studies, such as serum immunoelectrophoresis, serum complement, blood lipids and sugar, are indicated when suggested by clinical findings. Special diagnostic procedures such as bone marrow aspiration, muscle or lymph node biopsy, and arteriography may be required.

Management

Raynaud's disease and Raynaud's phenomenon often respond to various symptomatic measures. Patients should be cautioned to avoid exposure to cold. Light cotton gloves are useful for this purpose and should be worn during routine household activities. Warm outer clothing should be utilized as well, because symptoms result from cold exposure to the body in general. Patients with severe symptoms may benefit from a move to a warm climate. Various vasodilator agents are valuable in the nonspecific symptomatic approach to therapy. Phenoxybenzamine hydrochloride (Dibenzyline), an adrenergic blocking agent, may be tried in an initial dose of 10 mg twice daily. The dose is slowly increased to 10 mg four times a day, if tolerated and required. The patient should be cautioned regarding sudden postural changes because orthostatic hypotension is a bothersome side reaction. Reserpine may have a salutary effect in a dose of 0.25 to 0.5 mg daily by mouth. Intra-arterial administration of reserpine has been utilized,[2,3] but its efficacy is uncertain.[4] This drug should generally be avoided in patients with a history of depression; other agents may be effective alternatives. In particular, methyldopa, 250 mg three or four times daily, or guanethidine, 10 to 40 mg daily, are worthy of trial. Nitroglycerine ointment, 2%, is helpful in some patients. The ointment is spread on the hands in a dose beginning with one to two inches of the agent. (This dose can be measured with the applicator provided with the preparation.) It is used three or four times daily in gradually increasing amounts. The patient should be cautioned about nitroglycerine-induced headaches, which may occur early in use; headaches usually disappear as the drug is continued.

Sympathectomy should be considered in patients with severe disease who do not respond to a conservative medical regimen. This procedure is usually more effective in patients with Raynaud's disease than in those with Raynaud's phenomenon, in whom an underlying disorder is present. Prior improvement with stellate ganglion block should be demonstrated before sympathectomy is considered.

Specific therapy directed to the associated disorder often has a beneficial effect on the vascular symptoms of patients with Raynaud's phenomenon. Corticosteroids are particularly effective in patients with associated connective tissue disease; their use should be reserved, however, for severe cases not controlled by more conservative measures. Management of Raynaud's phenomenon secondary to non-connective tissue diseases should be directed to the underlying medical problem in addition to symptomatic measures.

OTHER SMALL VESSEL DISEASE

Other vascular abnormalities may be associated with connective tissue disease. *Livedo reticularis* is characterized by a peculiar mottled appear-

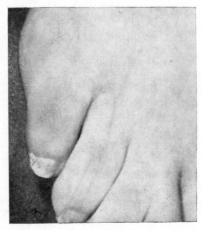

Figure 13-2. Livedo reticularis. Note mottled appearance of skin. (Courtesy, Dr. B. Michel)

ance of the skin (Fig. 13-2). The condition is usually benign and produces few or no symptoms. *Acrocyanosis* is manifested as a persistently cool extremity with bluish discoloration. Mild ulceration is a complicating finding in severe disease. *Erythermalgia* is an interesting and distressing disorder characterized by red, hot extremities that are extremely painful. The condition may be idiopathic or secondary in etiology. Symptoms are often relieved by elevating the extremities or by immersing them in cold water. Aspirin is frequently beneficial.

THROMBOPHLEBITIS

Thrombophlebitis occurs more frequently in patients with connective tissue diseases, particularly in systemic lupus erythematosus. Sometimes phlebitis is the initial manifestation of the underlying disease. Both superficial and deep phlebitis occur and attacks may be isolated single occurrences or recurrent. Thrombophlebitis occurs more frequently with long-term corticosteroid therapy, possibly related to changes in mechanisms of coagulation. Management of the thrombophlebitis associated with connective tissue disease is similar to that for idiopathic thrombophlebitis and includes rest, heat and the use of anticoagulants. Unfortunately, both the acute attack and prevention of recurrences may be more recalcitrant to therapy than phlebitis related to other causes. Vena caval ligation or insertion of a vena caval umbrella may be indicated in recurrent cases associated with pulmonary emboli not controlled by long-term anticoagulant therapy. Control of the underlying disorder may be beneficial but is not always effective. The use of anticoagulant therapy in patients with connective tissue disease is complicated by the frequent associated use of anti-inflammatory agents that augment the anticoagulant effect or predispose to gastrointestinal bleeding.

SYSTEMIC VASCULITIS

Patients with systemic connective tissue disease may have ischemic changes due to vasculitis of small or large vessels.[5,6] Such lesions are characteristic of periarteritis nodosa and the various forms of allergic angiitis. Similar lesions may be a complication in patients with systemic lupus erythematosus and rheumatoid arthritis, with or without a history of steroid therapy. Symptoms and signs are variable and depend on the size and location of the involved vessel. Involvement of large vessels of the extremities results in severe rest pain and claudication and a cool, cyanotic skin. Small vessel involvement produces focal areas of skin infarction with lesions strikingly similar in appearance to those seen in subacute bacterial endocarditis. Splinter hemorrhages beneath the nails and paronychial infarctions are common (Fig. 10-9). Involvement of vasa nervosum may result in

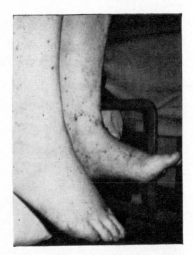

Figure 13-3. Right foot-drop due to necrotizing vasculitis with ischemic neuropathy. Purpuric lesions of the skin are readily apparent.

ischemic neuropathy. Mononeuritis multiplex is particularly characteristic. In this syndrome, scattered large nerves such as the peroneal, radial and median nerves are involved. Onset of symptoms is often sudden with the patient complaining of foot-drop (Fig. 13-3) or wrist-drop.

Steroid therapy is presently the most effective agent available for management. Dosage required to control the inflammatory changes is often large; doses of prednisone as high as 80 to 120 mg per day in divided doses are not unusual. Some patients with vasculitis associated with systemic lupus erythematosus or rheumatoid arthritis benefit from the use of antimalarial drugs in addition to steroids. Hydroxychloroquine (Plaquenil) is given in a dose of 200 mg BID for three or four months, following which a daily maintenance dose of 200 mg daily is instituted. Appropriate periodic eye examinations should be carried out to avoid ophthalmic side reactions. Immunosuppressive agents may benefit certain patients with vasculitis not responding to the usual therapeutic program.[7] D-penicillamine has been described as useful in the treatment of vasculitis associated with rheumatoid arthritis.[8,9] These methods of treatment are still *investigational* but should be considered in progressive life-threatening disease.

TEMPORAL ARTERITIS (CRANIAL ARTERITIS, GIANT CELL ARTERITIS)

Temporal arteritis is characterized by granulomatous inflammation of vessels associated with systemic constitutional symptoms and ischemic vascular changes.[10] The disease occurs most frequently in persons over 50 years of age. Although temporal arteries are involved most frequently, the process may affect other large arteries, such as the carotid, subclavian, femoral, coronary, renal and mesenteric vessels. Onset of symptoms may

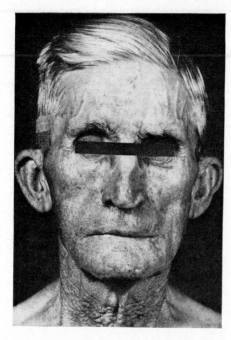

Figure 13-4. Temporal (cranial) arteritis. Note thickened enlarged vessels bilaterally, best seen over the lateral aspects of the forehead. (Courtesy, Dr. A. Mackenzie)

be acute or insidious. Throbbing headaches are associated with tenderness and swelling of the temporal arteries. The vessels are nodular to palpation (Fig. 13-4) and the overlying skin is erythematous. Pulsations may disappear as the disease progresses. Malaise, anorexia, fever and weight loss are frequent findings. Symptoms of polymyalgia rheumatica (see Chapter 9) occur in a high percentage of patients. Muscle pain involving the shoulders, hips and trunk may be severe. Limitation of function is due to pain rather than weakness. Ischemic changes may lead to claudication in the jaws and extremities. Involvement of vessels to the eye results in symptoms of transient diplopia or loss of vision, which may be irreversible.

Laboratory findings reveal mild anemia and leukocytosis. The erythrocyte sedimentation rate is characteristically elevated, often exceeding 80 to 100 mm/hour. Serum alpha-2 globulin is frequently elevated. Temporal artery biopsy is the most important diagnostic procedure. Pathologic findings include intimal proliferation with narrowing of the lumen. Thrombosis is often present and the internal elastic lamina is disrupted. Inflammatory infiltrates with lymphocytes and foreign-body giant cells are seen (Fig. 13-5). Temporal arteriography performed prior to biopsy may provide diagnostic information and help in selecting the optimal site for biopsy.[11] A positive study reveals stenotic and dilated segments of the vessel.

Although temporal arteritis is a self-limited disease, early diagnosis is important because the risk of blindness is significant. Steroid treatment is

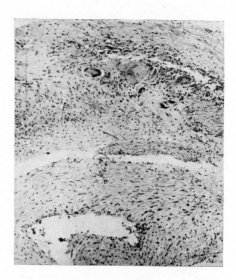

Figure 13-5. Cross-section of temporal artery from patient with temporal (cranial) arteritis. Intimal proliferation is associated with inflammatory infiltrates of lymphocytes and foreign-body giant cells in the vessel wall. (Hematoxylin, and eosin) (Courtesy, Dr. A. Mackenzie)

effective in preventing blindness and in suppressing local and systemic symptoms (see Chapter 18).

TAKAYASU'S DISEASE (AORTIC ARCH ARTERITIS, PULSELESS DISEASE)

This syndrome is characterized by vasculitis of large elastic arteries. In contrast to temporal arteritis, it is primarily a disease of young females. Pulses are absent in the neck, head and upper extremities. Blood pressure in the arms is usually unobtainable. Claudication of the upper extremities is common. Many patients have systemic symptoms such as malaise, fever, anorexia and weight loss. In some patients these systemic manifestations antedate objective changes in the pulses (prepulseless phase). Ischemic manifestations elsewhere lead to cerebrovascular insufficiency, jaw claudication, angina and myocardial infarction.

Laboratory studies reveal an elevated erythrocyte sedimentation rate during acute phases of the disease. Mild anemia and leukocytosis are common. Angiograms show irregular segmental stenosis localized to large arteries near their origin. Corticosteroid therapy is frequently beneficial. Surgery to correct chronic vascular occlusion may be indicated.

CASE HISTORIES

History 13-1. Idiopathic Raynaud's Disease

R.S., a 50-year-old white female, was first seen for rheumatologic evaluation in December, 1970. She gave a history of color changes in the hands beginning approximately 15 years prior. Fingers of both hands became white or blue with mild exposure to cold temperatures. Erythema of the fingers developed with rewarming. Color changes were associated with some itching and paresthesia of involved areas. She gave no history of joint symptoms nor any history of frostbite or injury to the hands. There were no ancillary symptoms of hair loss, pleurisy, skin rash, drug allergy, sun sensitivity, dry mouth or dry eyes, alopecia or dysphagia. The patient had been in otherwise generally good health and no chronic intake of medications was noted. On physical examination, blood pressure was 110/70 mm Hg. The skin of the hands and feet was cold and had a mottled red appearance. Exposure of the hands to cold running water induced pallor. No thickening of the skin of the hands or feet was seen. Peripheral pulses and joints were normal. Cervical spine motions were full and nonpainful. Thoracic outlet maneuvers were negative.

Urinalysis, hematocrit, white blood cell count and differential, erythrocyte sedimentation rate and serologic test for syphilis were normal or negative. Serum protein electrophoresis was normal, as were serum protein-bound iodine, calcium and phosphorus studies. Serum uric acid was 4.6 mg/100 ml and serum studies for rheumatoid factor, antinuclear antibody, cryoglobulins and cold agglutinins were negative. No cryofibrinogens were seen. Roentgenograms of the chest and hands were unremarkable. A diagnosis of idiopathic Raynaud's disease was made on the basis of the long history of color changes in the absence of any secondary disorder. The patient was placed on therapy with reserpine, 0.5 mg daily at night, with moderately good relief of symptoms. In addition, she was instructed to keep her hands and body warm. The patient has shown no subsequent evidence of underlying systemic disease on repeated clinical and laboratory study.

Discussion: This patient demonstrated characteristic color changes of Raynaud's disease. Repeated clinical examination and laboratory studies failed to reveal the presence of any systemic disorder. Prolonged observation is often required before a diagnosis of idiopathic Raynaud's disease can be made with assurance, because Raynaud's phenomenon may precede other clinical manifestations of associated diseases by months or years. Prognosis in this patient was good and she could be reassured regarding the relatively benign nature of her disorder.

History 13-2. Raynaud's Phenomenon Secondary to Systemic Lupus Erythematosus

F.R., a 68-year-old white female, was seen in consultation in January, 1974. The patient was in good health until four weeks previously, when she noted sudden discoloration of the fingertips with associated numbness of the hands. Discoloration was characterized by a persistent cyanosis at the distal aspects of the second and third fingers of the right hand and the second finger of the left hand. Symptoms were aggravated by exposure to cold, at which time the involved digits would become white. There were no other notable symptoms and the patient considered herself in good health otherwise. The patient was taking no medications. System review revealed no evidence of arthritis, myalgia, pleurisy, sun sensitivity, hair loss, dryness of the eyes or mouth, drug allergy or skin rash. Past medical history was noncontributory.

Hematocrit was 36%, white blood cell count was 3600/mm^3 with a normal differential, and urinalysis was normal. Routine serologic test for syphilis was weakly positive; FTA-Abs study was negative. Serum rheumatoid factor study was negative, but serum antinuclear antibody was present in a titer of 1:1000. LE cell determinations were consistently positive. Prothrombin time was normal but partial thromboplastin time was prolonged. Reticulocyte count was 1.1% and Coombs test was negative. Creatinine clearance was 83 ml/min. Total serum hemolytic complement was 60% of normal. A diagnosis of systemic lupus erythematosus was made. The patient was placed on prednisone, 10 mg BID, with moderately good relief of vascular symptoms.

Discussion: Raynaud's phenomenon was the initial clinical manifestation of systemic lupus erythematosus in this patient. Multiple laboratory abnormalities related to systemic lupus erythematosus were present. Subsequent studies revealed the presence of circulating anticoagulant as an explanation for her prolonged partial thromboplastin time. Vascular symptoms are a frequent manifestation of systemic lupus erythematosus, as this case well illustrates.

History 13-3. Raynaud's Phenomenon Secondary to Scleroderma

M.R., a 47-year-old white female, was first seen in consultation in January, 1972. She was in good health until March, 1969, at which time she noted color changes in both hands on exposure to cold. Pallor and whitening of the hands was followed by blue discoloration. Color changes involved several fingers of each hand and were associated with numbness and tingling. The patient did not seek medical help for this complaint until approximately six months later when she noted progressive tightening of the skin of her hands and forearms with limitation in finger range-of-motion. The skin of the hands had become darker and she noted a grating sensation when she flexed her right middle finger. System review was negative for symptoms of dysphagia, hair loss, sun sensitivity, drug allergy, pleurisy or dryness of the mouth or eyes.

Physical examination revealed blood pressure 130/80 mm Hg. The skin over both hands and forearms was erythematous and blanched slightly on pressure. Moderate thickening of the skin of the hands and forearms, and resorption of the tips of several fingers were noted. Telangiectases were absent.

Hematocrit was 39%, the white blood cell count was 6300/mm^3 with a normal differential, the erythrocyte sedimentation rate was 12 mm/hour (Wintrobe) and urinalysis was normal. Serum rheumatoid factor test was negative. Serum antinuclear antibody titer was positive 1:20. Roentgenograms of the chest showed interstitial fibrosis at the bases of both lungs. Pulmonary function studies were normal. Barium swallow and roentgenograms of the upper gastrointestinal tract were unremarkable. X-rays of the hands revealed resorption of several ungual tufts. Electrocardiogram was normal. Histopathologic study of skin obtained by punch biopsy from the dorsal aspect of the left distal forearm revealed thinning of the epidermis, loss of rete pegs and atrophy of dorsal appendages. A diagnosis of scleroderma was made on the basis of the clinical and pathologic findings.

The patient was placed on reserpine, 0.5 mg daily, for treatment of her Raynaud's phenomenon. In addition, she was advised to avoid cold exposure, to use gloves and to dress warmly. Improvement in the Raynaud's phenomenon was noted over a period of several weeks. She was also placed on potassium para-aminobenzoate (Potaba) in progressively increasing doses to 12 gm daily. Therapy was associated with softening of involved areas of skin over a period of six months. The dose of potassium para-aminobenzoate was slowly reduced and discontinued over the subsequent two years. No change in the pulmonary interstitial fibrosis was noted. The patient was maintained on no specific therapy except for reserpine, which she used during the winter to control the Raynaud's symptoms. There was no clinical or laboratory evidence of further progression of her disease.

Discussion: Raynaud's phenomenon was the initial clinical manifestation of scleroderma in this patient. Underlying associated disease states must always be excluded when patients appear initially with Raynaud's phenomenon. Clinical and laboratory evidence of the primary disorder is often absent for a long period of time.

REFERENCES

1. DeTakats, G. and Fowler, E. F.: Raynaud's phenomenon. JAMA 179:108, 1962.
2. McFayden, I. S., Housley, E. and MacPherson, A. I. S.: Intra-arterial reserpine administration in Raynaud syndrome. Arch Int Med 132:526, 1973.
3. Paolino, J. et al.: Arteriographic evaluation of intra-arterial reserpine in Raynaud's phenomenon. Arth Rheum 15:448, 1972.
4. Siegel, R. C. and Fries, J. F.: Double-blind cross-over study of intra-arterial reserpine and saline in scleroderma. Arth Rheum 15:454, 1972.
5. DePalma, R. G., Moskowitz, R. W. and Holden, W. D.: Peripheral ischemia and collagen disease. Arch Surg 105:313, 1972.
6. Bywaters, E. G. L. and Scott, J. T.: The natural history of vascular lesions in rheumatoid arthritis. J Chron Dis 16:905, 1963.
7. Mitchell, M. S. Malawista, S. E. and Bertine, J. R.: Successful therapy of disseminated vasculitis by methotrexate despite severe renal impairment. Arth Rheum 14:175, 1971.
8. Jaffe, I. A.: Rheumatoid arthritis with arteritis: Report of a case treated with penicillamine. Ann Int Med 61:556, 1964.
9. _____: The treatment of rheumatoid arthritis and necrotizing vasculitis with penicillamine. Arth Rheum 13:436, 1970.
10. Healey, L. A., Parker, F. and Wilske, K. R.: Polymyalgia rheumatica and giant cell arteritis. Arth Rheum 14:138, 1971.
11. Gillanders, L. A., Strachan, R. W. and Blair, D. W.: Temporal arteriography: a new technique for the investigation of giant cell arteritis and polymyalgia rheumatica. Ann Rheum Dis 28:267, 1969.

Chapter 14

LOCALIZED MUSCULOSKELETAL SYNDROMES

Localized musculoskeletal symptoms may be a manifestation of relatively circumscribed disorders or systemic disease. Accurate delineation of the problem is required for most effective therapy. When due to benign disease, the patient's anxiety regarding the presence of a more generalized disorder can be appropriately allayed. In other cases, the symptoms serve as a clue to the diagnosis of a more serious illness.

BURSITIS

Bursae are closed sacs lined with synovial-like cells. Interposed between bony prominences and tendons or muscles, they facilitate motion. Numerous bursae are present throughout the body and may be the site of localized inflammation, frequently associated with amorphous deposits of calcium. Among the bursae most commonly affected are the subdeltoid and subacromial bursae at the shoulder, the olecranon bursa at the elbow, the greater trochanteric bursa at the lateral aspect of the hip and the anserine bursa at the medial aspect of the upper tibia. Other bursae frequently involved are those related to the Achilles tendon, the ischial tuberosity, the first metatarsophalangeal joint and the prepatellar area.

Patients with shoulder bursitis usually give a history of acute pain and limitation of motion. The shoulder is tender to palpation; pain with passive motion may be excruciating. Although roentgenographic study often reveals evidence of calcification (Fig. 14-1), such deposits are frequently absent. Many cases of shoulder bursitis are associated with a concomitant inflammation of the tendon of the supraspinatus muscle. Bursitis of the shoulder may represent a secondary reaction to tendinitis, when tendinous deposits of calcium rupture into underlying bursae. Symptoms specifically related to shoulder bursitis must be differentiated from inflammation of shoulder area tendons and from tears of the musculotendinous rotator cuff (see following).

Olecranon bursitis produces swelling, pain, heat and redness at the posterior aspect of the elbow. Although most frequently a manifestation of

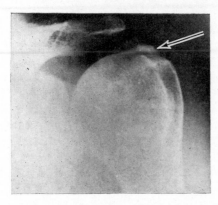

Figure 14-1. Roentgenogram of the shoulder from a patient with recurrent attacks of acute bursitis shows a large calcific deposit (arrow). (Courtesy, Dr. V. Goldberg)

chronic nonspecific trauma, it is also seen in association with connective tissue diseases or gout. Patients with greater trochanteric bursitis complain of pain and tenderness at the lateral aspect of the hip; pain is exaggerated by weight-bearing. Hip motion is usually normal, which helps to differentiate this entity from intrinsic disorders of the hip joint. Ischial bursitis involves the bursa between the gluteus maximus muscle and ischial tuberosity. Patients with inflammation of the anserine bursa have pain at the medial aspect of the knee, with localized tenderness readily demonstrable at the upper end of the medial tibial plateau. Prepatellar bursitis causes pain and swelling at the anterior aspect of the knee. Chronic trauma associated with occupations that require frequent kneeling is an important etiologic factor in many cases. Achilles bursitis involves the bursa at the lower end of the attachment of the Achilles tendon to the os calcis. Nonspecific cases are often caused by excessively tight shoes. In other cases, symptoms are related to systemic connective tissue diseases such as rheumatoid arthritis and ankylosing spondylitis. Painful bursitis may be seen overlying the first metatarsophalangeal joint at its medial aspect; tight shoes or hallux valgus are often predisposing factors.

Treatment of bursitis varies with the location of the disorder. Mild cases of shoulder bursitis may be managed with heat and mild anti-inflammatory agents such as aspirin or indomethacin. Local injections of various corticosteroid preparations with 1% lidocaine (see Chapter 20) are extremely efficacious and usually provide rapid relief. Physical therapy should be vigorously instituted when diminished pain allows increased joint use. Exercises of several types are utilized: pendulum exercises, for which the patient leans forward and gently rotates the arm in a circle, are helpful. Range of motion may be further aided by stringing a rope over a door or a shower bar; the patient grasps the ends of the rope and uses the good extremity to assist range of motion of the involved extremity. Another valuable exercise involves grasping the hands together behind the neck and forcefully moving the elbows and shoulders posteriorly. Phenylbutazone often aids patients who do not respond to local steroid therapy. An initial dose of 100 mg QID for two or three days is followed by gradually diminishing doses over a period of four to seven days. Severe cases with large calcium deposits evident on x-ray may be aided by "needling" the deposit with an 18-gauge needle under local anesthesia. Lidocaine or saline is used to lavage the involved area, followed by injection of steroid with lidocaine. Some patients who do not respond to conservative measures benefit from a short course of x-ray therapy to the involved area. An exposure dose of 150 rads (ortho voltage) is given every other day for three doses. Large calcific deposits may be recalcitrant to all the foregoing measures and require surgical excision. Fortunately, the need for surgery is not frequent.

Mild cases of bursitis in other areas similarly respond to heat and mild anti-inflammatory agents. Response to local injections of steroid with lidocaine is usually excellent. Phenylbutazone therapy, as described for shoulder bursitis, is often an effective therapeutic alternative. Recurrent bursitis may require excision of the bursa for permanent relief.

TENDINITIS AND TENOSYNOVITIS (TENOVAGINITIS)

Inflammation with resultant pain and tenderness commonly involves tendons (tendinitis) or tendon sheaths (tenosynovitis, tenovaginitis) in the area of the shoulder, elbow, hands and heel. Supraspinatus tendinitis probably results from an abnormal response of the tendon to chronic trauma. Fibrillary changes of degeneration are seen histologically, and secondary calcification is common. Symptoms, differential diagnosis, and management are similar to those described for shoulder bursitis.

Tenosynovitis at the long head of the biceps muscle as the tendon passes through the bicipital groove of the humeral head is common. Pain and tenderness are severe at the anterior aspect of the shoulder. Maximal pain may be reproduced by forced supination of the hand with the elbow in 45° flexion, because the biceps muscle is the primary supinator of the hand in this position. Shoulder motion is often limited. Roentgenographic studies are usually normal. Symptoms respond to local injections of steroid with lidocaine or to oral phenylbutazone. Surgical excision of the tendon sheath may be indicated if symptoms are chronic.

The common term for inflammation near tendon origins at the elbow is tennis elbow. However, symptoms may be idiopathic in origin or related to chronic trauma induced by other activities or occupations that produce stress at the elbow. Symptoms occur at either the lateral or medial epicondyle. The extensor muscles to the hand originate at the lateral epicondyle and this area is involved more frequently. Symptoms at the medial epicondyle are caused by involvement of flexor muscle tendons. Roentgenograms may reveal small calcific deposits in symptomatic areas. Management depends on the severity of the symptoms. Mild cases respond to heat, aspirin and the avoidance of activities that cause stress to the involved tendons. Other cases require local injections of steroid with lidocaine into the tender areas of the epicondyle. Injections should generally not be repeated more than every three to six months to avoid chronic damage and atrophy of tissue. Some patients benefit from splinting, which puts the elbow at rest. Other therapeutic approaches include periodic courses of phenylbutazone, or x-ray therapy. Recalcitrant cases may require surgery such as fasciotomy.

Tenosynovitis of the abductor pollicis longus and extensor pollicis brevis tendons at the wrist is common (DeQuervain's tenosynovitis). In most patients this disorder is primary and related to chronic nonspecific trauma. However, it may be associated with systemic connective tissue disease. The patient complains of pain with use of the thumb or wrist. Physical examination reveals severe tenderness and occasionally signs of inflammation over the tendon. Tenderness is usually maximal in the "snuff-box" area between the tendons of the abductor pollicis longus and extensor pollicis brevis muscles. Maximal pain is induced by forced ulnar deviation after the thumb has been placed in the palm of the hand and grasped by the fingers (Finkelstein's sign) (Fig. 14-2). Treatment with local injection of steroid and lidocaine usually results in satisfying relief. Activities that might have precipitated the tenosynovitis should be avoided. Chronic low-grade symptoms may require splinting for various periods of time.

Tendinitis or tenosynovitis of the hands occurs as a primary disorder resulting from chronic nonspecific trauma, or from inflammatory changes produced by the connective tissue diseases, particularly rheumatoid arthritis. Flexor tendons are affected most often. Involvement of the thumbs (snapping thumbs) is common. Examination reveals tenderness and a sensation of crepitus as the tendon moves. Swelling, which is often present, may be diffuse or localized in the form of a nodule. Locking, in which the patient

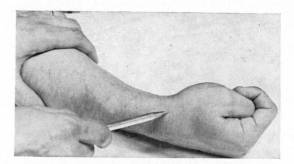

Figure 14-2. Finkelstein's sign. Acute pain and tenderness were localized to the "snuff-box" area when forced ulnar deviation was performed. Symptoms of tenosynovitis were relieved by local injection of steroid and lidocaine.

is able to flex the involved finger but unable to bring it back to its original position, occurs with chronic lesions. This symptom has given rise to the term "trigger finger." Locking results when the flexor muscles pull the tendon through the tendon sheath and the extensor muscles are unable to return the tendons to their original position. Patients often localize the locking to the finger area, but close observation usually reveals that the trouble site is at the distal palmar crease where the palmar fascia is tight and the tendon most subject to impingement.

Locking may occur if inflammation or fibrosis of the sheath causes stricture. In patients with rheumatoid arthritis, locking is related to diffuse rheumatoid inflammation of the sheath, of the tendon or both. In addition, rheumatoid patients may have locking when rheumatoid nodule formation on the sheath or tendon restricts tendon motion.

Most patients with tenosynovitis in the hand respond to local injections of steroid with lidocaine into the involved tendon sheath. Stressful activities should be avoided. In patients with chronic tenosynovitis, surgical release of the tendon sheath and removal of any nodules is indicated.

Inflammation of the Achilles tendon is common. Pathologic changes may result from chronic nonspecific trauma, such as that induced by tight shoes, or may be associated with various connective tissue diseases, especially rheumatoid arthritis, ankylosing spondylitis and Reiter's syndrome. Pain, especially with walking, and localized tenderness are present. Treatment includes removal of local traumatic factors, rest and anti-inflammatory agents. Phenylbutazone given over a period of four to five days is often efficacious. Local injections of steroid with lidocaine are also effective but should be used with caution because they predispose to tendon rupture. The injection should be made in a paratendinous location rather than the tendon or tendon sheath itself. The patient should be cautioned to avoid stressful activity for several days following injection.

ROTATOR CUFF TEAR OF THE SHOULDER

Tears of the musculotendinous rotator cuff of the shoulder most frequently involve the supraspinatus tendon. Partial rupture is more common than complete rupture. A history of injury is usually present; the patient may feel an actual snap, followed by pain and limitation of motion. Tenderness is noted over the greater tuberosity. Symptoms and physical findings may be difficult to differentiate from those of bursitis and tendinitis. Frequently the patient cannot initiate abduction. The tear may be demonstrated by contrast arthrography (Fig. 14-3). Complete rupture requires surgical management. Partial tears usually respond to conservative measures including heat, analgesics, and mild anti-inflammatory agents. A short course of phenylbutazone therapy is frequently effective. Local steroid therapy is

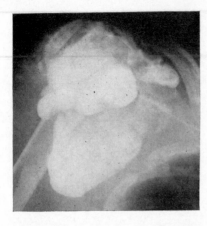

Figure 14-3. Contrast arthrogram of right shoulder in a patient with a rotator cuff tear reveals diffuse spread of dye beyond the normal confines of the shoulder.

beneficial in selected cases. Physical therapy exercises should be instituted early to maintain range of motion.

ADHESIVE CAPSULITIS OF THE SHOULDER (FROZEN SHOULDER)

Adhesive capsulitis may follow as a sequela of bursitis, tendinitis, or rotator cuff tear when therapy of the acute process has been inadequate or ineffective. Limitation of motion and occasionally pain are severe. Therapy with analgesic and anti-inflammatory agents is less effective at this stage of shoulder disease. Intensive physical therapy to promote increased range of motion is usually rewarding, although improvement may be slow. Surgical manipulation to release adhesions may be necessary in unresponsive cases.

MULTIPLE CALCIFIC PERIARTHRITIS

Acute episodes of tendinitis or bursitis are frequently associated with deposition of calcium apatite. In most patients, the lesions are localized to one or two joints such as the shoulders or epicondyles of the elbows. Some patients, however, demonstrate multiple areas of calcification of tendons, ligaments or bursae associated with recurrent attacks of acute periarthritis.[1,2] Clinical symptoms resemble acute attacks of gout or pseudogout. Structures in the areas of the shoulders, elbows and hips are commonly involved, but other areas such as the wrists and hands may be affected.

Pain and evidence of inflammation are most notable over the area of calcific deposit. Roentgenograms show mottled calcification in soft tissues at the site of the acute attacks. Aspiration of the affected area reveals a chalky, milky material. On study by phase microscopy, numerous round, globular bodies that have a shiny coin-like appearance are seen. Weakly birefringent particles may be present. Interestingly, the acute attack may be followed by disintegration and gradual disappearance of the calcium deposit.

Whether tendon degeneration precedes calcium deposition is uncertain. It has been suggested that deposition of calcium in these patients may be a primary event related to some systemic disorder. No abnormality in mineral or hormonal metabolism has yet been demonstrated. Treatment is symptomatic. Rapid improvement frequently follows oral administration of phenylbutazone, or administration of corticosteroids orally or by direct local injection. Splinting of involved areas helps to relieve pain.

A condition somewhat similar to the foregoing has been described in association with periarticular and para-articular deposition of calcium apatite in patients undergoing periodic hemodialysis for chronic renal failure.[3] Colchicine appears to be effective in managing acute attacks. Treatment with aluminum hydroxide gel to reduce serum phosphorus levels is associated with clinical and roentgenologic improvement. Prophylactic use of this agent in patients undergoing periodic hemodialysis is effective in preventing the syndrome.

SHOULDER-HAND SYNDROME (CAUSALGIA, REFLEX DYSTROPHY, SUDECK'S ATROPHY)

This interesting and often distressing syndrome is characterized by pain, swelling and limitation of the hand, wrist and shoulder. Symptoms may be

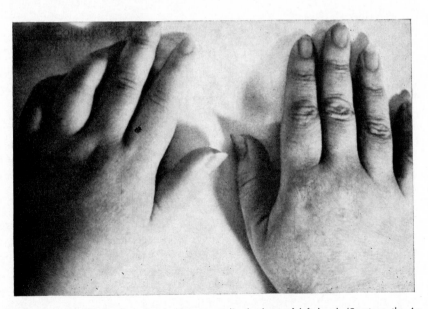

Figure 14-4. Shoulder-hand syndrome. Note generalized edema of left hand. (Courtesy, the Arthritis Foundation)

unilateral or bilateral. The syndrome is divided into three clinical phases: Phase one is associated with pain, tenderness and diffuse swelling of the hand (Fig. 14-4). Synovitis with localized swelling of proximal interphalangeal and metacarpophalangeal joints and the wrist is common. Shoulder motions are painful and limited. The first phase usually lasts three to six months. In phase two, swelling diminishes but limited movement of the joints of the hand, wrist and shoulder persists. Chronic changes are characteristic of phase three. The skin of the hand becomes cool and atrophic and soft tissue contractures ensue. Wrist motion is limited and adhesive capsulitis leads to a frozen shoulder. Raynaud's phenomenon is common. Radiologic examination reveals bone atrophy with patchy osteoporosis of the hand, wrist and shoulder at any phase of the disorder.

The etiology of this syndrome is unknown. It may result from instability of the autonomic nervous system with an abnormal outflow of neurogenic stimuli from the spinal cord. Many cases are idiopathic. Some cases follow trauma to the involved extremity; the injury may be relatively mild. Other cases are secondary to disorders such as cervical osteoarthritis, cervical disk herniation, esophageal disorders, and diseases of the heart such as chronic angina or myocardial infarction. Less commonly, the syndrome occurs in association with stroke, brain tumor or pulmonary neoplasm.

Management of shoulder-hand syndrome involves prevention as well as treatment. Prolonged immobilization of the upper extremity should be avoided; early mobilization is particularly valuable in patients following myocardial infarction. Mild cases often respond to intensive physical therapy, anti-inflammatory agents such as aspirin, indomethacin and phenylbutazone, and injection of trigger areas of tenderness with local steroids and lidocaine. More severe cases frequently respond to treatment with oral corticosteroids. Doses of 30 to 60 mg of prednisone or its equivalent are given daily, depending on disease severity. Steroids at these dose levels should be continued until moderate relief is obtained, after which the medication is gradually decreased and finally discontinued as improvement allows. An alternative method of treatment is the use of stellate ganglion blocks with lidocaine, given daily or every other day. Symptomatic response is almost immediate. Therapy should be discontinued if no relief occurs after four such blocks have been given; on the other hand, eight to twelve blocks may be required for complete remission. Pneumothorax is a possible complication of this therapeutic modality. Physical therapy exercises are vital in all cases. In general, the earlier treatment is instituted, the better the results. Resistant cases may respond to surgical sympathectomy. In late, chronic stages of the disease, measures other than physical therapy to maintain range of motion are usually unsuccessful.

Reflex dystrophy is also seen in the lower extremities, although with less frequency. Symptoms and physical findings in the involved foot are similar to those described in cases involving the hand. The foot is diffusely warm, tender and swollen. Therapy with systemic steroids or lumbar sympathetic blocks usually is efficacious.

THORACIC OUTLET SYNDROME

This term is used to describe several neurovascular compression syndromes that produce symptoms in the shoulder and upper extremity. Symptoms include paresthesia, pain, and occasionally swelling of the involved extremity. Muscle weakness may occur and Raynaud's phenomenon is common. Thoracic outlet syndrome may result from several specific mechanisms.

Cervical Rib Syndrome

Approximately 0.5% of individuals have cervical ribs originating from the seventh cervical vertebrae. Musculoskeletal symptoms result from compression of neurovascular structures between the rib and the scalenus anticus muscle. The degree to which symptoms occur depends largely on the size and shape of the rib. Diagnosis is based on clinical symptoms supported by the roentgenographic finding of a prominent cervical rib on the side of the involved extremity. A trial of therapeutic exercises may be helpful in management. Severe cases are managed by surgical resection of the first thoracic and cervical ribs.

Scalenus Anticus Syndrome

Pressure on the neurovascular bundle may be due to compression of the bundle between the scalenus anticus muscle and a normal first rib. Hypertrophy and spastic irritability of the muscle are often present. Pain extends from the neck to the hand, usually in an ulnar distribution. Tiredness or weakness of the extremity may follow. Paresthesia and vasomotor disturbances such as Raynaud's phenomenon are common. Applying pressure over the scalenus anticus muscle reproduces symptoms.

Diagnosis is aided by demonstrating occlusion of radial pulsation by the Adson maneuver (Fig. 14-5). The physician's fingers are held on the radial pulse of the seated patient. The patient takes a deep breath and holds it while fully extending the neck and turning the head toward the involved side. Occlusion of the pulse represents a positive result; in some patients, occlusion occurs only when the head is turned to the opposite side. Since many normal persons demonstrate a transient or persistent diminishing of the pulse by this maneuver, a positive test is merely suggestive and not diagnostic. Auscultation of a systolic bruit just below the proximal and medial portions of the clavicle as the radial pulse decreases and reproduction of symptoms during performance of the maneuver strongly corroborate the diagnosis.

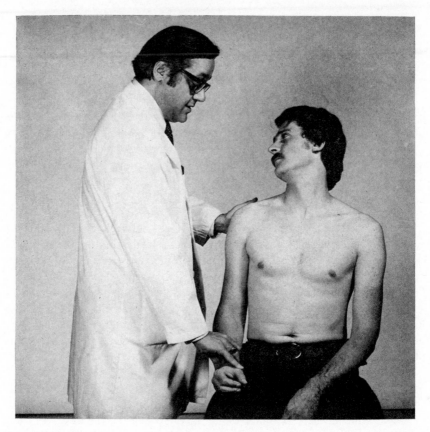

Figure 14-5. Adson maneuver. Partial or complete occlusion of the radial pulse may occur in patients with cervical rib or scalenus anticus syndromes.

Partial relief of symptoms by injection of a local anesthetic into the scalenus anticus muscle is diagnostically helpful. As in cervical rib syndrome, therapeutic exercises may be useful in relieving symptoms. Resection of the first thoracic rib should be considered in severely symptomatic cases.

Costoclavicular Syndrome

In some patients, neurovascular compression between the clavicle and first rib occurs when the shoulders are braced backward and downward, as in an exaggerated military posture (Fig. 14-6). This position is associated with a diminished radial pulse, but a similar response can be seen in normal people, as with the Adson maneuver. Reproduction of symptoms or demonstration of a loud bruit over the subclavian artery as the pulse diminishes are strong supportive findings. Symptoms are relieved by avoid-

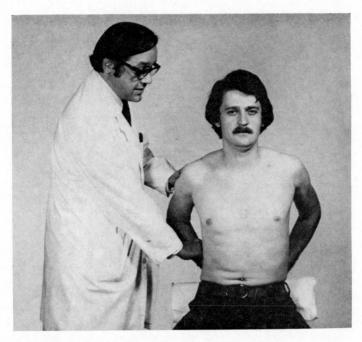

Figure 14-6. Costoclavicular maneuver. Auscultation over the subclavian artery may reveal a systolic bruit.

ing this posture. Resection of the first thoracic rib may be required for relief.

Hyperabduction Syndrome

In this condition, the neurovascular bundle is compressed by the pectoralis minor muscle, the coracoid process, the clavicle and first rib. Symptoms are precipitated by laterally circumducting the arms and clasping the hands over the head (Fig. 14-7). The radial pulse diminishes although positive results are noted frequently in normal individuals. This syndrome is induced by an abnormal persistent hyperabduction position of the extremity. It is particularly apt to occur in some persons during sleep, but is also seen in ballet dancers or mechanics as a result of positioning during occupational activities. Avoidance of hyperabduction is therapeutically indicated.

The diagnosis of thoracic outlet syndrome requires a careful history and physical examination to investigate the presence of various disorders at fault. The specific postural tests for the various syndromes are helpful. At times, a bruit may be heard over partially compressed vessels. Roentgenographic studies of the cervical spine are indicated. Venograms performed

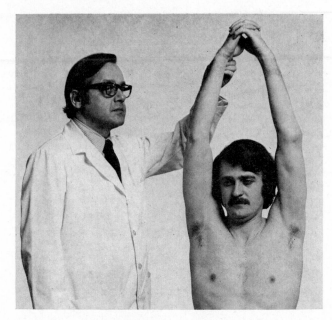

Figure 14-7. Hyperabduction maneuver. Partial or complete occlusion of the radial pulse supports a diagnosis of hyperabduction syndrome.

with the upper extremity in the precipitating postural positions may demonstrate compression abnormalities.

Other diseases that cause pain in the same area, such as cervical degenerative joint disease, cervical disk herniation, and infectious or neoplastic diseases of the lung, should be excluded.

CARPAL TUNNEL SYNDROME

Compression of the median nerve at the wrist occurs when pathologic abnormalities compromise the nerve as it passes under the rigid transverse carpal ligament.[4,5] Paresthesia and pain characteristically involve the first three fingers of the hand; in many patients, however, symptoms are localized to any one or a combination of the first three fingers. Occasionally, symptoms involve the forearm as well, or the ulnar aspect of the hand when branches of the ulnar nerve are affected. Symptoms are often worse at night when the patient sleeps with the hand forcibly flexed; they are also precipitated by long periods of driving, knitting, reading with the hands flexed, or carrying packages. At times, joint swelling occurs. Physical examination early in the disorder is often negative except for a positive Tinel's sign, in which paresthesia of the hand and forearm is precipitated by tapping the median nerve at the wrist. Similar accentuation of symptoms follows holding the wrist in forced flexion or extension. Decreased sensation over the distribution of the median nerve and atrophy of the thenar eminence are associated with late disease.

Carpal tunnel syndrome may have several local or systemic causes. Frequently it is due to chronic trauma sustained by repetitive flexion of the wrists at work. In some patients it results from nerve compression by callus formation or malunion following fracture of the wrist. Benign tumors or tophaceous gouty deposits of monosodium urate are other causes. Not infrequently, carpal tunnel syndrome occurs when wrist structures are compressed by swelling of the tendon sheaths or synovium by rheumatoid arthritis; at times, this syndrome may be the initial manifestation of the rheumatoid state.[4] Other systemic diseases associated with the syndrome include myxedema, amyloidosis, acromegaly and various hematologic disorders, such as polycythemia vera and the hemolytic anemias. It is seen more frequently in patients with diabetes mellitus, and is a common complaint in pregnant women in association with edema of soft tissues.

Diagnosis is directed not only toward defining the symptoms as carpal tunnel syndrome, but also toward demonstrating the presence of any associated disorder. In most cases, the history and physical findings are typical and strongly support the diagnosis. Roentgenograms of the wrists are indicated to exclude the presence of local pathology. Nerve conduction studies are generally diagnostic; they demonstrate prolonged motor and sensory median nerve conduction velocities across the wrist and a prolonged distal motor latency time. Although positive in most cases, these studies are occasionally normal despite the presence of proved compression.

Local injection of steroid with lidocaine into the carpal tunnel area is successful in a high percentage of cases, whether primary or secondary in etiology. A therapeutic trial is valuable when the diagnosis is in doubt. In chronic recurrent cases, a full diagnostic workup to exclude underlying etiologies should be performed. Indicated studies include a complete blood count, erythrocyte sedimentation rate, serum rheumatoid factor and antinuclear factor studies, serum protein electrophoresis (and, later, immunoelectrophoresis), serum uric acid, fasting blood sugar and protein bound iodine. When acromegaly is suspected, appropriate diagnostic studies should be performed.

Effective measures are available for management. Although immobilizing the wrist in a splint for several weeks may provide relief, symptoms are more consistently and rapidly relieved by local injections of steroid and lidocaine under the transverse carpal ligament superficial to the median nerve (see Chapter 20). This reduces inflammation and swelling and relieves symptoms for a prolonged time. Occupational stresses that aggravate symptoms should be avoided. Correction of local abnormalities should be considered when feasible. Systemic disorders related to the syndrome should be simultaneously treated. If symptoms are not completely relieved or recur following local steroid injection, a repeat injection may be given. Further recurrence is best treated surgically unless response to management of associated systemic disease is anticipated. Surgical division of the transverse carpal ligament, with or without neurolysis, gives definitive relief in almost all cases. When surgery has been unduly delayed, muscle weakness and sensory changes may resolve only slowly or persist indefinitely.

It is not unusual to see patients with pain, paresthesia and weakness of the upper extremity in whom it is difficult to differentiate carpal tunnel syndrome, compression of the ulnar nerve at the elbow, thoracic outlet syndrome and symptoms originating in the cervical spine. Symptoms may actually represent a composite of several entities present at the same time. Special attention to details of history is obviously important. In many cases therapeutic trials directed at various diseases that might be contributing to symptoms is indicated. Local steroid injection into the carpal tunnel area is valuable to exclude carpal tunnel syndrome if diagnostic studies are inconclusive. Similarly, a cervical collar and traction may be tried in excluding symptoms due to disease of the cervical spine. Therapy directed toward thoracic outlet syndrome should be considered in patients unresponsive to these approaches. In some patients, treatment directed at all these entities may be required to bring about significant relief of their symptomatology.

Tarsal tunnel syndrome[6] is an interesting disorder similar to carpal tunnel syndrome. Pain and paresthesia of the foot result from compression of the tibial nerve as it passes behind the medial malleolus. Treatment is similar to that described for carpal tunnel syndrome. Local injections of steroid with lidocaine are usually effective. Surgical decompression may be required in resistant cases.

COSTOCHONDRITIS (TIETZE'S SYNDROME)

Inflammation and enlargement of the costal cartilages may cause severe annoying chest pain.[7] Tenderness is localized to specific areas of involvement. Swelling due to cartilaginous hypertrophy may be present. The etiology of the syndrome is unknown; symptoms are occasionally preceded by mild trauma such as vigorous coughing. In most patients, a single cartilage is involved, but multiple unilateral and bilateral areas may be affected. The second and third costal cartilages are involved most frequently. Pain may be acute or insidious in onset. Symptoms are aggravated by motion and may radiate to the shoulder and arm. Duration of symptoms varies from weeks to years; spontaneous remission is common. Management includes use of heat, analgesics and anti-inflammatory agents; giving reassurance relative to the benign nature of the disease is helpful. Injections of involved areas with steroid and lidocaine are often beneficial; multiple, repeat injections may be necessary. Some patients demonstrate a similar syndrome that involves the xiphoid process, with tenderness and pain localized to this area. Management is similar to that described for costochondritis.

GANGLION

Ganglia are cystic swellings that contain a thick mucinous material. Quite common, they usually occur along tendon sheaths or joint capsules, particularly on the dorsum of the wrist. They may represent synovial membrane herniation through tears in the tendon sheath or retention cysts. The lesions respond well to aspiration and local introduction of steroids. Recurrent cases require surgical excision.

POPLITEAL CYSTS

Cystic tumors of the popliteal space (Baker's cysts) are common. They frequently reflect other primary knee pathology, such as rheumatoid arthritis,[8] osteoarthritis, or internal mechanical derangements. Cyst formation is caused by posterior herniation of synovial membrane through the posterior capsule or bursal swelling. Lesions may be large and dissect through fascial planes down the calf. Cysts may be asymptomatic but pain and stiffness are common. Physical examination reveals swelling and tenderness in the popliteal area. Popliteal aneurysms and enlarged popliteal nodes must be excluded in differential diagnosis. Symptoms frequently simulate thrombophlebitis of the calf, although secondary phlebitis may actually be present due to venous compression and hemostasis. Arthrograms of the knee are diagnostic and delineate the presence and extent of cyst formation (Fig. 2-8).

The cysts usually respond to local injections of steroid with lidocaine. In patients with rheumatoid arthritis, injection of steroid directly into the knee may alleviate the cyst swelling as well. Surgical ligation of the neck of the cyst followed by excision is required when cysts are large and unresponsive to a conservative therapeutic approach.

PELLEGRINI-STIEDA SYNDROME

This disorder is characterized by para-articular calcification at the medial aspect of the knee in the area of the medial collateral ligament. Stiffness and pain occur over the area of involvement. Para-articular calcification is seen on roentgenologic study (Fig. 14-8). Various etiologic possibilities include osseous metaplasia, presence of a detached bone fragment, ossification of a hematoma or calcification of soft tissues. Symptoms may simulate those seen in bursitis in this area. Therapy includes use of aspirin, indomethacin or phenylbutazone. Local injections of corticosteroids with lidocaine are often helpful. Surgical excision is occasionally indicated.

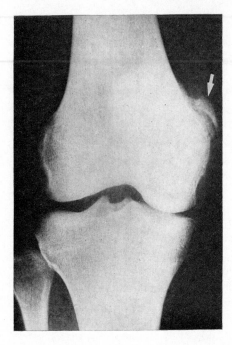

Figure 14-8. Roentgenogram of right knee in patient with Pellegrini-Stieda syndrome. A large para-articular calcification appears at the medial aspect of the femur (arrow). (Courtesy, Dr. V. Goldberg)

CASE HISTORIES

History 14-1. DeQuervain's Stenosing Tenosynovitis

J.R., a 23-year-old black female, was well until February, 1973. At that time she noted pain, slight redness, and swelling at the radial aspect of the left wrist. The patient was a piano major at the Institute of Music and symptoms were aggravated by her routine of three to four hours of piano practice daily. She was seen at the school infirmary where treatment with aspirin, 640 mg QID, splinting of the left wrist, and advice to limit her piano practice was instituted. Symptoms resolved only partially, and acute exacerbations were noted over the ensuing months. Pain and limitation of motion were aggravated by attempts to return to a more full practice schedule in her piano studies. She was referred for evaluation in November, 1973. System review was negative other than her chief complaint, and past medical history was noncontributory.

Physical examination revealed tenderness and slight swelling along the abductor pollicis longus and extensor pollicis brevis tendons. Grip strength was diminished due to pain and the patient had a positive Finkelstein test. The remainder of the joint examination was negative. Laboratory studies revealed normal hematocrit, white blood cell count, serum uric acid and erythrocyte sedimentation rate. Serum rheumatoid factor and antinuclear antibody determinations were negative. No abnormalities were noted on roentgenologic study of both wrists. A diagnosis of DeQuervain's tenosynovitis was made. Local injection of the area with steroid and lidocaine produced excellent relief of symptoms after several days. No recurrence of symptoms was noted despite gradual resumption of piano practice on a limited basis.

Discussion: In this patient DeQuervain's tenosynovitis was probably related to chronic trauma associated with intensive prolonged periods of practice on the piano. Unfortunately, recurrences may be anticipated if chronic trauma is continued. Although a relatively benign disease, this disorder represents a real threat to this patient who has serious goals of achievement as a concert pianist.

History 14-2. Shoulder-hand Syndrome

D.H., a 67-year-old white female, was seen in consultation in December, 1973. She gave a history of radical mastectomy for carcinoma of the left breast in 1969. Metastatic disease to the dorsal spine produced symptoms of spinal cord compression in April, 1973. Decompression laminectomy followed by trans-sphenoidal hypophysectomy provided symptomatic relief. Replacement therapy with cortisone acetate, 25 mg BID by mouth, and l-thyroxine, 0.2 mg daily, was begun. The patient did satisfactorily until December, 1973, when she developed subacute pain and limitation of the right shoulder, and pain and swelling of the right hand. System review was otherwise noncontributory, and past medical history revealed no other significant illnesses.

Physical examination showed extensive limitation of the right shoulder in all directions. The right hand and wrist were diffusely swollen and tender and the proximal interphalangeal and metacarpophalangeal joints of the right hand were slightly swollen. Right hand grasp was weak and fist formation was limited. Cervical spine motions were within normal limits. No other musculoskeletal abnormalities were noted. The remainder of her general physical examination showed no evidence of recurrence of carcinoma.

Hematocrit was 46%, the white blood cell count was $4000/mm^3$ with a normal differential, the erythrocyte sedimentation rate was 31 mm/hour (Wintrobe) and urinalysis was normal. Serum electrolytes were normal. Fasting blood sugar was 115 mg/100 ml (normal, up to 100 mg/100 ml). Serum calcium was 9.3 mg/100 ml, serum phosphorus, 3.1 mg/100 ml, and serum alkaline phosphatase, 9 King-Armstrong units (normal, 3 to 13 units). Serum glutamic oxaloacetic transaminase and creatine phosphokinase were normal. Serum uric acid, serologic test for syphilis, and studies for serum rheumatoid factor and antinuclear antibody were normal or negative. Serum protein electrophoresis revealed a mild increase in alpha-2 globulin.

Chest x-ray showed no abnormalities except for bony changes secondary to previous surgery. Roentgenograms of the shoulders were normal. Hand x-rays revealed hypertrophic spur formation at the margins of the distal interphalangeal joints. Cervical spine x-rays revealed mild degenerative changes. A diagnosis of right shoulder-hand syndrome was made.

The patient was placed on prednisone, 10 mg QID, and a physical therapy program was instituted. Within 48 hours, symptoms involving the right upper extremity improved greatly. Swelling of the right hand and wrist had diminished, and range of motion of the right shoulder, fingers and wrist was improved. After four days, prednisone dosage was decreased to 30 mg daily. The patient was discharged from the hospital one week later. Physical therapy instructions were given for home use and plans were made for reducing steroid dosage according to clinical response.

Discussion: The history and physical findings in this case were consistent with shoulder-hand syndrome. No specific precipitating cause was noted. The patient had no evidence of recurrence of breast carcinoma. The excellent clinical response to steroid therapy supported the diagnosis. No evidence of other forms of connective tissue disease was detected. Repeated stellate ganglion blocks are an alternative form of therapy when steroid therapy is contraindicated or unsuccessful.

History 14-3. Thoracic Outlet Syndrome

J.S., a 34-year-old white female, was first seen for evaluation in June, 1969. She was well until approximately six months prior, when she noted pain and weakness of the left upper extremity. Pain was aggravated by carrying heavy baskets elevated in front of her, by driving, or by reaching up to shelves. Pain later involved not only the left upper extremity but also the left postero-lateral aspect of the cervical spine and the left infrascapular area. Prolonged use of the left arm caused increased pain and tingling of the fourth and fifth fingers of the left hand. Daily activities became severely restricted. Physical examination at the time of consultation revealed normal and equal blood pressures in both arms. There was tenderness over the left brachial plexus and complete occlusion of the left radial artery pulse with Adson's maneuver. Deep tendon reflexes were normal. Several tender trigger areas of spasm of the left shoulder girdle muscles were observed. Sensory examination revealed mild hypalgesia of the medial aspect of the left hand.

X-rays of the chest were normal. Roentgenologic examination of the cervical spine showed mild spondylosis in the area of the C5 and C6 vertebrae. No cervical ribs were seen. Thoracic spine x-rays were normal. Laboratory studies including hematocrit, white blood cell count, erythrocyte sedimentation rate, urinalysis, serum electrolytes, serum calcium, phosphorus and alkaline phosphatase, serum uric acid and fasting blood sugar were normal. Routine serologic test for syphilis was negative, as were serum studies for rheumatoid factor and antinuclear antibody. A diagnosis of left thoracic outlet syndrome was made and the patient was placed on therapy with aspirin, 960 mg QID, muscle relaxants, and physical therapy. Intermittent injections with steroid and lidocaine were made into tender trigger areas of muscle spasm.

The patient failed to respond to therapy and had progressive increase in symptoms. She was admitted to hospital for evaluation later in the year. Clinical evaluation revealed normal cervical spine motions. Hyperabduction and Adson maneuvers resulted in a notably diminished left radial pulse. No carotid or subclavian bruits were heard. Nerve conduction studies of the upper extremities and spinal fluid examination were within normal limits. Roentgenograms of the cervical and dorsal spine were unchanged. Cervical myelogram was normal. Venograms of the left upper extremity revealed sub-clavian vein compression when hyperabduction and Adson maneuvers were performed. The patient was again placed on a full program of conservative therapy which included aspirin, analgesic medications, muscle relaxants, use of a cervical collar, cervical traction and local steroid injections into tender trigger areas. Deep heat was administered to symptomatic regions. Left trans-axillary resection of the first thoracic rib and section of the insertion of the anterior scalene muscle was performed when conservative measures failed to relieve symptoms. The patient had an excellent clinical response.

Discussion: Most patients with various forms of thoracic outlet syndrome will respond to conservative therapeutic measures. Continuous severe or progressive symptoms warrant consideration of surgery, as was eventually performed in this patient. Section of the insertion of the anterior scalene muscle and resection of the first thoracic rib on the side of involvement was associated with excellent relief of symptoms. Diseases of the cervical spine and carpal tunnel syndrome may sometimes simulate symptoms seen with thoracic outlet disorders. These other entities should be excluded by appropriate clinical and laboratory studies before definitive surgical therapy for thoracic outlet syndrome is contemplated.

History 14-4. Carpal Tunnel Syndrome

A.G., an 80-year-old white female, had a history of joint symptoms for many years characterized by mild swelling of the knees, ankles, wrists and proximal interphalangeal joints of the hands. Generalized morning stiffness that lasted two to three hours was a prominent complaint. Treatment with aspirin, 640 mg QID, and indomethacin, 25 mg TID, provided good relief of symptoms. When first seen in consultation in October, 1971, she was particularly troubled by paresthesia and burning sensations in the second and third fingers of the right hand. Physical examination revealed mild swelling of both knees, ankles and the left wrist. The right wrist was moderately swollen and limited in range of motion. Pressure over the right carpal tunnel area produced paresthesia of the second and third fingers. No muscle atrophy was noted and sensory neurologic examination was normal. Elbow and shoulder examinations were unremarkable. Thoracic outlet maneuvers were negative. Cervical spine motions were slightly limited but movement was unassociated with pain. Deep tendon reflexes in the upper extremity were present and equal bilaterally.

Hematocrit was 36%, white blood cell count and differential were normal, and erythrocyte sedimentation rate was 32 mm/hour (Wintrobe). Serum latex fixation test for rheumatoid factor was positive in a titer of 1:160. Serum uric acid was 3.2 mg/100 ml and serum antinuclear antibody was negative. Roentgenograms of the chest were normal. X-rays of the hands and wrists revealed periarticular demineralization of bone and joint space narrowing involving several proximal interphalangeal joints and both wrists. Cervical spine x-rays showed mild spur formation. Nerve conduction studies revealed prolonged motor and sensory nerve conduction velocities and a prolonged distal latency time of the median nerve across the right wrist. A diagnosis of rheumatoid arthritis with associated right carpal tunnel syndrome was made.

Local injection of steroid with lidocaine into the right carpal tunnel area produced relief of hand symptoms within 24 hours. Relief lasted approximately three months; at that time symptoms of right carpal tunnel disease recurred. The patient refused definitive surgery for her median nerve compression and was again treated with local injection of steroid. Injections were repeated as required four times over the ensuing two years. Surgery was repeatedly advised and the patient finally acceded. Surgery revealed moderate synovial swelling at the volar aspect of the right wrist with compression of the right median nerve. Histopathologic study of synovium showed nonspecific synovitis consistent with rheumatoid arthritis. The patient had persistent good relief of her carpal tunnel symptoms.

Discussion: Carpal tunnel syndrome was a major manifestation of rheumatoid arthritis in this patient. Conservative therapy with intermittent injections of local steroid is a reasonable interim approach to management while efforts to suppress generalized disease are carried out. Surgical management is indicated when conservative management is ineffective. Prolonged median nerve compression may lead to chronic disability. Delay in surgical decompression is often associated with incomplete postoperative response of symptoms.

History 14-5. Costochondritis (Tietze's Syndrome)

L.P., a 46-year-old white female, was first seen in consultation in November, 1972. She was well until approximately two months prior, when she noted soreness and tenderness of the upper left anterior chest wall. There was no history of trauma and the patient had no other musculoskeletal complaints. Pain was moderately severe and often awakened the patient at night. Therapy with low-dose salicylates gave inconsistent relief. On physical examination no abnormal findings were noted except for marked tenderness in the area of the second and third costochondral junctions of the left anterior chest wall. Slight swelling was seen. Laboratory studies revealed normal white blood cell count and differential and erythrocyte sedimentation rate. Serum rheumatoid factor and antinuclear antibody studies were negative, and serum uric acid was 3.4 mg/100 ml. Roentgenograms of the chest and rib cage and electrocardiogram were normal. A diagnosis of Tietze's syndrome (costo-chondritis) was made.

The patient was treated with local injections of steroid and lidocaine into the tender areas of costochondritis. She had almost complete relief of symptoms within 24 hours with sustained improvement for approximately one month. A mild recurrence of similar symptoms occurred at this time and local steroid injections were repeated. The patient was subsequently completely asymptomatic and no evidence of other disease states was noted on followup evaluation.

Discussion: This patient gave a history consistent with costochondritis, characterized by local tenderness of several costochondral areas. She responded well to local steroid therapy and was reassured regarding the benign nature of her symptomatology. Although recurrences are not uncommon, complete remission may be anticipated in most cases after a variable period of time.

REFERENCES

1. McCarty, D. J. and Gatter, R. A.: Recurrent acute inflammation associated with focal apatite crystal deposition. Arth Rheum 9:804, 1966.
2. Pinals, R. S. and Short, C. L.: Calcific periarthritis involving multiple sites. Arth Rheum 9:566, 1966.
3. Moskowitz, R. W. et al.: Crystal-induced inflammation associated with chronic renal failure treated with periodic hemodialysis. Am J Med 47:450, 1969.
4. Phalen, G. S.: The carpal-tunnel syndrome. J Bone Joint Surg 48A:211, 1966.
5. Chamberlain, M. A. and Corbett, M.: Carpal tunnel syndrome in early rheumatoid arthritis. Ann Rheum Dis 29:149, 1970.
6. Lloyd, K. and Agarwal, A.: Tarsal-tunnel syndrome, a presenting feature of rheumatoid arthritis. Brit Med J 3:32, 1970.
7. Levey, G. S. and Calabro, J. J.: Tietze's syndrome. A report of two cases and review of the literature. Arth Rheum 5:261, 1962.
8. Jayson, M. I. V. et al.: Popliteal and calf cysts in rheumatoid arthritis. Ann Rheum Dis 31:9, 1972.

Chapter 15

NECK PAIN

Neck pain is a common complaint. Although most frequently due to local disease, it may reflect a number of systemic disorders.

DIFFERENTIAL DIAGNOSIS

Fibrositis (myofascitis) is a common cause of neck distress (see Chapter 9). Stiffness and pain on motion may be severe. Onset of symptoms is usually subacute and they may become increasingly severe. Continuous low-grade symptoms are associated with more severe exacerbations of acute pain. The patient will often describe localized areas of maximal pain from which more diffuse pain and stiffness seem to radiate. Symptoms are most prominent in the posterior and posterolateral cervical areas and at the upper aspects of the trapezius muscles. Muscle spasm and pain limit cervical spine motion. Symptoms can frequently be reproduced or exaggerated by applying pressure over localized trigger areas of pain. The cervical myofascial syndrome is frequently caused by chronic tension that causes continuous muscle spasm. A vicious cycle occurs, because spasm causes pain and pain causes more spasm. Although essentially a benign disorder, this syndrome can be quite disabling. Systemic disorders that produce similar symptomatology and physical findings must be differentiated.

Degenerative joint disease of the cervical spine is characterized by degeneration of intervertebral disks and osteophytic spur formation from the vertebral bodies (Fig. 15-1). In addition, a true osteoarthritis of the articulating apophyseal joints between vertebrae often exists (Fig. 15-1). Localized and radicular pain and stiffness are the usual symptoms. Localized pain results from spasm and secondary inflammatory reactions. Radicular pain occurs when nerve roots are compressed by degenerative spurs or by a prolapsed degenerated disk as the roots exit through the vertebral foramina. Paresthesia and weakness of areas of the extremities innervated by these roots is common. Deep tendon reflexes in the upper extremity may be diminished. Large posterior spurs cause spinal cord compression. In these cases, hyperactive deep tendon reflexes and pathologic reflexes such

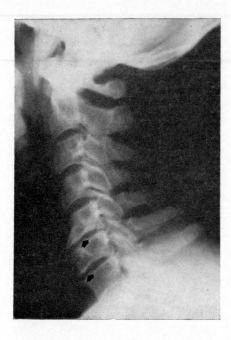

Figure 15-1. Degenerative joint disease of cervical spine. Note narrowing of the intervertebral disk spaces between C5-C6 and C6-C7 vertebrae (arrows). Osteophytic spur formation is seen at the anterior and posterior aspects of these vertebral bodies. Apophyseal joints reveal narrowing and sclerosis.

as the Babinski are seen in the lower extremities. If the anterior spinal artery is compressed, a central cord syndrome results. Compression of the vertebral arteries by spurs may also compromise the blood supply to the brain, causing transient symptoms of vertigo and visual impairment. Neck motion is usually limited by the osteoarthritic joint changes and by associated pain and spasm.

Herniated intervertebral cervical disks produce pain similar to that caused by degenerative joint disease. Symptoms vary depending upon whether protrusion of disk material occurs posteriorly or laterally. Disk herniation frequently occurs in association with degenerative changes typical of osteoarthritis but it may occur separately. As in cervical osteoarthritis, spinal cord compression can result from posteriorly protruded disks.

Involvement of the cervical spine is common in patients with *rheumatoid arthritis;* it occurs so frequently in juvenile rheumatoid arthritis (JRA) that its presence is a clue to diagnosis. Roentgenologic changes in JRA are characterized by atlantoaxial subluxation and a tendency toward ankylosis of apophyseal joints (Fig. 15-2). Atlantoaxial subluxation is also common in adults with rheumatoid arthritis of the cervical spine (Fig. 15-3).[1] Inflammatory erosions in bone may result in partial or complete dissolution of the odontoid process. Subluxation may go undetected if only routine lateral roentgenograms are obtained. Lateral roentgenograms taken with the neck in gentle flexion are necessary for complete evaluation. However, these should be performed only with great care if clinical symp-

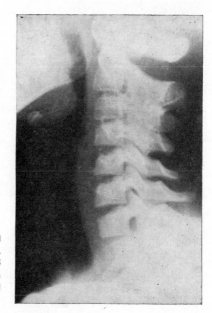

Figure 15-2. Lateral roentgenogram of cervical spine, juvenile rheumatoid arthritis. Irregularities in contour of the C5 and C6 vertebrae are associated with fusion of the upper apophyseal joints. (Courtesy, Dr. V. Goldberg)

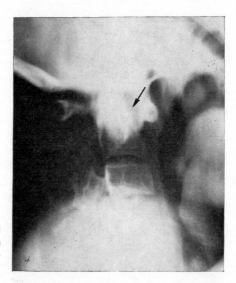

Figure 15-3. Lateral tomogram, cervical spine. Atlantoaxial subluxation (arrow) in a patient with rheumatoid arthritis.

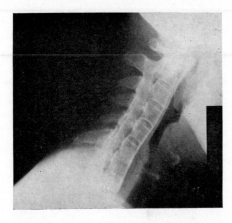

Figure 15-4. Calcification of the paravertebral ligaments, as seen in this lateral neck x-ray, was associated with severe limitation of cervical motion in patient with ankylosing spondylitis. (Courtesy, Dr. A. Mackenzie)

toms suggestive of neurologic compression are present. Lateral tomograms (Fig. 15-3), and cineradiograms help to demonstrate detailed abnormalities that might be present. The atlanto-odontoid interval in adults should not exceed 3.0 mm and should be constant in neutral, flexion and extension positions.

Rheumatoid changes in the cervical spine produce local pain and spasm. Occipital headaches are common and the patient may hear a clunking noise when flexing the head. Severe cases are associated with neurologic signs and symptoms due to compression of vascular and neurologic structures. Upper extremity weakness and long tract signs may be present. Quadriplegia may occur but is fortunately uncommon.

Ankylosing spondylitis most commonly produces symptoms in the low back and sacroiliac areas (see Chapter 16). However, upward progression of the disease into the dorsal and cervical spine is common. The patient

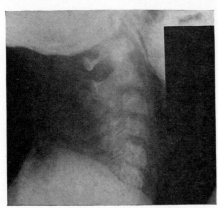

Figure 15-5. Diffuse lytic lesions of the cervical spine caused by bony metastases from a carcinoma of the breast.

complains of pain and stiffness. Cervical spine motions are limited. Roentgenograms show calcification and ossification of paravertebral ligaments (Fig. 15-4).

Metastatic carcinoma of the cervical spine is usually characterized by severe, continuous pain. In its early stages it may simulate nonspecific myofascial syndrome or degenerative joint disease. Careful evaluation of neck x-rays is important in differential diagnosis (Fig. 15-5).

Benign local tumors that arise in bone or neurologic structures must be excluded as a cause of neck pain. Bone tumors such as giant cell tumor and osteochondroma are fortunately uncommon; hemangiomas and osteoid osteomas are more frequent. Roentgenograms may reveal vertical striations and partial vertebral collapse when hemangioma is present. Osteoid osteomas are characterized by an area of sclerotic bone that surrounds a small central radiolucent nidus. Tomograms help in diagnosis. Pain is severe, especially at night. Aspirin provides dramatic relief of symptoms. Removal of the central nidus is associated with lasting relief.

Tumors of nerve tissue origin, such as neurofibromas and meningiomas, may cause severe neck symptoms. Radiating pain related to motion is common. Myelograms are often necessary for diagnosis.

Osteoporosis occurs earliest and most severely in the dorsal and lumbar spine, but cervical spine involvement often occurs as the disease progresses. This disorder most frequently affects older patients. Symptoms may be vague and nonspecific. Diagnosis is based on roentgenographic findings of decreased bone density, "fishmouth" deformities of the vertebral bodies and, when changes are severe, vertebral collapse and fracture.

Whiplash injury occurs most commonly after automobile accidents. The patient usually gives a history of being in a car that was hit suddenly from behind by a second vehicle. This results in a forceful movement of the neck forward with posterior recoil. Neck pain and spasm may occur shortly after injury, but symptoms may be delayed for several days to a week. Symptoms include neck pain, stiffness and limitation of motion; they often spread to the upper trapezius muscle, causing pain and spasm. Neck roentgenograms are often negative; straightening of the cervical spine due to spasm may be noted.

Temporal arteritis (cranial arteritis, giant cell arteritis), a disease of older age, is associated with severe temporal headaches and polymyalgia rheumatica (see Chapter 13). The occipital vessels are also commonly affected, which may cause pain in the occipital and upper cervical regions. The temporal arteries are usually tender, nodular and irregular. Aching and stiffness in the shoulders and hips, fever, weight loss and depression are common associated findings. Laboratory studies show an elevated erythrocyte sedimentation rate, anemia, and a reversal of the albumin/globulin ratio.

DIAGNOSTIC STUDIES

History and physical examination will often define whether the basic problem is local or systemic. All patients should have adequate radiologic examination of the neck, with PA, lateral and oblique views. Oblique views are extremely important to adequately view foraminal openings through which nerve roots exit (Fig. 15-6). Lateral views in flexion and extension are necessary to demonstrate vertebral body subluxation and lesions in the odontoid area. They should be performed with caution. Spot films and tomograms (Fig. 15-3) allow further characterization of suspected pathologic changes. Cineradiography is helpful in detailing functional structural abnormalities, but it is not frequently required.

Spinal fluid examination should be performed when myelopathy is present. Manometric studies to evaluate patency of the subarachnoid space should be considered when intracranial lesions can be reasonably excluded. Subsequently, cervical myelography may be indicated.

The foregoing routine studies will usually be adequate in the diagnosis of degenerative joint disease, cervical disk disease, metastatic carcinoma, rheumatoid arthritis, ankylosing spondylitis and osteoporosis. Negative studies are reassuring to those patients whose symptoms are related to myofascial syndrome. Other studies may be indicated to exclude systemic disease; these include erythrocyte sedimentation rate, rheumatoid factor

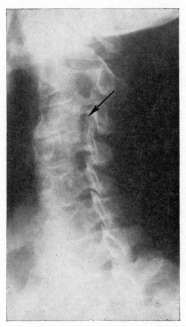

Figure 15-6. Oblique view of cervical spine reveals narrowing of foraminal spaces by osteophytic spurs of degenerative joint disease. Changes are most marked at the C3-C4 foramen (arrow).

test, serum alkaline phosphatase, and roentgenograms of the lumbar spine and sacroiliac joints. Temporal artery biopsy and arteriograms should be performed when temporal arteritis is suspected.

THERAPY

Symptomatic Measures

Conservative symptomatic measures may be instituted even before a specific diagnosis has been made. Aspirin, 640 to 960 mg four times a day, may relieve pain and inflammation. Local heat applied as hot packs, a warm shower, or heating pad similarly relieve pain and spasm. Mild analgesics such as acetominophen, 300 to 600 mg, propoxyphene hydrochloride, 65 mg, or ethoheptazine citrate (Zactane), 75 mg, used on a PRN or regular basis are helpful. A soft cervical collar limits excessive motion and protects against irritation of neurologic structures. Tranquilizers such as diazepam (Valium), 5 mg TID, provide various degrees of relief from spasm and associated pain.

Specific Therapeutic Measures

Patients with *fibrositis* should avoid tension-producing factors if possible. The patient should be reassured that no serious underlying disease exists and that a reasonable amount of relief can be obtained by simple conservative measures. Emotional support is an important element of the therapeutic approach. Aspirin in maximally tolerated dosage should be instituted in addition to mild analgesics. In more severe cases, trials of more potent anti-inflammatory agents, such as indomethacin, 25 mg three to four times a day with meals, should be considered. Phenylbutazone, 100 mg QID for three or four days, with gradually decreasing doses over a period of seven to 10 days, is beneficial in treating acute episodes. Local injections of trigger point areas of pain and spasm with steroids and lidocaine are frequently effective; several areas may have to be injected. Injections should be repeated after several weeks if certain areas have been missed or symptoms are relieved incompletely. Heat and mild range-of-motion exercises are advisable. Tranquilizers help to relieve tension.

A soft cervical collar limits neck motion. This should be worn throughout the night and as frequently as possible during the day when symptoms are severe. Use of the collar can be gradually decreased as symptoms improve. Cervical traction is instituted by the physical therapist and instructions given for home use. Traction should be utilized at least 20 minutes twice a day when symptoms are severe.

Management of *cervical degenerative joint disease* and *herniated cervical disk* is similar to the program outlined for fibrositis syndrome. Therapeutic measures include analgesic and anti-inflammatory agents and muscle relaxants. Heat, use of a cervical collar and traction are beneficial. Local steroid and lidocaine injections relieve muscle spasm. Surgery should be considered when symptoms are severe and not responding well to a conservative medical program over a reasonable period of time. Anterior fusion has less morbidity and a shorter convalescence than fusion performed by a posterior approach. Posterior fusion and laminectomy may be required, however, in patients with cord compression.

The usual therapeutic programs for *rheumatoid arthritis* and *ankylosing spondylitis* should be instituted in patients with neck pain due to these disorders (see Chapter 18). However, severe involvement of the spine in rheumatoid arthritis requires additional special measures to prevent cord compression. A soft cervical collar should be worn at night and as much as possible throughout the day. It is particularly important to wear the collar when driving because even mild neck injuries may result in severe neurologic damage. A more firm cervical collar made of leather or plastic is required in severe cases. Cervical fusion should be considered if neurologic involvement is severe; unfortunately, failure of fusion is not uncommon. Patients with ankylosing spondylitis find great relief from the usual anti-inflammatory measures such as aspirin, indomethacin or phenylbutazone (see Chapter 18). Physical therapy measures are extremely important.

Patients with *metastatic carcinoma* to bone may obtain relief from radiation therapy if the tumors are radiation-sensitive. Appropriate therapy to the primary tumor is indicated when feasible. A cervical collar helps to avoid damage to neurologic structures.

Surgery is usually necessary in the management of benign *local tumors*. Hemangiomas of bone frequently respond to radiation therapy. Failure to rapidly diagnose and treat local neoplasms may result in irreversible neurologic defects.

Although *osteoporosis* is frequently difficult to treat, presently accepted methods of management are worthy of a trial period. Estrogenic and androgenic hormones, and calcium lactate powder, 4 gm TID, may be helpful. In severe cases, vitamin D, 50,000 units twice a week, and sodium fluoride, 22 mg BID, may provide additional benefit.[2] Use of the latter agent is still *investigational. Whiplash* syndrome is treated by measures similar to those described for fibrositis syndrome. Unfortunately, ongoing litigation often obscures therapeutic results until an adequate settlement has been made.

Prednisone, 15 mg QID, usually relieves symptoms of *temporal arteritis* rapidly, often within two or three days. A good response supports the diagnosis. Steroid therapy is valuable not only in relieving headache and polymalgia but also in preventing blindness that can occur as a complication of vasculitis involving the ophthalmic artery and vessels to the optic nerve.

CASE HISTORIES

History 15-1. Cervical Spine Degenerative Joint Disease

C. G., a 54-year-old white male, was first seen in consultation in December, 1967, with the chief complaint of acute pain in the right side of the neck of several weeks' duration. Pain radiated down the arm to the wrist and was associated with paresthesia. Pain was also prominent over the dorsal aspect of the right shoulder. Past history revealed a short bout of similar distress in 1962, which had been treated with cervical traction and a soft cervical collar. The symptoms had resolved completely after several weeks, but the patient was troubled with recurrent episodes of neck pain over the ensuing years. On physical examination at time of consultation, cervical spine motions were moderately limited by pain and spasm. Tenderness was present over the right posterior cervical muscles and lateral flexion of the neck to the right produced paresthesia of the right upper extremity. The right grip was diminished in strength and sensation was diminished over the dorsolateral aspect of the forearm. Deep tendon reflexes were normal.

Cervical spine x-rays revealed moderately severe degeneration of the C5-C6 and C6-C7 disks. Severe spur formation compromised the intervertebral foramina in the C5-C6 and C6-C7 areas bilaterally. Symptoms and radiologic findings were consistent with a diagnosis of cervical degenerative joint disease. The patient was treated with cervical collar, cervical traction, aspirin, 640 mg QID, and propoxyphene hydrochloride, 65 mg, as needed for pain. Symptoms progressively improved over a period of several weeks and objective neurologic abnormalities disappeared.

Discussion: Cervical degenerative joint disease is a common disorder. In most patients, symptoms are minimal and objective neurologic findings absent. However, acute symptoms may be associated with major disability. Intensive therapy with neck immobilization and traction and the use of mild anti-inflammatory agents and analgesics helps to relieve distress. More serious disorders as a cause of this pain syndrome should be routinely excluded.

History 15-2. Metastatic Carcinoma of the Cervical Spine

S.R., a 73-year-old white male, was first seen in consultation in December, 1970. The patient had a long history of cervical spine pain of mild to moderate degree. Roentgenograms of the cervical spine performed several years earlier had revealed extensive changes of degenerative joint disease. The patient had been treated intermittently with a cervical collar, cervical traction, aspirin, and mild analgesics with good relief. Several months prior to referral the patient had noted increased pain in the cervical spine. The symptoms were considered an exacerbation of his cervical degenerative joint disease; x-rays of the cervical spine were not obtained. Therapy with aspirin, analgesics, cervical collar and cervical traction were again instituted. Symptoms did not respond to this program of management and the patient was referred for evaluation.

System review was significant in that the patient had suffered a 15-pound weight loss over the previous two months. On physical examination there was slight tenderness over the cervical spine, and cervical spine motions were moderately limited. Cardiorespiratory examination revealed a Grade 2/6 systolic ejection murmur. Prostatic enlargement without nodules or tenderness was noted. Cervical spine x-rays taken at this time revealed multiple lytic lesions consistent with metastatic carcinoma. Additional roentgenographic studies revealed destructive bone lesions in the left rib cage and infiltrative changes at the apical segment of the left lower lobe of the lung. Hematocrit was 40%, white blood cell count was 7900/mm³ with a normal differential, the serum alkaline phosphatase and acid phosphatase values were within normal limits, and tuberculin skin test was positive. Rib biopsy was performed under local anesthesia. Histopathologic study revealed metastatic, poorly differentiated adenocarcinoma. The bone lesions were considered to be metastatic from a primary adenocarcinoma of the lung. The patient was treated with radiation therapy to the cervical spine, with no improvement in pain. A large left pleural effusion, noted on subsequent chest x-rays, was treated with instillation of 5-fluorouracil into the pleural cavity. The patient had a progressive downhill course and died after the thirty-sixth hospital day.

Discussion: Pain is a prominent component of the clinical presentation of metastatic carcinoma of the spine. In this patient, recent cervical spine symptoms were attributed to degenerative joint disease that had been demonstrated previously. A notable increase in symptoms associated with a 15-pound weight loss suggested the presence of a more serious disorder. The presence of degenerative joint disease is often a "red herring" in the clinical evaluation of patients with symptoms related to the musculoskeletal system.

History 15-3. Temporal (Cranial) Arteritis

M.S., a 70-year-old white female, was first seen in December, 1966, for evaluation of pain and swelling of the proximal interphalangeal and metacarpophalangeal joints of the hands, both knees and ankles. Physical examination and laboratory studies were consistent with a diagnosis of rheumatoid arthritis and the patient was placed on a conservative program of aspirin, analgesics and physical therapy. The patient responded well with little progression of joint manifestations. In December, 1967, she noted moderately severe pain in the left side of her neck and scalp. Pain was aggravated by applying pressure to involved areas. The patient increased her dose of aspirin, which provided partial relief of symptoms. She was seen in the office in January, 1968, when pain in the posterior cervical area and over the posterior aspect of the scalp became more severe. She now complained of pain and tenderness in the left temporal area as well. Examination revealed tenderness to palpation over the posterior cervical spine, the posterior aspect of the scalp and the left temporal region. Temporal artery pulsations were normal and no thickening of the vessels was noted. The patient was admitted to hospital for general studies and temporal artery biopsy.

Erythrocyte sedimentation rate was 48 mm/hour (Wintrobe). Hematocrit was 36%, white blood cell count was 12,600/mm³, and urinalysis was normal. Serum protein electrophoresis revealed a slight elevation in gamma globulin. Roentgenograms of the skull and cervical spine showed mild degenerative arthritis. Left temporal artery biopsy was performed. Histopathologic examination showed intimal proliferation and an inflammatory infiltration of the vessel wall with mononuclear and giant cells. A diagnosis of temporal arteritis was made. The patient was begun on prednisone therapy, 15 mg Q6H. Symptoms responded rapidly over 36 hours. The patient was subsequently maintained on progressively lower doses of prednisone for several years. After this time, her symptoms completely resolved and no further therapy was required.

Discussion: Early symptoms of temporal arteritis in this patient consisted of pain in the posterior cervical and occipital areas. Only after a period of one month did symptoms occur in the temporal area as well. The posterior cervical and occipital areas are occasionally the site of prominent symptomatology in patients with temporal arteritis.

REFERENCES

1. Mathews, J. A.: Atlanto-axial subluxation in rheumatoid arthritis. A 5-year follow up study. Ann Rheum Dis 33:526, 1974.
2. Jowsey, J., et al.: Effect of combined therapy with sodium fluoride, vitamin D
   and calcium in osteoporosis. Am J Med 53:43, 1972.

Chapter 16

LOW BACK PAIN

Diagnosis and treatment of low back pain often tax the ingenuity of the physician. Although in many patients a diagnosis can be made after appropriate history, physical examination and laboratory studies, a specific diagnosis is not always possible and management must be based on an empiric symptomatic approach.

DIFFERENTIAL DIAGNOSIS

One of the most common causes of low back pain is *abnormal posture*. In most cases, the postural defect is functional; in others, structural bony changes result in fixed postural abnormalities. In the latter, secondary degenerative changes are often noted on roentgenographic examination; the postural abnormalities are not readily reversible. Pain associated with functional postural abnormalities is usually relatively mild and results from muscular imbalance and spasm. In patients with fixed changes, severe pain may result from compression of nerve roots; this tends to occur especially when secondary degenerative changes are severe.

Herniation of a nucleus pulposus in the lumbar area is a common cause of low back pain. Unfortunately, this diagnosis is often overused as a "wastebasket" diagnosis when studies are inconclusive. Pain may be acute or chronic. Acute pain results from posterior or lateral herniation of a nucleus pulposus causing compression of contiguous neurologic structures. Chronic symptoms usually result from degeneration of the annulus fibrosus with eventual prolapse or protrusion of degenerated material. In the latter cases, degenerative changes in the vertebral body and apophyseal joints are a common associated finding.

The patient complains of low back pain. Spasm and tenderness of associated muscles are noted in the involved area. Radicular pain in the distribution of the sciatic nerve is often prominent. Straight-leg-raising is limited due to muscle spasm and nerve root irritation. The patient walks with a list, and secondary functional scoliosis is common. Chronic com-

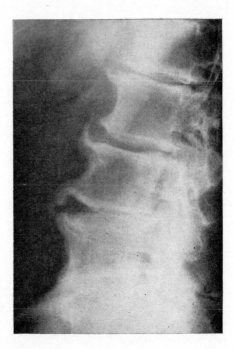

Figure 16-1. Osteoarthritis of lumbar spine. Note florid spur formation, narrowed disk spaces and sclerosis of apophyseal joints. (Courtesy, Dr. F. Bishko)

pression of nerve roots results in neurologic abnormalities such as loss of reflexes, muscle weakness and sensory deficits.

Low back pain may result from *primary degenerative joint disease* of the spine. Degenerative changes are characterized by osteophyte spur formation of the vertebral bodies, degeneration of the annulus fibrosus with eventual prolapse, and joint space narrowing and spur formation involving the apophyseal joints (Fig. 16-1). Pain is usually subacute or chronic; acute symptoms occur if nerve root compression complicates the picture. Clinical findings are generally similar to those described in patients with herniated nucleus pulposus.

Spondylolysis, a defect in the pars interarticularis of the neural arch (Fig. 16-2), may be congenital or acquired and traumatic in origin. Symptoms are not usually common unless *spondylolisthesis,* a forward displacement of one vertebra on the other, ensues (Fig. 16-3). The latter condition may be asymptomatic, but mild to moderate pain and spasm are not uncommon. Symptoms resemble those seen in herniated disk disease and, in fact, secondary disk disease may also develop. Vertebral displacement is usually anterior. Posterior displacement may compress the cauda equina; fortunately, this is uncommon. Spondylolisthesis sometimes occurs in the absence of spondylolysis. Displacement in these cases results from a congenitally large pedicle or from severe degenerative joint disease of the apophyseal joints with dislocation.

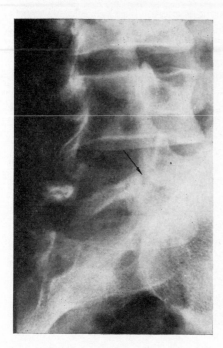

Figure 16-2. Spondylolysis, lumbar spine. A defect (arrow) is seen in the pars interarticularis in this oblique roentgenographic view. (Courtesy, Dr. V. Goldberg)

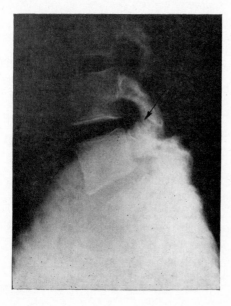

Figure 16-3. Spondylolisthesis. Early forward displacement of L5 vertebra on S1 is seen. A defect, seen in the pars interarticularis (arrow), was better demonstrated on oblique roentgenographic view. (Courtesy, Dr. V. Goldberg)

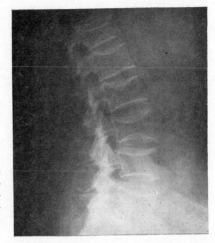

Figure 16-4. Osteoporosis of spine. All vertebrae appear extensively demineralized. Additional diagnostic features include accentuation of cortical bone outlines and codfish
deformities.

Osteoporosis produces mild to moderate pain that usually parallels the
degree of disease (Fig. 16-4). Pain may be continuous, increasing with
activity. Compression fracture should be suspected when there is a sudden
increase in pain with or without a history of trauma. Trauma may be mild,
such as a slight fall, tripping or stressful motion. Neurologic abnormalities
occur when structural changes associated with fracture produce compression of adjoining neurologic structures.

Primary bone disease such as *multiple myeloma* is a cause of persistent
low back pain (Fig. 16-5). *Metastatic carcinoma* frequently involves the
lower spine (Fig. 16-6). Pain, usually persistent, is present at rest and
aggravated by motion. Night pain is common.

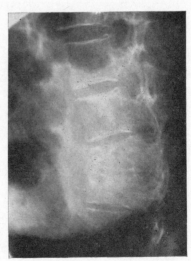

Figure 16-5. Lesions of multiple myeloma seen on
lateral spine roentgenogram. Note
demineralized appearance of vertebral bodies and compression fracture.

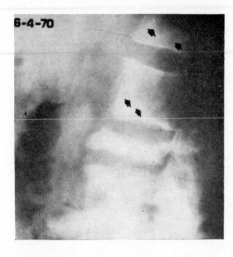

Figure 16-6. Metastatic carcinoma, lumbar spine. Complete collapse of L3 vertebra is associated with metastases to other areas (arrows). (Courtesy, the Arthritis Foundation)

Paget's disease frequently involves the spine and pelvis. Pain resembles that seen in several other low back disorders. The diagnosis depends on demonstrating typical radiologic changes characterized by sclerosis and a coarsening of the trabecular pattern of bone (Fig. 16-7). The serum alkaline phosphatase level is characteristically elevated. Superimposition of an osteogenic sarcoma should be considered in the presence of severe pain.

Initial symptoms in *ankylosing spondylitis* characteristically involve the area of the sacroiliac joints and lumbosacral spine.[1] This disease, most commonly seen in young males, may cause very mild symptoms with minimal or absent objective findings early in its course. A diagnosis of ma-

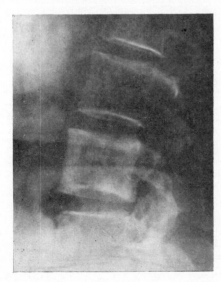

Figure 16-7. Paget's disease, lumbar spine. Sclerosis and a coarsening of the trabecular pattern are seen in the lower lumbar vertebrae. (Courtesy, Dr. V. Goldberg)

lingering or psychiatric illness is often entertained when stiffness and pain are present in the absence of positive physical and laboratory findings. Low back symptoms are often accompanied by pain in a sciatic distribution to the buttocks and knees. Sciatic pain not infrequently alternates from side to side. Peripheral joint involvement occurs in one-third of patients. Heel pain is common. As the disease progresses, pain, stiffness and limitation of motion involve the dorsal and cervical spine. Chest pain occurs when costovertebral joints are affected. Systemic manifestations include pericarditis, cardiac conduction abnormalities, aortic insufficiency and iritis. Physical examination shows tenderness and limitation of affected areas of the spine and spasm of paravertebral muscles. Chest expansion may be severely limited. Progression of the disease leads to severe kyphosis and forward protrusion of the neck (Fig. 16-8).

Laboratory findings other than roentgenologic changes are frequently minimal. The erythrocyte sedimentation rate is elevated during active disease. Serum studies for rheumatoid factor and antinuclear antibody are negative. However, 90% of patients with ankylosing spondylitis have HLA-W27 histocompatibility antigen.[2] Roentgenologic studies may be negative for several years after disease onset, but eventually characteristic changes

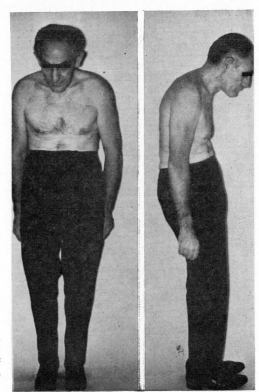

Figure 16-8. Ankylosing spondylitis, showing kyphosis and forward protrusion of the neck. (Courtesy, the Arthritis Foundation)

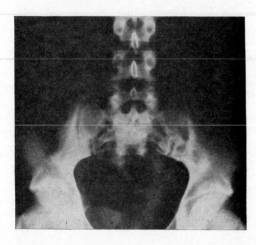

Figure 16-9. Ankylosing spondylitis, pelvic x-rays. Sacroiliac joints reveal apparent widening of joint spaces and bony sclerosis.

in the sacroiliac joints and spine appear. Early, sacroiliac joints reveal juxta-articular bony osteoporosis and apparent joint space widening (Fig. 16-9); later, joint space narrowing, sclerosis and fusion appear (Fig. 16-10). Spinal x-rays show syndesmophytes or calcified spurs. These spurs lie in a vertical direction, which differentiates them from osteophytes of degenerative joint disease, which characteristically lie in a horizontal direction and are less likely to be fused. Granulomatous changes at the anterosuperior and anteroinferior aspects of the vertebral bodies produce a squared appearance of the vertebrae (Romanus sign) (Fig. 16-11). Calcification and ossification of paravertebral ligaments lead to classic bamboo spine changes (Figs. 16-10, 16-11). Destructive lesions of intervertebral disks and ad-

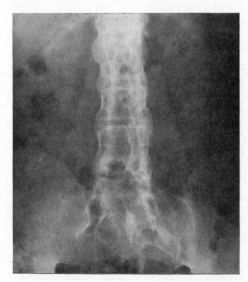

Figure 16-10. Ankylosing spondylitis. Sacroiliac joints are fused. Calcification of paravertebral ligaments has led to development of bamboo spine.

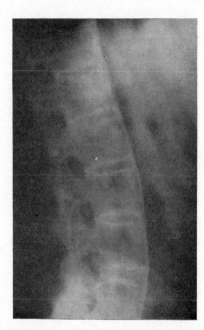

Figure 16-11. Ankylosing spondylitis. Note squared appearance of vertebrae (Romanus sign) in this lateral lumbar roentgenogram. Paravertebral calcification of ligaments is extensive.

joining vertebral bodies may be seen; these lesions may be confused with tuberculous or pyogenic infection.

Spondylitic changes occur in other disease states, such as psoriasis, ulcerative colitis, regional enteritis and Reiter's syndrome.[3] Syndesmophyte spur formation in patients with ulcerative colitis and regional enteritis is similar to that seen in idiopathic ankylosing spondylitis. The spurs are usually relatively thin, regular, bilateral and lie close to the intervertebral disk. In patients with psoriasis and Reiter's syndrome, the syndesmophytes tend to be larger, more irregular and are often unilateral.

Osteitis condensans ilii occurs most commonly in young women of childbearing age. Symptoms are characterized by pain and stiffness in the area of the sacroiliac joint. At times, mild radicular pain is present. Radiologic changes are usually easily differentiated from those of ankylosing spondylitis. In osteitis condensans ilii, a condensing sclerosis of iliac bone is seen, and no changes in the sacroiliac joint or sacrum are noted (Fig. 16-12).

Acute spinal infections affect the intervertebral disk spaces or sacroiliac joints. Bone involvement is usually secondary. Spinal infection usually emanates from foci elsewhere, such as genitourinary, pulmonary or cutaneous areas. Radiologic changes may be slow in developing but serial examination eventually reveals gradual destruction of vertebral margins and obliteration of the disk space. Diagnosis is confirmed by culture of aspirates from the disk space. A positive blood culture is helpful in diagnosis, because bacteremia is frequently present.

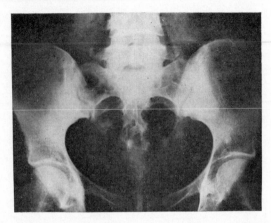

Figure 16-12. Osteitis condensans ilii. Sclerotic changes involve the iliac sides of both sacro-iliac joints. Oblique views showed that the joints themselves were normal. (Courtesy, Dr. V. Goldberg)

The most common cause of chronic infection of the spine is *tuberculosis*. Symptoms are often insidious in onset. Systemic evidence of tuberculous infection such as fever, chills and night sweats is helpful in diagnosis. A negative tuberculin test militates against the diagnosis; a positive tuberculin test, however, is only supportive and not conclusive. The erythrocyte sedimentation rate is usually elevated. Radiologic examination reveals narrowing of the disk space, the site of initial tuberculous involvement (Fig. 16-13).[4] Soft tissue abscesses are typical. Diagnosis should be pur-

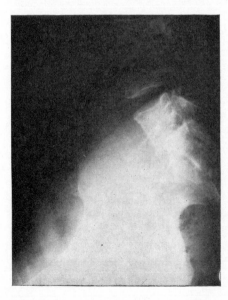

Figure 16-13. Tuberculosis of the lumbosacral spine resulted in loss of the L5-S1 disk space and destructive changes in contiguous bone.

sued by aspiration and culture of the abscessed area. Sacroiliac joint involvement is not uncommon. *Fungal infections* and *brucellosis* cause similar lesions. Diagnosis is based on fungal complement-fixation studies, brucella agglutination titer and culture of involved areas.

Vertebral epiphysitis (Scheuermann's disease) causes back pain in adolescents. It is more common in males and most frequently involves the dorsal spine. Rounding and limitation of the dorsal spine is seen on physical examination. Tight hamstrings are common. Pain may be minimal or absent and the patient's primary complaint is poor posture. The condition is self-limited. Roentgenologic study reveals wedging of the vertebrae, narrow disk spaces and irregular vertebral margins (Fig. 16-14).

Coccygodynia, pain in the area of the coccyx, results from direct trauma with fracture of the coccyx or strain of the sacrococcygeal joint. It may also occur as a result of visceral disease in organs anterior to the area of the coccyx itself. Rectal examination reveals tenderness of the coccyx and associated ligamentous and muscular structures.

Subarachnoid hemorrhage of intracranial origin is an uncommon cause of low back pain but should be considered diagnostically in cases with atypical symptoms. Pain, due to irritation by blood in the spinal fluid, may simulate acute disk herniation or vertebral fracture. Headache and pain and limitation of the cervical spine are frequent associated findings.

Herpes zoster may cause severe low back pain when localized to nerves in this area. The diagnosis is often missed until the characteristic vesicular eruption is seen.

Benign local tumors, such as neurofibroma, meningioma, osteoid osteoma and hemangioma, should be considered in the differential diagnosis of low back pain. Diagnosis requires full use of radiologic techniques includ-

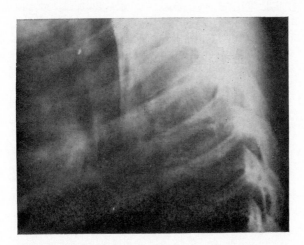

Figure 16-14. Vertebral epiphysitis (Scheuermann's disease). (Courtesy, Dr. V. Goldberg)

ing routine x-rays, spot films, tomograms and myelograms. Tomograms are particularly helpful in the diagnosis of osteoid osteoma, which usually involves the posterior aspects of the vertebrae and may not be seen on routine radiologic studies. The typical lesion consists of a zone of dense bone surrounding a small radiolucent nidus. Pain is severe and usually more prominent during the night. Relief of pain by aspirin is often dramatic; this is a helpful diagnostic test.

Although *fractures* of the vertebral bodies are associated most commonly with osteoporosis, they may occur secondary to trauma in otherwise normal spines. Fractures of the posterior elements of the spine are complicated by severe neurologic damage; rapid neurosurgical intervention is indicated. Pathologic fractures occur in patients with metastatic malignancy, primary neoplasms or metabolic bone dyscrasias.

Idiopathic scoliosis is associated with various degrees of back pain. Osteoarthritis, a frequent secondary finding, contributes to the symptomatology. At times, nerve compression with radicular pain is prominent.

Not infrequently, low back pain is a manifestation of *visceral disease,* such as carcinoma of the uterus, kidney, pancreas or bowel. Large aortic aneurysms that impinge upon the vertebral column cause persistent boring back pain. Adequate investigation of the patient by history and physical examination and appropriate laboratory studies is mandatory, particularly when back symptoms are atypical.

DIAGNOSTIC STUDIES

PA, lateral and oblique roentgenograms of the lumbosacral spine should be performed routinely. Disk disease is not excluded by normal findings, however, since the soft tissue herniation does not show and narrowing of the disk space may appear only late. Oblique views are necessary to demonstrate spondylolysis because the pars interarticularis cannot be outlined adequately in routine PA and lateral views. Spondylolisthesis, a displacement of one vertebra on the other, is best seen on the lateral view. Lesions due to osteoporosis, fracture, metastatic carcinoma, Paget's disease, spondylitis, osteitis condensans ilii, acute or chronic infection, epiphysitis, and scoliosis are usually detected readily. Special oblique views of the sacroiliac joints should be performed in patients suspected of having ankylosing spondylitis when changes on routine PA views are absent or nonspecific. Tomograms may be helpful. Coned-down spot films and tomograms of other areas of the lumbosacral spine are indicated to exclude subtle abnormalities readily missed on routine study.

Lumbar myelograms may be necessary in patients with severe persistent disease if the diagnosis cannot be made otherwise. Myelograms are not usually performed in patients with suspected herniated disks unless symptoms are severe and unresponsive to conservative therapy and surgery is being contemplated. Radioactive scans are helpful in delineating early otherwise nondemonstrable lesions of bone.

Other studies frequently necessary in diagnosis include chest x-ray, complete blood count, erythrocyte sedimentation rate, serum calcium, phosphorus and alkaline phosphatase, serum protein electrophoresis, urine for Bence Jones protein, bone marrow study, and skin testing for tuberculosis and fungal diseases. Histocompatibility antigen studies to demonstrate the presence of HLA-W27 antigen may be diagnostically helpful when ankylosing spondylitis is suspected. Appropriate radiologic studies of viscera are indicated when symptoms are deemed most likely nonosseous in origin. Aortic aneurysms, if calcified, are usually visible on lateral views of the lumbar spine.

THERAPY

Nonspecific therapy with rest and analgesic and anti-inflammatory agents is utilized until a diagnosis is made, when specific measures can then be instituted. The latter vary with the diagnosis, as follows.

Postural low back pain often responds to a program of strengthening exercises for abdominal and spine muscles and directions for better posture. Mild analgesic and anti-inflammatory agents and muscle relaxants are helpful. A lumbosacral corset is valuable for acute or severe symptoms. *Structural abnormalities* such as scoliosis may require corrective immobilization or surgery.

Acute symptoms due to *herniation of a nucleus pulposus* frequently require complete bed rest. Toileting should be limited to use of a bedpan or bedside commode. Rest is aided by pelvic traction, which keeps the patient from moving about excessively and relieves some of the spasm of involved muscles. Pelvic traction is used throughout the day and night. Local heat, such as Hydrocollator packs applied for 30 minutes twice daily, is helpful. Analgesic and anti-inflammatory agents relieve pain and secondary muscle spasm. Occasionally, mild narcotics are required. Muscle spasm is further decreased by the use of tranquilizers such as diazepam, 5 mg three to four times a day. The patient must understand the nature of the disease and the goals of management. Response may be slow; hospitalization to assure complete bed rest may be required. In patients with *degenerative joint disease of the spine,* a similar program of analgesic and anti-inflammatory agents, muscle relaxants, adequate rest, heat, exercise and avoidance of physical stress are all indicated. A lumbosacral corset should be prescribed when symptoms require; continued physical therapy must not be neglected.

Management of *spondylolysis and spondylolisthesis* is similar to that described for chronic degenerative joint disease. Surgical fusion with or without prior decompression may be indicated in severe cases.

Osteoporosis frequently does not respond to medical management, but a trial of presently accepted regimes is worthwhile. Theoretically, anabolic hormones are helpful. In addition, calcium lactate or gluconate, 4 gm TID, is prescribed if no contraindications exist. In severe cases, vitamin D, 50,000 units twice a week, and sodium fluoride, 22 mg BID, may be beneficial.[5] Sodium fluoride is available on an *investigative* basis only. Patients should be given a lumbodorsal corset to relieve pain and to prevent vertebral fractures resulting from excessive stress on the spine. Compression fractures are treated with bed rest for four or five days. Analgesic agents including narcotics are usually required temporarily. Progressive ambulation is permitted when pain is diminished or absent and a lumbosacral corset available. The corset should be used during the waking hours and may be needed for a long period of time or indefinitely.

In patients with metastatic *carcinoma* of the spine, x-ray therapy may relieve pain. Treatment of the primary neoplasm is indicated when feasible.

Most patients with *Paget's disease* do not require treatment; others respond to full doses of aspirin and mild analgesic drugs. Severe cases may require trials of more recent therapeutic agents including mithramycin,[6] thyrocalcitonin[7] or diphosphonates.[8] These agents are available for use in this disease on an *investigative* basis only. Their administration is limited to patients with severe disease who are being treated by physicians with a specific interest and expertise in managing this disorder.

Ankylosing spondylitis usually responds well to current programs of management (see Chapter 18). *Osteitis condensans ilii* usually responds to conservative therapy that includes salicylates, heat and rest. More potent anti-inflammatory agents such as indomethacin or phenylbutazone may be indicated occasionally.

Spondylitis of *acute infectious* etiology requires treatment with chemotherapeutic agents directed toward the causative organism. Bed rest and immobilization are often indicated. Surgery is not usually necessary because the involved vertebrae frequently fuse spontaneously. *Tuberculosis* of the spine is treated with appropriate antituberculous regimens, utilizing isoniazid, ethambutol and rifampin. Triple therapy is given for approximately six months, at which time rifampin can usually be discontinued. Therapy with isoniazid and ethambutol is continued for at least another six to twelve months. Brace immobilization is indicated to promote fusion. Surgical arthrodesis is sometimes necessary. Drainage of abscesses may be required. Fungous infectious are treated with specific antifungal agents if available. Brucellosis usually responds to tetracycline, 500 mg QID, given in combination with streptomycin, 1 gm daily for three weeks.

Vertebral epiphysitis (Scheuermann's disease), when symptomatic, is treated conservatively with rest and salicylates. Physical activity should be limited. A lumbodorsal corset or brace may be required for a prolonged period for relief of symptoms and prevention of kyphosis.

Benign *coccygodynia* due to sprain or old fracture will often respond to local injections of steroid with lidocaine. A soft foam rubber pad is advisable for prolonged sitting in patients with chronic symptoms.

Surgery of the offending tumor is usually required for pain relief in patients with *benign local neoplasms*. Orthopedic and neurosurgical consultation should be sought in most cases of *fracture* of the spine. Treatment includes immobilization and appropriate surgical procedures.

Management of *scoliosis* requires extensive evaluation of the nature and etiology of the scoliosis and the structural changes that are present. In younger patients, appropriate extraspinal or intraspinal bracing should be considered. In older patients, management is conservative and similar to that prescribed for degenerative joint disease. Management of low back pain of *visceral origin* is directed to the primary disease process.

CASE HISTORIES

History 16-1.   Herniated Nucleus Pulposus

S.C., a 40-year-old white female, was first seen in consultation in September, 1972, with a history of low back pain beginning approximately three years before. Low back symptoms occurred in intermittent episodes that had become progressively more frequent, severe, and prolonged. Pain was worse after sitting for a long period on a soft chair. Past treatment for acute attacks had included pelvic traction, bed rest, heat, and salicylates. Hospital admission was required in September, 1972, for an acute attack of severe low back pain with posterior radiation of pain to the left heel. Symptoms were worse with coughing, sneezing and straining at stool. The patient was unable to perform routine activities. Symptoms were not relieved by therapy with bed rest, pelvic traction and salicylates instituted at home.

Upon physical examination at the time of consultation, the patient was in acute distress, with pain aggravated by twisting and turning motions of the back. The left sacroiliac area was tender. Flexion of the lumbosacral spine was limited and the patient was able to sit only with pain. Straight-leg-raising was accomplished to 85° on the right side but to only 45° on the left side. Sensory examinations were normal but the left ankle jerk was diminished and slight weakness of left foot dorsiflexion was noted. The remainder of her physical evaluation including pelvic and rectal examination was unremarkable. Routine laboratory studies were normal. Erythrocyte sedimentation rate was 12 mm/hour (Wintrobe). X-rays of the lumbosacral spine revealed narrowing of the L5-S1 interspace. No evidence of spondylitis was seen. A diagnosis of acute herniation of the lumbosacral intervertebral disk was made.

The patient was placed on bed rest. Therapy with continuous pelvic traction, hot packs, aspirin and analgesic medications was instituted. Symptoms gradually improved over the next three to four days and gradual ambulation was begun. The patient improved on this program and was discharged from hospital after ten days. She was instructed in a physical therapy program of exercises to strengthen the abdominal muscles.

Discussion: The history and clinical course in this patient was typical of that seen in patients with herniated nucleus pulposus. Other causes of low back pain were excluded by appropriate clinical and laboratory studies. Most patients with this disorder will respond satisfactorily to an intensive program of conservative therapy. Although treatment at home is often effective, hospitalization is frequently necessary to provide a full program of management.

History 16-2. Spondylolysis and Spondylolisthesis

L.R., a 17-year-old white male, was first seen in consultation in December, 1973. He gave a history of mild back symptoms for several years. He tolerated these without great difficulty until he began work as a clerk in a grocery store six months prior to consultation. Pain, located in the low back, was aggravated by twisting and turning motions. There was no history of morning stiffness, sciatica, heel pain, urethritis, iritis, conjunctivitis, psoriasis or bowel symptoms. There was no family history of arthritis nor back difficulties. Other joints were asymptomatic and his general health was otherwise good. There was no history of back trauma.

On physical examination, abnormal findings were limited to the lumbosacral spine. Flexion was slightly limited and the lower lumbar area was tender. Straight-leg-raising was 85° on the right and 80° on the left. Height was 68″ and chest expansion 3½″. Laboratory studies revealed normal urinalysis and complete blood count. Erythrocyte sedimentation rate was 12 mm/hour (Wintrobe). Serum rheumatoid factor and antinuclear antibody studies were negative. Serum uric acid was 5.5 mg/100 ml. PA, lateral and oblique views of the lumbosacral spine revealed bilateral spondylolysis of L5. Anterior displacement of L5 on S1 was approximately 1 cm. Sclerotic changes were seen bilaterally in the region of the apophyseal joints of the L4-L5 articulation. Sacroiliac joints were roentgenographically normal.

Discussion: This patient complained of back pain aggravated by activity. Initial diagnostic considerations at the time of his examination included ankylosing spondylitis or lumbar disk herniation. Although symptoms were consistent with a diagnosis of spondylolysis and spondylolisthesis, ankylosing spondylitis should still be considered as a diagnostic possibility, because roentgenographic abnormalities may become apparent long after the onset of clinical symptoms in this disease. The patient was placed on a program of aspirin, 640 mg QID as needed for pain, heat, and exercises to strengthen his abdominal muscles. Use of a lumbosacral corset might be considered if he has more acute exacerbations and distress. Clinical observation and followup x-rays will be helpful in determining whether ankylosing spondylitis is present.

History 16-3. Osteoporosis

M.P., an 85-year-old white female, was first seen in consultation in December, 1973, for low back pain that had begun three days earlier. Pain was sudden in onset and radiated from the L4 area of the spine bilaterally in a transverse direction. There was no radiation to the legs. Motion made symptoms worse and walking was painful. History revealed the presence of rheumatoid arthritis of one year's duration, for which she was being treated with aspirin, 960 mg QID and prednisone, 2.5 mg QID.

On physical examination there was evidence of rheumatoid deformities involving the small joints of the hands, both wrists and both knees, with swelling and limitation of motion. The patient lay uncomfortably in bed and was fearful of moving lest she precipitate low back pain. Neurologic examination was within normal limits. There was moderate tenderness to percussion over the L4 area of the spine.

Hematocrit was 34%, white blood cell count was 4700/mm³ and the differential was normal. Serum calcium was 9.9 mg/100 ml and serum phosphorus was 3.7 mg/100 ml. Serum alkaline phosphatase was 9 King-Armstrong units (normal, 3 to 13 units). Serum electrolytes were normal. Erythrocyte sedimentation rate was 22 mm/hour (Wintrobe). Urinalysis was normal except for trace albumin; urine was negative for Bence Jones protein. Serum protein electrophoresis revealed essentially normal findings. Chest x-ray was normal. X-rays of the lumbar spine showed moderately severe diffuse osteoporosis and compression of the vertebral body of L4. A diagnosis of vertebral fracture secondary to osteoporosis was made.

The patient was placed on a program of Myochrysine therapy for her rheumatoid arthritis. Gradual decrease in steroid therapy was begun. Indomethacin, 25 mg QID with food, was added as an anti-inflammatory agent. Treatment of the osteoporosis included calcium lactate, 4 gm TID, androgenic hormones, sodium fluoride, 22 mg BID, and vitamin D, 50,000 units twice weekly. The patient was maintained on bed rest for several days until a lumbodorsal corset was obtained, at which time gradual ambulation was instituted.

Discussion: Osteoporosis is a common complication of steroid treatment in rheumatoid arthritis, likely to be seen earlier and with greater severity in older patients who already have postmenopausal or senile osteoporosis. Vigorous efforts to decrease and discontinue steroid therapy are important in the treatment of the osteoporosis. Other disorders, such as multiple myeloma, hyperparathyroidism and metastatic carcinoma, may produce a similar clinical picture. Accurate diagnosis requires exclusion of these other entities as part of the routine evaluation.

History 16-4. Multiple Myeloma

A.L., a 34-year-old white male, was first seen in January, 1969, for a routine physical examination. He had no specific complaints and system review and past medical history were unremarkable. Clinical and laboratory studies revealed no evidence of significant disease. The patient was seen again for his annual examination in January, 1970. He once again felt in good general health except for a feeling of cracking sensations in the neck and low back. Symptoms were aggravated by long hours of driving in his occupation as a salesman. Physical examination was completely negative. X-rays of the cervical and lumbosacral spine were normal. Symptoms were relieved by use of a firm seat support while driving.

The patient was seen again at annual intervals. He had no notable complaints and routine laboratory studies were normal. In April, 1973, he appeared with a complaint of moderately severe pain and spasm in the muscles of the low back with pain radiating to the left leg. System review revealed dysuria with frequency of urination. He had no eye symptoms nor symptoms in peripheral joints. Physical examination was normal except for the presence of a slightly boggy prostate gland. Lumbosacral spine motions were completely normal. Initial clinical impressions included prostatitis, degenerative disease of the lumbar spine, incomplete Reiter's syndrome, or ankylosing spondylitis.

Urinalysis was normal, hematocrit was 33%, white blood cell count was $3900/mm^3$ with 45% neutrophils, and erythrocyte sedimentation rate was 44 mm/hour (Wintrobe). Repeat leukocyte counts ranged from 2900 to $4000/mm^3$. Roentgenograms of the lumbosacral spine were reported to be within normal limits. Hematology consultation was requested to evaluate the leukopenia and anemia. Bone marrow aspiration study revealed numerous plasma cells, many of which were binucleated. Serum protein electrophoresis showed a monoclonal peak in the gamma globulin region. Roentgenographic bone survey revealed numerous punched out lesions in the skull and long bones consistent with multiple myeloma. Retrospective review of his lumbosacral spine films showed very early lytic lesions.

9

Discussion: This patient had a history of intermittent mild low back and neck pain of several years' duration. Clinical examination and laboratory studies, including x-rays, were negative for any serious underlying disorder and the patient responded to symptomatic therapy. Diagnostic considerations did not include multiple myeloma. Lumbosacral spine films were initially interpreted as normal. Hematologic abnormalities were the clue to the presence of serious systemic disease.

History 16-5. Acute Leukemia

S.R., a 24-year-old white male, was well until three weeks prior to consultation, at which time he had noted pain in the low back and thighs, and stiffness in the region of the cervical spine. Pain was aggravated by motion and was worse at night. Aspirin, 640 mg TID, provided mild symptomatic help. Approximately two weeks after the onset of symptoms, the patient developed low-grade fever and night sweats. There was no prior history of musculoskeletal symptoms. System review revealed no evidence of Raynaud's phenomenon, conjunctivitis or iritis, urethritis, colitis, or skin rash. He had been treated for gonococcal urethritis six months prior. The patient worked as a car salesman and had not left this area of the country for the previous two years.

On physical examination, blood pressure was 120/90 mm Hg. Temperature was 38° C, pulse was 90/minute, and respirations were 22/minute. The patient appeared pale and acutely ill. He lay quietly in bed and was afraid to move lest he precipitate more severe pain. The remainder of the examination was normal except for decreased mobility of the lumbar spine and tenderness over the sacroiliac joints. No peripheral joint abnormalities were noted. Muscles were strong and nontender. Clinical diagnostic considerations included ankylosing or infectious spondylitis, regional enteritis with spondylitis, vasculitis, or unusual infections such as brucellosis or trichinosis.

Hematocrit was 42%, white blood cell count was 10,200/mm^3, and erythrocyte sedimentation rate was 38 mm/hour (Wintrobe). Differential white blood count showed 49% neutrophils, 25% lymphocytes, 5% monocytes, 1% eosinophils, 15% band forms, 1 myelocyte and 4% metamyelocytes. Studies for serum rheumatoid factor and antinuclear antibody and LE cell determinations were negative. Urinalysis, serum electrolytes, fasting blood sugar, serum protein bound iodine and serum calcium and phosphorus studies were normal. Serum alkaline phosphatase was 25 King-Armstrong units (normal, 3 to 13 units). Serum creatine phosphokinase was normal. Heterophile antibody titer was negative. Brucella agglutination, cold agglutinin and febrile agglutinin studies were negative. Australia antigen was absent in the serum. Cultures of blood, throat, and urine were nonrevealing. X-rays of the chest and lumbosacral spine were normal. The patient continued to run a febrile course with temperatures up to 39° C. On the basis of the abnormal differential blood cell count, hematologic consultation was requested. Sternal marrow aspiration study revealed uniform replacement of the marrow with immature blast cells, probably granulocytic in origin. A diagnosis of acute myeloproliferative disease, probably acute granulocytic leukemia, was made.

Discussion: This patient had a history suggestive of primary musculoskeletal disease. Ankylosing spondylitis was considered on the basis of his severe low back pain and sacroiliac tenderness. Although fever is not common in ankylosing spondylitis, moderate temperature elevation occasionally occurs. Other causes of spondylitis more frequently associated with fever, such as infectious spondylitis or spondylitis associated with regional enteritis or chronic ulcerative colitis, were also considered. Leukemic involvement of the marrow produced symptoms highly suggestive of a primary rheumatic disorder.

The patient was placed on an intensive therapeutic program including prednisone, vincristine sulfate, cytosine arabinoside and cyclophosphamide. Response to therapy was poor, and other antimetabolic agents were added. The patient died from his primary disease about four months later.

History 16-6. Paget's Disease

O.B., a 65-year-old white male, was first seen in consultation in February, 1969. He gave a history of having been well until two years prior, when he noted pain in the low back. Pain was worse in the morning and was associated with moderate stiffness. Pain was not accentuated with cough, sneeze or other strain, and no sciatic radiation of pain was observed. Twisting or turning in bed during the night awakened him at times. There was no history of specific back injury. He was treated with aspirin, 640 mg QID, with little relief. Symptoms continued with slow progression in severity. Further treatment with various anti-inflammatory and analgesic agents gave limited help. The patient considered himself to be in otherwise good health. System review was negative and past medical history was noncontributory. The patient had worked as an accountant and was now retired.

On physical examination, abnormal findings were limited to the spine. The lumbar spine was slightly tender to percussion and moderately limited in all directions. Cervical spine motions were also slightly limited. Rectal examination was negative. Hematocrit was 40%, white blood cell count was 9500/mm³ with a normal differential, erythrocyte sedimentation rate was 18 mm/hour (Wintrobe), and urinalysis was normal. Serum studies for rheumatoid factor and antinuclear antibody were negative. Serum uric acid was 6.1 mg/100 ml. Serum alkaline phosphatase was 36 King-Armstrong units (normal, 3 to 13). Serum calcium, phosphorus and acid phosphatase were normal. Serum protein electrophoresis was within normal limits. Urine was negative for Bence Jones protein. Chest x-ray was normal. Roentgenograms of the lumbosacral spine and pelvis revealed Paget's changes in the pelvic bones, the proximal end of the left femur, and the third, fourth and fifth lumbar vertebrae. Bone changes were characterized by coarsening of trabecular structure. The patient was placed on therapy with aspirin, 960 mg QID, on a regular basis. Symptoms were moderately improved but later gradually increased in severity. The patient was referred to participate in an investigative program evaluating the effects of thyrocalcitonin in the management of severe Paget's disease.

Discussion: At first, degenerative joint disease in the lumbar spine was considered the most likely diagnosis for this patient. Radiologic studies revealed severe diffuse bone involvement with Paget's disease. Symptoms were consistent with this radiologic finding. Other causes of bone disease such as neoplasm, multiple myeloma and osteoporosis appeared unlikely on the basis of typical radiologic appearance, general good health and otherwise normal laboratory results.

History 16-7. Ankylosing Spondylitis

M.D., a 32-year-old white male, was first seen for evaluation in January, 1972. He gave a history of low back pain of approximately five years' duration. Low back symptoms were associated with radiation of pain from the low back to both knees. Pain radiation involved the left and right side separately, and at times both sides simultaneously. Morning stiffness lasting 15 to 30 minutes daily had been noted in the low back for the past several years. During the past year the patient had pain and stiffness of the proximal interphalangeal (PIP) joint of the right index finger, and mild stiffness of the PIP joint of the left index finger. No other joint symptoms were noted. The patient was seen by a neurosurgeon who made a clinical diagnosis of herniated disk disease. PA, lateral and oblique roentgenographic views of the lumbosacral spine were read as normal. Lumbar myelogram demonstrated a possible extradural defect at L4-L5 on the right, consistent with a herniated disk. At surgery, minimal abnormalities were noted. The patient was referred for rheumatologic evaluation when low back pain persisted. Review of preoperative x-rays of the pelvis and lumbosacral spine revealed that the sacroiliac joints had poorly defined margins and sclerotic borders. The changes were consistent with a diagnosis of ankylosing spondylitis. The patient was placed on buffered aspirin, 640 mg QID, with excellent relief of back pain. He was instructed in a full exercise program for ankylosing spondylitis. In addition, he was advised to have adequate rest and to use a firm mattress and no pillow for sleeping. The patient did well on this program.

Discussion: In this patient, low back pain due to ankylosing spondylitis was initially misdiagnosed as herniated disk disease. Chronic low back pain and morning stiffness associated with incomplete bilateral sciatica are typical findings in patients with ankylosing spondylitis. Roentgenographic changes may be minimal or absent early, in which case the diagnosis remains presumptive. The extradural defect seen on lumbar myelography in this case was equivocal in appearance and did not adequately explain the patient's symptoms.

History 16-8. Tuberculous Spondylitis

M.L., a 33-year-old Iranian male, was well until November, 1970, when he noted mild but persistent low back pain. Aching was associated with pain radiating into both upper gluteal areas. He attributed his symptoms to physical exertion associated with moving heavy furniture about his office. Low-grade symptoms continued and he was treated with mild analgesic medications. Radiologic examination of the lumbosacral spine was normal. Symptoms were not especially disabling except for occasional mild episodes, at which time he obtained relief by increased rest and regular intake of aspirin. Approximately one year after onset, symptoms became more persistent and severe. In addition to low back pain, morning stiffness lasting 15 to 30 minutes was noted. The patient was referred at that time for rheumatologic evaluation. System review was otherwise negative, except for his low back complaints. There was no associated history of other joint symptoms, Raynaud's phenomenon, psoriasis or other skin rash, iritis, urethritis, pleurisy, alopecia, oral lesions, dry mouth or eyes, or other joint symptoms. He denied symptoms of anorexia, weight loss, fever or night sweats. Past medical history was noncontributory. He had emigrated to the United States from Iran in 1967, following which he had attended college and started his own business.

Physical examination revealed mild limitation of the lumbar spine, with tenderness to percussion over the L5-S1 area. The remainder of his examination was otherwise normal. Initial diagnostic considerations included ankylosing spondylitis or degenerative disease of the intervertebral disk. Hematocrit was 44%, white blood cell count was 8600/mm³ with a normal differential, erythrocyte sedimentation rate was 27 mm/hour (Wintrobe), and urinalysis was normal. Serum electrolytes, calcium, phosphorus, glutamic oxaloacetic transaminase, and serologic test for syphilis were normal or negative. Serum protein electrophoresis showed slight elevation of gamma globulin. Serum alkaline phosphatase was normal. Studies for serum rheumatoid factor, antinuclear antibody, and antibodies to Brucella were negative.

Roentgenograms of the lumbosacral spine revealed a pathologic fracture at the anterior inferior portion of the body of the L5 vertebra. In addition, there was irregular sclerosis of the inferior aspect of the body of L5 and the superior aspect of the body of S1. The L5-S1 interspace was narrowed. A bulging mass was seen in the right parapsoas region. Tuberculin skin test was strongly positive. Skin tests for histoplasmosis and coccidioidomycosis were negative. Urine cultures for tuberculosis were negative. Culture of material obtained by closed needle aspiration of the L5 region was negative for tuberculous infection. Open biopsy of the L5-S1 area was performed by a retroperitoneal approach. Study of biopsy material revealed caseating necrosis and granulomatous inflammation of bone and fibrous connective tissue consistent with tuberculosis. Acid fast stains were negative. Positive cultures for Mycobacterium tuberculosis were subsequently reported.

Discussion: This case demonstrates the insidious manner in which tuberculous spondylitis frequently develops. Symptoms were initially attributed to physical trauma; when evaluated later, they were attributed to ankylosing spondylitis or degenerative disease of the intervertebral disks. Diagnosis was made when the disease was already in advanced state. The patient was treated with isoniazid, ethambutol and rifampin, and a Knight spinal brace was prescribed. Subsequent studies showed progressive healing of the lesion with an excellent clinical response. Rifampin was discontinued after six months and the patient was continued on isoniazid and ethambutol. Therapy for a total of one to two years is contemplated.

History 16-9. Coccygodynia

B.G., a 59-year-old white female, was first seen in consultation in September, 1971. She was in good health until approximately two months previously, when she noted severe pain and tenderness at the base of the spine when sitting. There was no history of trauma to the sacrococcygeal area and no history of joint symptoms elsewhere. Physical examination was negative except for moderate tenderness on pressure over the coccygeal area. Rectal examination revealed a moderately mobile coccyx and tenderness over the coccygeal area and paracoccygeal soft tissue attachments. Pelvic examination was normal. Roentgenograms of the lumbosacral spine were normal. A diagnosis of coccygodynia was made and steroid with lidocaine was injected into the tender area over the coccyx. The patient was advised to use soft chairs or a foam rubber cushion when sitting. The patient had excellent relief of symptoms following local steroid injection. No recurrence of symptoms over a period of several months was noted.

Discussion: This patient had symptoms consistent with coccygodynia characterized by pain in the coccygeal area on sitting and local tenderness to pressure and palpation over the coccygeal area. Frequently, such cases have a prior history of trauma. Although the diagnosis is readily made in most cases, disorders in the pelvic and rectal area and other diseases of bone must be excluded as part of the routine clinical and laboratory evaluation.

REFERENCES

1. Sigler, J. W. et al.: Clinical features of ankylosing spondylitis. Clin Orthop 74:14, 1971.
2. Schlosstein, L. et al.: High association of an HL-A antigen, W27, with ankylosing spondylitis. N Eng J Med 288:704, 1973.
3. McEwen, C. et al.: Ankylosing spondylitis and spondylitis accompanying ulcerative colitis, regional enteritis, psoriasis and Reiter's disease: A comparative study. Arth Rheum 14:291, 1971.
4. Berney, S., Goldstein, M. and Bishko, F.: Clinical and diagnostic features of tuberculous arthritis. Am J Med 53:36, 1972.

5. Jowsey, J. et al.: Effect of combined therapy with sodium fluoride, vitamin D and calcium in osteoporosis. Am J Med 53:43, 1972.
6. Condon, J. R. et al.: Treatment of Paget's disease of bone with mithramycin. Brit Med J 1:421, 1971.
7. Haddad, J. F., Birge, S. J. and Avioli, L. V.: Effects of prolonged thyrocalcitonin administration on Paget's disease of bone. N Eng J Med 283:549, 1970.
8. Altman, R. D. et al.: Influence of disodium etidronate on clinical and laboratory manifestations of Paget's disease of bone (osteitis deformans). N Eng J Med 289:1379, 1973.

Chapter 17

THE PAINFUL FOOT

Foot pain of musculoskeletal origin is a common cause of disability. It is frequently the primary complaint of the patient coming into the physician's office. Although often benign and seemingly unimportant, the symptoms are distressing to the patient. Careful study and appropriate therapy to relieve symptoms can be rewarding.

DIFFERENTIAL DIAGNOSIS

The differential diagnosis of foot pain varies with the area of the foot involved. The following diagnostic considerations are divided on the basis of location of symptoms, proceeding from the anterior to the posterior aspect of the foot.

Painful Swollen Great Toe (First Metatarsophalangeal Joint)

Acute gouty arthritis characteristically produces acute pain, tenderness and swelling of the first metatarsophalangeal (MTP) joint at the base of the great toe. Not all gouty attacks, however, occur in the big toe. In many patients, the first attack occurs in another joint such as the tarsal area, ankle or knee. Similarly, other disorders may cause acute painful swelling of the great toe. A diagnosis of gout, although primarily suspected when acute symptoms develop in this joint, should not be made without considering other possible diagnoses.

The patient with acute gouty arthritis usually gives a rather characteristic history. Acute onset occurring during the night is common. The pain may be so exquisite that even movement of the bed covers or someone walking heavily about the room may increase the already severe throbbing pain. As swelling and inflammation progress, cutaneous changes of inflammation are noted. Skin desquamation occurs as the attack reaches its crest or begins to wane. The inflammation often simulates cellulitis and misdiagnosis is common. On physical examination the inflammation is obvious. Pain and tenderness in gout are likely to be more pronounced medially, in contrast to rheumatoid arthritis, in which tenderness is often maximal at the inferior aspect of the joint.

Pseudogout is characterized by calcifications in hyaline or fibroarticular cartilage and the presence of calcium pyrophosphate crystals in synovial fluid. Acute attacks of crystal-induced arthritis are common. The most common site of attack is the knee. Podagra, or first MTP joint involvement, occurs much less frequently than in true gout.

Rheumatoid arthritis may produce acute inflammation of the metatarsophalangeal joints. Although the first MTP joint is frequently involved, other MTP joints are often affected simultaneously. This is in contrast to gout, in which the acute attack is usually localized to the first MTP joint alone. Acute inflammation of the toes is characteristic of the episodic form of rheumatoid arthritis (see Chapter 8). Acute attacks of pain resolve over several days. A clinical syndrome similar to episodic rheumatoid arthritis is *palindromic rheumatism* (see Chapter 8), which also is characterized by acute attacks of arthritis. Because several connective tissue diseases may simulate palindromic rheumatism during their early phases, diagnosis depends on continued observation.

Acute joint symptoms may result from *trauma*. This often poses a problem in differential diagnosis, because both acute gout and rheumatoid arthritis may be precipitated by trauma. In patients with arthritis due to trauma alone, pain usually develops immediately after the injury and symptoms are proportional to the extent of the injury. In patients in whom gout or rheumatoid inflammation are precipitated by trauma, pain is usually delayed in onset and the severity of symptoms is out of proportion to that anticipated from the injury.

Cellulitis may simulate acute arthritis because it also is characterized by pain, tenderness, increased warmth and swelling. Search for local entry sites of infection should be carried out if this diagnosis is suspected. Blood cultures are frequently positive as a supportive corollary finding. Symptoms respond to appropriate antibiotic therapy based on culture and sensitivity studies.

Pain and swelling in the first MTP joint due to *osteoarthritis* are extremely common; however, symptoms are low-grade and chronic in contrast to the foregoing diseases. Ill-fitting shoes or mild trauma aggravate the symptoms. X-rays reveal joint space narrowing, bony sclerosis and osteophyte formation. Treatment is usually conservative; well-fitting bunion-last shoes and mild anti-inflammatory drugs are prescribed. Surgery is indicated in patients who do not respond to a conservative program. Excellent relief is anticipated.

Occasionally, acute symptoms may occur with osteoarthritis of the great toe when there is acute inflammation of the overlying bursa. The bursa is usually readily outlined and fluid can be obtained on aspiration. Response to injection of local steroid with lidocaine into the bursa is good.

Symptoms Involving Interphalangeal Joints

Any form of arthritis that affects peripheral joints may involve inter-phalangeal joints of the toes. Involvement of these joints is particularly characteristic of *psoriatic arthritis,* the arthritis of *ulcerative colitis* and *regional enteritis,* and the arthritis of *Reiter's syndrome.* The history should specifically include questions concerning skin rash consistent with psoriasis, chronic diarrheal symptoms, or evidence of the typical triad of arthritis, urethritis and conjunctivitis seen in Reiter's syndrome.

Symptoms Involving Other Metatarsophalangeal Joints

These joints may also be involved in any of the systemic arthritides that produce peripheral joint symptoms. *Rheumatoid arthritis* classically involves these joints and may produce severe disability early in the course of the disease. Hammer-toes and subluxation of the joints are common. In addition to the usual systemic management, the use of transverse metatarsal pads inside the shoes or transverse metatarsal bars on the soles aids relief. Pads are usually tried first, because if they give relief, they can be conveniently transferred to various pairs of shoes. If the patient does not respond, transverse metatarsal bars are then prescribed. These often provide more effective relief but have to be placed on each pair of shoes separately. Local injection of steroids is valuable when one or two joints are especially bothersome.

Metatarsal Pain

Morton's metatarsalgia produces severe cramping pains in the anterior part of the foot. Pain is usually precipitated by weight-bearing and walking. The patient gets relief by removing the shoe and rubbing the toes. The syndrome occurs most frequently in the third and fourth interspaces. Although originally attributed to pinching of the plantar nerve between the metatarsal heads, the syndrome may result from ischemia of the plantar nerve induced by traumatic degeneration of the plantar digital artery. Ischemia may eventually lead to fibrosis and neuroma formation. In uncomplicated Morton's metatarsalgia, pain occurs only on weight-bearing and use. Constant pain suggests the presence of a neuroma, in which case a mass often can be palpated between the metatarsal heads when the heads have been squeezed together.

Therapy of simple metatarsalgia is conservative. Well-fitting shoes and a transverse metatarsal pad or metatarsal bar should be prescribed. Local injection of the tender area with steroids and lidocaine provides relief for acute symptoms. In patients in whom the diagnosis of neuroma is fairly

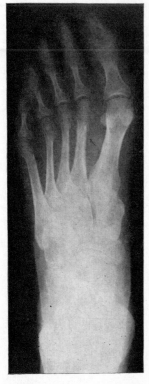

Figure 17-1. Fatigue fracture, second metatarsal bone of left foot. Fracture with callus formation was not visible until several weeks after onset of foot pain.

well corroborated and who do not respond to conservative measures, excision of the neuroma should be considered.

Fracture of a metatarsal bone near its neck may occur in the absence of definitive trauma, the so-called *fatigue* or *march fracture*. Fracture most often involves the necks of the second or third metatarsals. The propensity for this site may be related to congenital shortening of the first metatarsal bone, since dorsiflexion then occurs across the necks of the second and third metatarsals. This type of fracture is not uncommon following continual stress on long military marches; thus the name "march fracture." Tenderness is followed by swelling due to callus formation in healing. Roentgenograms of the foot are required for diagnosis, although the fracture may not be evident until days or weeks following onset of symptoms (Fig. 17-1). Periodic re-examination should be performed if the diagnosis is suspected. The fracture is treated by immobilizing the limb in a plaster cast that extends up to the knee until healing.

Sudeck's atrophy (post-traumatic osteoporosis) is closely related to shoulder-hand syndrome seen in the upper extremity (see Chapter 14). Of unknown etiology, it is characterized by a vasomotor disturbance with hyperemia and atrophy of bone. Precipitating causes include trauma, which

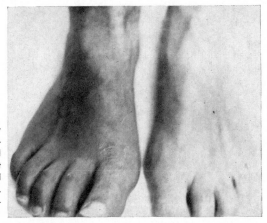

Figure 17-2. Sudeck's atrophy (post-traumatic osteoporosis). Erythema and edema of the right foot were associated with severe pain. (Courtesy, Dr. F. Bishko)

is often minimal, local infections, or neoplasm. Pain, edema and local heat are the earliest manifestations (Fig. 17-2). Later, the skin becomes cold, cyanotic and atrophic. Severe secondary trophic changes eventually ensue. Roentgenographic studies show a patchy bone atrophy after four to six weeks (Fig. 17-3). Later, the osteoporosis becomes diffuse.

Mild cases respond to aspirin, analgesic agents and physical therapy. Contrast baths, warm soaks, or sometimes cold applications are particularly helpful. More severe cases require a trial of systemic corticosteroids such as prednisone in a dose of 20 to 40 mg a day. As symptoms are relieved, the dose is gradually diminished and then discontinued over a period of six to seven weeks. In patients in whom steroids have failed or are contraindicated, a trial of lumbar sympathetic blocks repeated every other day for a series of four to eight injections may be effective. Lumbar sympathectomy should be considered when local blocks are only temporarily successful.

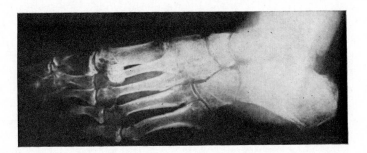

Figure 17-3. Sudeck's atrophy. Roentgenogram reveals osteoporotic changes throughout tarsal, metatarsal and phalangeal areas.

Tarsal Pain

Sudeck's atrophy (see preceding discussion) frequently involves the tarsal as well as metatarsal bones.

Various forms of *flat feet* (pes planus) cause pain in the tarsal area. Weakness, aching and cramps may occur. Flat feet can be classified as flexible (flaccid) type with normal peroneal muscles, rigid type with normal peroneals, and rigid type with spastic peroneals (peroneal spastic flat foot). In all cases, the longitudinal arch is depressed in association with medial prominence of the foot. In the flexible type, the longitudinal arch is depressed with weight-bearing and assumes a normal shape at rest. The joints of the foot may be hypermobile and the Achilles tendon may be short. This type of flat foot is often asymptomatic, but may become painful during adolescence. Conservative therapy utilizing arch supports and corrective exercises is usually beneficial. Heat or contrast baths are helpful. In more severe cases, corrective shoes and medial heel wedges are prescribed. Surgery, including tendon transfers and arthrodesis, is occasionally required. Flexible flat foot is common in blacks and the American Indian; in these individuals, this condition can almost be considered physiologic. Symptoms related to anatomy are uncommon and no specific therapy is usually required.

Rigid flat foot with normal peroneal muscles may result secondary to infectious or rheumatoid arthritis or following injury to the tarsal areas. Triple arthrodesis is probably the most satisfactory form of therapy. Rigid flat foot with spastic peroneal muscles is most often due to congenital fusion (coalition) of the tarsal bones. Other cases result secondary to infectious or rheumatoid arthritis or traumatic malalignment of joints. Joint motion is limited and the peroneal muscles are spastic. The spasm probably represents reflex muscle spasm due to pain. Initial therapy should be conservative; arch supports alone are often effective. Immobilization in a plaster cast may be required for management of acute painful episodes. Excision of bony bars early is helpful in certain forms of congenital coalition syndrome. In other cases, treatment by triple arthrodesis must be considered.

Severe pain in the tarsal area may be due to *neuropathic (Charcot) joints.* Although any chronic neuropathy, such as that seen in tabes dorsalis or syringomyelia, may be the cause of this disorder, diabetic neuropathy is the most common etiology. Pain on walking is the earliest symptom; later, pain occurs even at rest. The tarsal area is warm, tender, and swollen. X-rays reveal extensive disorganization of joint structures in the area of involvement. Early changes are characterized by severe bone atrophy; later changes reveal a florid osteoarthritis. Periosteal reaction is common.

Heel Pain

Plantar fascitis is a common cause of heel pain. It may be localized or systemic in origin. The etiology of localized fascitis is primarily mechanical, the result of repeated microtrauma. The origin and insertion of the plantar fascia are such that it acts as a bowstring for the foot. Tension on the fascia exerts a pull at its origin, which eventually leads to an inflammatory periostitis at its attachment to the os calcis. Calcaneal spur formation results from stimulation of bone; accordingly, the calcaneal spur may be secondary to inflammation rather than a primary abnormality.

Pain is the primary symptom of localized fascitis. Physical examination reveals a tender spot about two inches from the point of the heel. Ossification of the fascia in the form of spur formation may be present on x-ray. Calcaneal spurs are usually asymptomatic unless associated with active fascitis. However, large spurs may contribute secondarily to pain by applying pressure on the plantar tissues.

Fascitis occurs as a manifestation of systemic diseases such as rheumatoid arthritis, ankylosing spondylitis (Fig. 17-4) and Reiter's syndrome. Symptoms may be most severe at the heels or they may be diffuse. The periosteal reaction is often less dense than that seen in idiopathic fascitis; a fluffy periostitis on x-ray is characteristic.

Calcaneal epiphysitis, a form of osteochondritis, usually occurs in younger patients. The child complains of pain at the back of the heel and usually limps to relieve distress. X-rays reveal areas of osteoporosis interspersed with areas of increased bone density. The disease is usually self-limited and responds to conservative symptomatic measures. In particular,

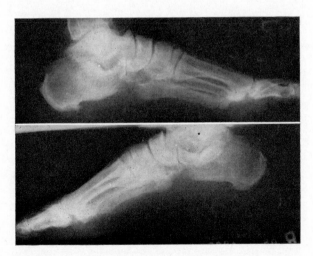

Figure 17-4. Periosteal reaction with new bone formation involves the attachments of the plantar fascia and Achilles tendon in this patient with ankylosing spondylitis.

rest, avoidance of excess weight-bearing, the use of foam rubber heel cushions, and mild anti-inflammatory medications are beneficial.

Inflammation of the bursa underlying the Achilles tendon (*Achilles bursitis*) or inflammation of the tendon itself (*Achilles tendinitis*) causes pain at the back of the heel. Inflammation may result from systemic disease or from local trauma, such as that caused by ill-fitting shoes. Diagnostic studies to rule out systemic connective tissue disease should be performed when symptoms are severe and persistent. In young males, symptoms in this area are often an early manifestation of ankylosing spondylitis.

Post-traumatic osteoporosis (Sudeck's atrophy) may cause heel pain, although, as noted earlier, pain usually occurs throughout the foot. *Paget's disease* is an uncommon cause of heel pain, but it may cause pain at night and after weight-bearing.

Ischemic vascular disease with claudication may cause foot pain. Symptoms are characteristically associated with walking and are relieved readily by standing or sitting. Physical examination demonstrates severely diminished or absent pedal pulses. Trophic changes associated with ischemia are often present. Laboratory evidence of diabetes mellitus or elevated serum lipids is frequently noted.

Neuropathies cause foot pain with burning and dysesthesia. They are usually related to systemic disorders, which should be sought by appropriate clinical and laboratory studies.

CASE HISTORIES

History 17-1. Gout

S.M.N., a 38-year-old white male, gave a history of joint pains beginning in February, 1970. At that time, on the second day of a skiing excursion, he was awakened during the night by moderately severe pain in the left tarsal area. There was no history of specific trauma. Roentgenographic study of the left foot taken the following morning was normal. He was treated with heat and a walking splint. Symptoms resolved after approximately ten days. He was completely asymptomatic until January, 1972, when he noted tenderness and slight swelling of the left tarsal area several hours following a game of paddleball. He attributed symptoms to a slight twisting injury suffered during the game. Pain and tenderness persisted. Roentgenograms of the foot performed the next morning were normal. Symptoms resolved after several days.

In June, 1973, he noted acute onset of pain in the dorsum of the right tarsal area. There was no history of trauma and the patient had not recently engaged in any athletic activities. Symptoms resolved after several days, but recurred on July 5th, 1973, when he was awakened with soreness and tenderness in the right tarsal area. He attributed his symptoms to a slight twist of the foot suffered while walking to his office that day. The patient was first seen for evaluation at this time. The history was negative for joint symptoms elsewhere. There was no history of renal stones nor family history of gout. The patient considered himself to be in generally good health and system review was otherwise negative. Physical examination was completely normal except for tenderness and a slight increase in temperature over the dorsum of the tarsal area of the right foot. Laboratory studies showed normal hematocrit, white blood cell count and differential, erythrocyte sedimentation rate and urinalysis. Serum rheumatoid factor and antinuclear antibody studies were negative. Serum uric acid was 11.7 mg/100 ml. Repeat serum uric acid study several days later revealed a level of 10.9 mg/100 ml. Twenty-four-hour urinary uric acid excretion was 650 mg on a normal diet. Roentgenograms of both feet were normal. A diagnosis of gouty diathesis with gouty arthritis was made and interval therapy with probenecid and colchicine was instituted.

Discussion: Gouty symptoms in this patient were interpreted for a long while as nonspecific reactions to trauma. Symptoms were disproportionate in severity to the trauma sustained and were usually delayed in onset for several hours after trauma occurred. Gout should be excluded in young males with a history of chronic recurrent tarsalgia or metatarsalgia, particularly when severe pain occurs as a delayed response to mild trauma.

History 17-2. Fatigue Fracture

H.H., a 46-year-old white male, had had rheumatoid arthritis for approximately 20 years. Past therapy included aspirin, 960 mg QID, indomethacin, 25 mg TID, and, for the previous six years, prednisone in an average dose of 2.5 mg TID. When the patient was first seen in referral in December, 1969, examination revealed rheumatoid swelling and deformities involving the small joints of the hands, left elbow, right knee, and left ankle. Serum rheumatoid factor was positive in a titer of 1:160. Other studies for complicating illness or other forms of connective tissue disease were negative or normal. Hydroxychloroquine, 200 mg BID, was added to his previous therapeutic program. This agent was discontinued after six months when no improvement in symptoms was noted. Gold therapy was instituted but was discontinued when severe bone marrow depression occurred at a total gold dose of 640 mg. Efforts to reduce his prednisone dosage were unsuccessful.

The patient was seen in October, 1972, with the chief complaint of severe tenderness and pain at the lateral aspect of the right foot. This symptom, of relatively recent origin, was aggravated by weight-bearing. There was no history of acute trauma. Examination revealed tenderness and slight swelling at the base of the fifth metatarsal bone. Differential diagnosis included rheumatoid changes at the tarsal-fifth metatarsal area, tendinitis of peroneal tendons, or fatigue fracture. Roentgenograms of both feet revealed moderate periarticular osteoporosis and marginal erosions at the metatarsophalangeal joints, unchanged from previous findings. There was no evidence of fracture. The patient was seen in consultation with an orthopedic consultant who recommended a short-leg plaster cast for relief of symptoms. Following removal of the cast three weeks later, tenderness and pain in the same area were unchanged. Repeat roentgenographic examination now revealed a fracture at the base of the fifth metatarsal bone with fragments in excellent position. The patient was treated with plaster cast immobilization for an additional six weeks. Good callus formation and relief of symptoms were subsequently noted.

Discussion: The clinical features of this patient's foot problem were consistent with fatigue fracture. As in this case, roentgenographic changes consistent with definitive fracture may not develop until several weeks after onset of symptoms. Osteoporotic changes related both to rheumatoid arthritis and to long-term corticosteroid therapy were probably associated with the development of fracture in this patient.

Part III
MANAGEMENT

Chapter 18

SPECIFIC TREATMENT OF COMMON RHEUMATOLOGIC DISORDERS

RHEUMATOID ARTHRITIS

Rheumatoid arthritis is a systemic disease that involves not only joints but other areas of the body. A multidisciplinary approach to therapy is required if all facets of disease manifestations and effects are to be adequately managed.

Systemic and Emotional Rest

Bed rest for a prolonged period of the day is required during acute phases of the disease. In patients with subacute or chronic disease, rest periods of 45 to 60 minutes following lunch and 30 to 45 minutes following supper are helpful. Emotional as well as physical rest is important. The home and family situation should be examined to allow maximal emotional support. In very severe cases, hospitalization is necessary for adequate physical and emotional rest.

Physical and Occupational Therapy and Supportive Appliances

A regular program of physical and occupational therapy (see Chapter 19) should be specifically prescribed for each patient. Adequate detailed instructions for use of heat and exercises must be given and the importance of the program stressed. Canes, crutches or walkers should be utilized when limited weight-bearing is desirable. Splints are helpful for pain relief and prevention of deformities. Periodic conferences by the physicians and allied health professionals involved in the patient's care are valuable. Past treatment programs can be evaluated and future therapeutic goals outlined.

Drug Therapy

Initial drug treatment is begun with aspirin administered on a regular basis in properly divided dosage. A reasonable starting dose is 640 mg, four to five times daily. The dose is gradually increased until symptoms are relieved or toxicity develops, such as tinnitus or impaired hearing. Determination of blood salicylate levels aids management when response to the usual doses is inadequate; a level of 20 to 30 mg% should be sought for clinical effectiveness. Hepatic abnormalities have been noted in association with high blood salicylate levels.[1] These changes have not been clinically significant in most cases, but close monitoring is advisable.

Aspirin is best tolerated when taken with food or antacids. For patients with aspirin intolerance, certain salicylate preparations such as enteric-coated aspirin, aspirin with insoluble alkali, choline salicylate liquid, time-release salicylate preparations, or salicylsalicylic acid may be better tolerated. Analgesic therapy with propoxyphene hydrochloride (Darvon), 65 mg, ethoheptazine citrate (Zactane), 75 mg, or acetominophen, 300 mg, given on a regular or PRN basis is a helpful adjunct. For patients with aspirin allergy, it may be necessary to use large amounts of analgesic agents or to proceed to more potent anti-inflammatory preparations.

If patients do not respond adequately to salicylates in full dosage, other anti-inflammatory agents should be considered. Indomethacin is helpful in some patients, but side effects unfortunately are common. An initial dose of 25 mg BID with food can be gradually increased to a total daily intake of 100 to 150 mg in divided doses. Higher doses have been used but the subsequent increase in side reactions is not worth the mild gain in therapeutic effect. Occipital headaches, gastrointestinal upset, peptic ulcers, aggravation of colitis, and vague psychic reactions occur. Initial observations of ocular abnormalities[2] have not been confirmed.[3]

Phenylbutazone has a good anti-inflammatory effect in many patients. It is particularly valuable in treating acute episodes because side reactions are minimal when this agent is used for a short period of time. A dose of 100 mg QID with food is given for several days; it is then gradually decreased and discontinued over 7 to 10 days. The drug is less attractive for long-term use because it may cause severe bone marrow depression. It should be used with caution in patients with a history of peptic ulcer disease, and it may cause fluid retention in patients with congestive heart failure. Phenylbutazone accentuates the prothrombin-lowering effect of coumarin agents and should be used cautiously in patients receiving such medications. Oxyphenbutazone (Tandearil), an almost identical drug, is used in similar fashion and identical dosage. [Ibuprofen (Motrin). See Addendum, p. 279.]

In patients who require additional therapy, the use of antimalarial drugs, such as hydroxychloroquine (Plaquenil) should be considered. Hydroxychloroquine is begun in a dose of 200 mg BID. Response is slow in onset; the drug should be given a three- to six-month trial before being discontinued for lack of effect. When improvement occurs, the dose is decreased to 200 mg once daily. Side effects, such as gastrointestinal upset, rash, headaches, nightmares, and psychic disorientation, may occur but are uncommon. Leukopenia sometimes occurs. The toxic reaction of major concern is visual impairment due to the effect of the drug on the retina.[4] Transient changes in visual acuity that occur early in treatment usually resolve and are not important. A baseline ophthalmologic examination should be performed at the outset of treatment and repeated at six-month intervals for the first several years. After two or three years, eye examinations at four-month intervals are advisable. A complete evaluation includes slit lamp and funduscopic examination and studies of visual fields, visual acuity and color vision. A defect in visual fields to a 3-mm red dot is the earliest manifestation of toxicity; visual loss is usually still reversible at this stage. Visual field cuts to a white dot occur late and reversal of visual loss is less likely. Visual abnormalities may worsen even after the drug is discontinued, owing to its prolonged persistence in body tissues. Antimalarial medications are contraindicated in patients with psoriasis because psoriatic lesions may be exacerbated.

Gold therapy is effective in inducing partial or complete remission in many patients with rheumatoid arthritis.[5,6] The most frequently used preparations are gold sodium thiomalate (Myochrysine), gold sodium thioglucose (Solganal), and gold sodium thiosulfate. Gold sodium thiomalate and gold sodium thiosulfate are prepared as aqueous solutions; gold sodium thioglucose is prepared as a suspension in oil. All three preparations can be used satisfactorily to initiate and maintain therapy. A leukocyte count, differential white blood cell count, hematocrit, platelet count and urinalysis should be obtained for baseline study and repeated at weekly intervals for the first 15 to 20 injections. After that time, laboratory studies may be performed following every second or third injection. The gold preparations are administered by intramuscular injection. Aqueous solutions may be given into the deltoid or gluteus muscle regions; oily suspensions are injected into the gluteal region only. Ten mg of gold salt is given the first week, 25 mg the second week, and 50 mg weekly thereafter.

Gold therapy is stopped in the presence of clinical side reactions or untoward laboratory abnormalities. Prior to each gold injection, the patient is queried for the presence of stomatitis, metallic taste in the mouth, itching of the skin, rash or diarrhea. Nitritoid vasomotor reactions, characterized by light-headedness, flushing, and syncope, are an unusual type of side reaction that occurs particularly with gold sodium thiomalate. Sometimes, mild reactions of this type are eliminated by using a lower dose of the drug. Symptoms may decrease and disappear after five or six injections. When severe, other gold preparations less likely to cause this reaction should be substituted.

Laboratory evidence of toxicity includes leukopenia, eosinophilia, thrombocytopenia, proteinuria, or the presence of formed elements in the urine. Symptoms may improve after a total dose of 600 to 800 mg of gold salt has been administered. At least 1 gm of gold salt should be given as a therapeutic trial. If improvement occurs, the maintenance dose can be administered at two-week intervals for several injections, then every three-weeks, and finally once a month to maintain remission. Gold injections are reinstituted at a more frequent interval if exacerbation occurs. Contraindications to gold administration are a history of prior gold reaction, systemic lupus erythematosus, severe hepatic or renal disease, and blood dyscrasias. Mild toxicity is treated by stopping gold therapy. More severe reactions are treated with prednisone in a dose of 20 to 60 mg daily, depending on the type and severity of the reaction. Chelating agents, such as dimercapto-propanol (British anti-Lewisite) or D-penicillamine which increase gold excretion, should be added in cases of severe toxicity.

Systemic corticosteroid agents are utilized at various stages in the treatment of rheumatoid arthritis, depending on disease severity, socioeconomic needs and response to other agents. In general, systemic corticosteroids should be avoided whenever possible, due to the many severe toxic side effects associated with their use. When utilized, the lowest dose possible should be used for the shortest period of time. Maximal doses for long-term use vary with the age and sex of the patient. If possible, long-term use should be limited to 10 mg per day in adult males, 7.5 mg per day in premenopausal females and 5 mg per day in menopausal females. Alternate day therapy may be associated with fewer side reactions[7]; unfortunately, it is therapeutically effective in a relatively small number of patients.

Although systemic corticosteroids should be utilized with caution in patients with rheumatoid arthritis, intra-articular administration of these agents is frequently useful and has limited hazard when used judiciously (see Chapter 20).

Systemic immunosuppressive agents such as chlorambucil, cyclophosphamide,[8] and azathioprine[9] are reported beneficial in protracted progressive disease. *The use of these agents remains investigative.* Even on an investigative basis, their use is limited to patients with chronic progressive disease who have not responded to other agents, or in whom other agents have been tried and are now contraindicated due to toxicity.

Surgical Management

Orthopedic surgery plays a major role in multidisciplinary treatment. Synovectomy is valuable early in the course of the disease to relieve pain and swelling when the inflammatory process has not been controlled adequately by medical means. Surgical procedures for more advanced disease include release of contractures, resection osteotomy, arthrodesis (fusion) and arthroplasty. Total hip prostheses are a notable advance in the treatment of severely involved hips. Total knee prostheses are being used with increased frequency, but results are less predictable and complete.

ANKYLOSING SPONDYLITIS

Management of ankylosing spondylitis involves a combined program of physical therapy and drugs. Exercises are directed toward maintaining a straight posture and preventing flexion deformity of the spine. Spinal hyperextension and breathing exercises are performed for 10 or 15 repetitions twice daily. Heat in the form of a warm tub bath or shower relieves pain and stiffness and allows the patient to exercise more effectively.

Drug therapy begins with aspirin, 640 to 960 mg QID. If necessary, the dosage is gradually increased to obtain therapeutic blood salicylate levels of 20 to 30 mg%. In patients whose response is inadequate, indomethacin, 100 to 150 mg daily in equally divided doses with food, is added. In more severe cases, phenylbutazone or oxyphenbutazone are often effective. An initial dose of 100 mg QID of either drug is instituted; the dosage is gradually decreased to the minimal daily maintenance dose required to produce reasonable relief of symptoms. A dose of 300 mg daily should rarely be exceeded on a long-term basis. Frequently, 100 to 200 mg daily is adequate for routine administration, with increases to 200 to 400 mg daily for acute episodes. Indomethacin should be discontinued when phenylbutazone or oxyphenbutazone are used, but a baseline dosage of aspirin should be maintained. In many patients, aspirin alone in adequate dosage will suffice to bring satisfactory comfort most of the time. Indomethacin or phenylbutazone can then be added for short periods to treat acute episodes. Oral steroids, such as prednisone, 2.5 mg TID, are effective in many patients. These agents can be tried if the other programs are inadequate or poorly tolerated. Roentgen therapy to the spine, once used with some frequency, has generally been abandoned due to associated complications of bone marrow aplasia or leukemia.

PSORIATIC ARTHRITIS

Psoriatic arthritis sometimes parallels the course of cutaneous lesions. Vigorous therapy of the psoriasis with crude coal tar and ultraviolet light or with local steroid creams and ointments is indicated. Mild cases of arthritis respond satisfactorily to the use of aspirin in full therapeutic dosage. Indomethacin, a particularly effective drug in psoriatic arthritis, should be added when the response to aspirin alone is inadequate. Daily doses of 100 to 150 mg administered in equally divided doses with food are often beneficial. Antimalarial drugs are contraindicated because they may aggravate the psoriatic rash and cause exfoliation.

Gold therapy may be considered but its effectiveness is less consistent in psoriatic arthritis than in rheumatoid arthritis. In addition, toxic skin rashes caused by gold may be difficult to differentiate from the basic psoriatic process. Systemic corticosteroid therapy is beneficial in many patients, but its use should be restricted to patients with severe progressive disease. Folic acid antagonists such as methotrexate[10] and purine antagonists such as azathioprine[9] and 6-mercaptopurine[11] are beneficial in severe uncontrolled cases of psoriasis and psoriatic arthritis. Serious side reactions preclude their use in all but the more advanced cases. Methotrexate in a single oral dose of 10 to 15 mg once a week is often effective. Hepatotoxicity and pulmonary fibrosis are major side reactions. Continued use of this drug requires periodic liver biopsy to detect early changes not evident on routine liver function laboratory profiles. Azathioprine, 2.0 to 3.0 mg/kg/day, or 6-mercaptopurine, 1.0 to 1.5 mg/kg/day, are effective alternatives. Physical therapy programs are important in the management of articular changes, as described in patients with rheumatoid arthritis.

GOUT AND PSEUDOGOUT

Gout

Management of gout is divided into treatment of acute gouty attacks and interval treatment designed to prevent recurrent attacks and chronic tophaceous gout.

Treatment of Acute Attacks. Although colchicine is regarded as specific for gout, it may be somewhat effective in other forms of arthritis. With onset of symptoms, one 0.6-mg tablet is given every hour until symptoms are relieved or until gastrointestinal side effects of nausea, vomiting or diarrhea occur. A maximum of eight to ten tablets is administered. Gastrointestinal side effects, if they occur, are usually controlled with paregoric or diphenoxylate hydrochloride. Intravenous colchicine is associated with fewer gastrointestinal side reactions; for this reason, intravenous administration is preferred when gastrointestinal symptoms are particularly to be avoided, as after surgery. A dose of 2 mg is given initially, followed by 1 mg at eight-hour intervals if needed; a daily dose of 4 mg should not be exceeded. Colchicine solutions are highly irritating to veins and soft tissues. The dose should be diluted with 10 cc of sterile saline and administered slowly. Infiltration of soft tissues around the vein should be avoided.

Phenylbutazone or oxyphenbutazone are highly effective in the treatment of acute gouty attacks. Four hundred to 600 mg a day in divided doses is given for several days, followed by gradually decreasing doses over six to eight days. These agents are contraindicated in patients with active ulcer disease. They should be used cautiously in patients with congestive heart failure because salt and water retention is a troublesome side reaction.

Indomethacin is frequently effective in the treatment of acute gout, but results are somewhat less consistent than those seen with colchicine or phenylbutazone. A dose of 150 to 200 mg daily in divided doses with food is recommended. Side reactions are common but are usually mild.

ACTH gel may be used in the management of acute attacks. The drug is given in a daily intramuscular dose of 40 to 80 mg for two or three days. Oral corticosteroids such as prednisone, 20 to 30 mg daily in divided doses, are often efficacious. The daily dose is then gradually decreased over a period of four to seven days. Acute gouty episodes following cessation of steroid therapy are not uncommon. It is wise to place the patient on maintenance colchicine, 0.6 mg BID, when the prednisone is discontinued. Aspiration of the involved joint followed by intra-articular injection of steroid with lidocaine is an effective therapeutic alternative when larger joints are involved.

Prevention of Recurrent Acute Attacks and Chronic Tophaceous Gout (Interval Therapy). Chronic manifestations of gout can be prevented by treatment programs that reduce the body pool of urates and serum uric acid. Indications for use of a preventive interval program include the presence of tophi, recurrent acute gouty arthritis or significant asymptomatic hyperuricemia. The level at which asymptomatic hyperuricemia should be treated is not universally agreed upon. Consistent hyperuricemia above 9 mg% probably deserves treatment because acute attacks of gouty arthritis and renal calculi are common. Patients who overexcrete uric acid similarly deserve initiation of an interval program, irrespective of the height of the serum uric acid, since many of these patients will develop renal stones.

In routine cases of gout uncomplicated by urate overexcretion or renal stones, probenecid is the treatment of choice. This drug has a proven record of safety and efficacy and can be taken lifelong with minimal hazard. Treatment is initiated in a dose of 0.5 gm daily. Dosage is increased by 0.5 gm weekly until the serum uric acid level, checked at periodic intervals, is brought into a normal range. Not all patients should be treated with a standard daily dosage, since the dosage required for adequate control varies. At times, a dose of 2 or 3 gm per day is required for adequate results. Sulfinpyrazone (Anturane) is an alternative uricosuric agent for use in patients who are intolerant or allergic to probenecid. One hundred milligrams are approximately equivalent to 0.5 gm of probenecid. Patients being treated with probenecid or sulfinpyrazone should avoid salicylate-containing compounds, which nullify the action of the uricosuric agents.

Allopurinol (Zyloprim), a xanthine-oxidase inhibitor, reduces serum uric acid by reducing uric acid formation. The fall in serum uric acid is accompanied by a drop in urinary uric acid excretion. Although it is a relatively safe drug, side effects are more serious than those occurring with uricosuric agents. Side reactions include fever, skin rash, elevations of serum glutamic oxaloacetic transaminase (SGOT), bone marrow depression, vasculitis and diarrhea. Xanthine stones, secondary to increased xanthine levels, may occasionally occur. Muscle deposits of hypoxanthine, xanthine, and oxypurinol have been described but no serious toxic effects on muscle have been reported. Long-term side effects resulting from inhibition of purine metabolism by this agent are theoretically hazardous; fortunately, none have yet been noted. Despite these considerations, allopurinol is a valuable and useful drug when used in appropriate situations. Indications for the use of allopurinol in the interval treatment of gout include allergy to the usual uricosuric agents, a history of uric acid stones, presence of renal impairment, or urinary uric acid overexcretion. In these situations, allopurinol is the drug of choice. It is given in a starting dose of 100 mg BID. The dose is gradually increased at increments of 100 mg every two to four weeks until the serum uric acid is brought to a normal level. Most patients are controlled on a total daily dose of 300 to 600 mg. The drug has a long duration of action and may be given in one daily morning dose.

Colchicine, 0.6 mg once or twice daily, should be given to patients who are beginning therapy with uricosuric agents or allopurinol, because onset of therapy with these agents may be associated with an increased frequency of acute gouty attacks. Colchicine therapy is continued for approximately six months, at which time it can be discontinued if the gouty attacks have been controlled. Scattered reports suggest that daily colchicine therapy may be associated with decreased male fertility[12] or with induction of congenital birth defects.[13] The drug should probably be discontinued two to three months before attempts at conception to avoid any possible hazard. In patients over 70 years of age who experience acute gouty attacks for the first time, interval therapy with a uricosuric agent or allopurinol is less mandatory. Tophaceous complications, which usually take years to develop, are unlikely to be troublesome. Prophylaxis of acute attacks in these patients can usually be attained by daily use of colchicine alone in a dose of 0.6 mg once or twice daily.

Pseudogout

Therapy of pseudogout syndrome is divided into the management of acute attacks and chronic arthralgia and the prevention of recurrent acute attacks. Joint aspiration followed by local intra-articular injection of steroids is efficacious for treatment of acute inflammation. In addition to the therapeutic effect of the steroids, prior aspiration is beneficial because offending crystals that perpetuate the inflammation are removed. Short courses of phenylbutazone or indomethacin, or systemic corticosteroids are effective therapeutic alternatives. Phenylbutazone is administered orally in a dose of 100 mg QID for two or three days, followed by gradually decreasing doses for five to seven days. Indomethacin is given in a daily dose of 100 to 150 mg, divided in equal doses with meals and at bedtime. The dosage is gradually decreased as symptoms diminish. Prednisone is administered in a dose of 5 mg QID for several days, followed by gradually decreasing dosages until the patient is asymptomatic. Colchicine, 0.6 mg given orally every hour until nausea, vomiting or diarrhea occur or symptoms are relieved, is effective at times, but less consistently than in the treatment of true gout.

Aspirin in daily doses of 640 to 960 mg QID is helpful in the management of low-grade chronic arthralgias. Indomethacin, 25 mg three or four times a day, can be used in more symptomatic cases. Colchicine, 0.6 mg BID, or indomethacin, 25 mg TID, are worthy of trial in the prevention of recurrent attacks. Therapy based on removal of calcium deposits has not yet been described.

DEGENERATIVE JOINT DISEASE (OSTEOARTHRITIS)

Osteoarthritis, the most common form of arthritis, is often undertreated owing to the misconception that it is always a benign disease. On the other hand, overtreatment is not unusual when it is misdiagnosed as some other more serious disorder.

Rest of involved joints is important for relief of pain and to delay disease progression. Bed rest is usually unnecessary. Physical therapy with heat and therapeutic exercise is a vital part of the therapy program, as in other types of arthritis.

No specific drug is presently available that consistently prevents or retards the basic degenerative disease process. Drug therapy is directed toward symptomatic relief. Aspirin is the preferred drug for basic management. Doses of 640 to 960 mg, three or four times a day, usually provide analgesic and anti-inflammatory effects. Analgesic agents such as propoxyphene hydrochloride, ethoheptazine citrate or acetaminophen can be added as needed. Other analgesic and anti-inflammatory agents such as indomethacin and phenylbutazone are effective in many patients. Indomethacin is given in a dose of 25 mg, three to four times a day, with meals. Phenylbutazone is used most safely on a short-term basis to treat acute episodes of symptoms. Long-term daily administration of phenylbutazone may be indicated at times, but careful monitoring for possible side effects is necessary. [Ibuprofen (Motrin). See Addendum, p. 279.]

Systemic corticosteroids are contraindicated in the management of osteoarthritis. They are minimally effective and toxic reactions may be severe. Intra-articular corticosteroid injections, on the other hand, are valuable when judiciously used in the treatment of acute episodes (see Chapter 20).

Appropriate supportive appliances are helpful in overall management. Cervical spine symptoms often benefit from use of a soft cervical collar and cervical traction. Traction is usually begun by the physical therapist and the procedure is taught for home use. Involvement of the lumbosacral spine is helped by abdominal muscle strengthening exercises and a lumbosacral corset. Canes, crutches or walkers are required for joint protection when weight-bearing joints are severely affected. Surgical procedures such as debridement, osteotomy, arthrodesis, and partial or total prosthetic replacement should be considered when indicated.

SYSTEMIC LUPUS ERYTHEMATOSUS

The treatment of systemic lupus erythematosus depends on which organ systems are involved. Adequate rest and good general health measures are valuable to increase resistance to stress. Mild cases require little specific therapy. When arthritis is the major manifestation of the disease, management is similar to that described for rheumatoid arthritis, although gold therapy is contraindicated. Severe manifestations of systemic lupus erythematosus, such as severe serositis, vasculitis or renal involvement, require the addition of corticosteroids to the therapeutic program. The dosage depends on the acuteness of the process and the critical nature of the organ involved.

Active progressive renal disease is treated with prednisose, 40 to 60 mg, or its equivalent, daily for weeks or months. The dosage is gradually decreased on the basis of clinical and laboratory response. Urinalysis, quantitative urinary protein, and creatinine clearance studies are important parameters in followup of therapeutic response. A fall in the serum anti-DNA titer, a rise in serum complement and a fall in urinary excretion of protein light chains indicate improvement. Therapy with immunosuppressive agents, such as azathioprine, 2 mg/kg/day,[14,15] cyclophosphamide, 2 mg/kg/day,[14,16] or chlorambucil, 4 to 8 mg/kg/day,[17] has been described in investigational studies as being beneficial. Although *their use remains investigational,* these agents should be considered for patients who do not respond to steroids.

Vasculitis is also an indication for high-dose steroid therapy. The dosage should be increased to whatever level necessary to bring this complication under control. Prednisone in doses of 60 to 80 mg per day is usually effective. However, doses of 150 to 200 mg per day or higher may be indicated.

Antimalarial drugs, such as hydroxychloroquine (Plaquenil) or quinacrine (Atabrine), are effective in the treatment of the arthritis and skin rash. Hydroxychloroquine is given in a dose of 200 mg BID until clinical response occurs; the dose is then reduced to 200 mg once a day for maintenance therapy. Periodic eye examination is mandatory to avoid irreversible eye toxicity. Atabrine is used in a dose of 100 mg BID for two weeks, followed by 100 mg daily. Yellowing of the skin can be controlled by periodic discontinuation of the drug. Skin rash is further helped by topical steroids. Excessive sun exposure should be avoided if there is a history of sun sensitivity; sun screen lotions are valuable as preventive agents in this regard.

SCLERODERMA (PROGRESSIVE SYSTEMIC SCLEROSIS)

Treatment of scleroderma is difficult since no agent has been proven effective for therapy. Potassium para-aminobenzoate (Potaba), 12 gm daily in divided doses, is helpful in some patients for cutaneous changes. The dosage is gradually decreased as response ensues. Reserpine, 0.5 mg daily, has also been associated with clinical improvement. It is particularly effective in the management of associated Raynaud's phenomenon. Depression, a significant side reaction, precludes its continued use. Favorable effects have been noted occasionally with antimalarial agents, such as hydroxychloroquine. The use of immunosuppressive agents remains *investigative*.

Symptomatic measures are beneficial in the treatment of various manifestations of the disease. Rest, maintenance of good nutrition, and an exercise program to avoid soft tissue contractures and joint limitation are important measures. Raynaud's phenomenon may be severe and trials with various agents known to be beneficial are indicated (see Chapter 13). Skin ulcers are difficult to manage, although local steroid applications may hasten healing. The ulcer should be kept clean and trauma avoided. Infection, if present, is treated with appropriate antibiotics.

Dimethylsulfoxide (DMSO), which has been helpful in some cases, is still *investigational*. Dysphagia caused by involvement of the esophagus may respond to bethanechol chloride (Urecholine). Tablets of 5 to 10 mg are chewed and swallowed 30 minutes before meals. Antacids prevent reflux esophagitis. Elevation of the head of the bed on 6- to 8-inch blocks is also valuable. Severe constipation is aided by the use of high fluid intake and bulk promoting agents. Diuretics lessen skin edema and are worthy of trial when this is a prominent symptom. Joint symptoms respond to mild anti-inflammatory agents, such as aspirin, 640 to 960 mg QID, or indomethacin, 25 mg three or four times a day with food. Pulmonary complications benefit from postural drainage and intermittent antibiotic therapy.

POLYMYOSITIS (DERMATOMYOSITIS)

Although previously considered a generally fatal disease, polymyositis can now be effectively treated in most patients with corticosteroids. The average patient usually responds to prednisone, 15 mg QID. Doses as high as 150 mg a day may be required, however, in patients with resistant disease. High doses are maintained until the patient has shown significant clinical improvement and serum muscle enzymes are approaching normal values. A decrease in creatinuria is also anticipated, but the response is generally slower than that seen with the enzyme levels. Prednisone dosage is then slowly decreased as clinical response and laboratory parameters allow. A dose of 7.5 to 15 mg/day is usually required for a prolonged period to maintain disease control. Close monitoring of the patient by clinical and laboratory study at regular intervals is important during periods of remission, because elevations in serum enzymes or the urinary creatine-creatinine ratio usually precede and signal a clinical episode. Increased doses of prednisone are then indicated.

Routine use of a low-salt diet, potassium supplements, and antacids are valuable in avoiding steroid side reactions. Periodic examination of stools for occult blood and checks for edema and weight gain are advisable. Precipitation of active clinical diabetes is not uncommon. In those few patients who do not respond to prednisone, immunosuppressive agents such as azathioprine[18] and methotrexate[19] may be helpful. The use of these drugs is currently *investigational,* but they should be considered in patients who respond poorly to appropriate doses of steroids or in patients in whom continued administration of high-dose steroids is contraindicated. Isoniazid, 300 mg per day, is added to the program in patients with a positive tuberculin test.

NECROTIZING VASCULITIS

High-dose prednisone therapy is the treatment of choice in the management of various forms of necrotizing vasculitis. The average starting dose is 60 mg per day. Higher doses are required in severe disease and the dosage should be increased to whatever level is required to be effective. Immunosuppressive agents are inconsistently effective in the treatment of necrotizing vasculitis,[20] except in patients with Wegener's granulomatosis. In the latter, immunosuppressive therapy may be life-saving. Azathioprine,[21] cyclophosphamide,[22] and methotrexate[23] have all been described as being efficacious. Cyclophosphamide is probably the drug of choice at this time.

TEMPORAL (CRANIAL) ARTERITIS AND POLYMYALGIA RHEUMATICA

Although temporal arteritis is a self-limited disease that usually remits spontaneously over a period of two to three years, symptoms may be disabling and blindness may occur in untreated cases. Corticosteroid therapy is effective in relieving symptoms and preventing blindness. The average starting dose of prednisone is 60 mg per day in divided doses. This dosage is continued until symptoms are relieved, and a fall in the erythrocyte sedimentation rate occurs. The dosage is then gradually decreased to the maintenance level required for suppression of symptoms; 5 to 10 mg of prednisone daily is usually adequate. Since temporal arteritis is a disease of older persons, special attention must be paid to possible complications of steroid therapy, such as diabetes and osteoporosis. The lowest dose possible to maintain control of symptoms should be used.

Polymyalgia rheumatica syndrome may be idiopathic or may be associated with temporal arteritis and rarely with carcinoma, lymphoma or rheumatoid arthritis. Idiopathic polymyalgia rheumatica can usually be managed with a more conservative program than that outlined for temporal arteritis. Although high-dose salicylate therapy, or indomethacin, 25 mg QID, may give relief, therapy with prednisone is generally preferred. An initial dose of 5 mg QID is usually effective. The dosage is gradually lowered to the minimal dose required to suppress symptoms and to maintain an essentially normal erythrocyte sedimentation rate. In patients with polymyalgia rheumatica associated with temporal arteritis, treatment is the same as that outlined for temporal arteritis alone. In patients with polymyalgia rheumatica associated with other disorders, treatment of the underlying disease may provide symptomatic relief. Additional therapy with salicylates, indomethacin or steroids is usually necessary.

GONOCOCCAL AND SEPTIC (INFECTIOUS) ARTHRITIS

Gonococcal arthritis responds to appropriate doses of penicillin. In acute cases, daily doses of 6 to 10 million units of aqueous penicillin G are given intravenously. Results are most effective if the daily dosage is divided into equal amounts and given as intermittent rather than continuous infusions. High-dose intravenous therapy is continued until clinical response occurs (usually within three to four days). Ampicillin in a dose of 500 mg QID orally can be substituted when acute symptoms have been brought under control. A total of 10 to 14 days of therapy is usually recommended. Bed rest, use of analgesic agents and splinting of acutely inflamed joints are helpful for symptomatic relief. Heat applications should be used with caution (if at all) because they may potentiate the inflammatory process. For patients who are allergic to penicillin, tetracycline is the drug of choice. A dose of 500 mg QID intravenously for two to three days is followed by 500 mg QID orally for the two-week course of therapy.

Management of septic arthritis requires specific identification of the offending infectious agent followed by institution of appropriate antibiotic therapy. The most commonly involved organisms are the gram-positive cocci, Staphylococcus aureus, Streptococcus pneumoniae (pneumococcus) and Streptococcus pyogenes. Less common causes are the gram-negative bacilli, Escherichia coli, Salmonella species and Pseudomonas. The gram-negative coccobacillus Hemophilus influenzae is a common cause of infectious arthritis in infants and children up to age three.

Antibiotic treatment can be divided into four phases: (1) therapy before the infecting organism has been identified, (2) therapy based on gram-stain identification of the etiologic agent, (3) therapy following specific culture identification of the organism and knowledge of the results

TABLE 18-1. Suggested Treatment Schedules for Management of Septic (Infectious) Arthritis

Drug	Dosage*	Alternative agents†
(1) Therapy before infecting organism has been identified or presumptive diagnosis, no organism eventually isolated		
Adults and older children:		
Penicillinase-resistant semisynthetic penicillins‡		Clindamycin, 20 to 30 mg/kg/day in equal doses q 4-6 h IV, or Cephalothin,§ 100 mg/kg/day in equal doses q 4-6 h IV
Nafcillin	100 mg/kg/day in equal doses q 4-6 h IV	
Oxacillin	100 mg/kg/day in equal doses q 4-6 h IV	
Methicillin	150 mg/kg/day in equal doses q 3-4 h IV	
Children under age three:		
Penicillinase-resistant semisynthetic penicillins	See above	
plus		
Ampicillin‖	150 to 200 mg/kg/day in equal doses q 4-6 h IV	Chloramphenicol, 25 to 60 mg/kg/day in equal doses q 4-6 h IV‖
(2) Therapy based on gram-stain identification		
Gram-positive cocci		Clindamycin, 20 to 30 mg/kg/day in equal doses q 4-6 h IV, or Erythromycin, 30 to 50 mg/kg/day in equal doses q 4-6 h IV
Penicillinase-resistant semisynthetic penicillins	See above	
Adults:		
Gram-negative cocci or coccobacilli		Tetracycline, 500 mg q 6 h IV, or Chloramphenicol, 0.5 to 1.0 gm q 6 h IV
Aqueous penicillin G	1.5 to 2.5 million units q 6 h IV	

Gram-negative bacilli	Children: Ampicillin‖	150 to 200 mg/kg/day in equal doses q 4-6 h IV	Chloramphenicol, 25 to 60 mg/kg/day in equal doses q 4-6 h IV¶‖
	Gentamicin	3.0 to 5.0 mg/kg/day in equal doses q 8 h IV	Chloramphenicol 0.5 to 1.0 gm q 6 h IV
(3) Therapy based on specific organism identification			
Penicillin-G resistant Staphylococcus aureus	Penicillinase-resistant semisynthetic penicillins	See above	Clindamycin, 20 to 30 mg/kg/day in equal doses q 4-6 h IV, or Erythromycin, 30 to 50 mg/kg/day in equal doses q 4-6 h IV
Penicillin-G sensitive Staphylococcus aureus	Aqueous penicillin G	1.0 million units q 6 h IV	
Streptococcus pneumoniae (pneumococcus)	Aqueous penicillin G	600,000 units q 6 h IV	
Streptococcus pyogenes	Aqueous penicillin G	600,000 units q 6 h IV	Tetracycline, 500 mg q 6 h IV
Gonococcus	Aqueous penicillin G	1.5 to 2.5 million units q 6 h IV	
Hemophilus influenzae	Ampicillin‖	150 to 200 mg/kg/day in equal doses q 4-6 h IV	Chloramphenicol, 25 to 60 mg/kg/day in equal doses q 4-6 h IV¶‖
Escherichia coli	Ampicillin	8 to 12 gm daily in equally divided doses q 4 h IV	
Pseudomonas	Gentamicin	3.0 to 5.0 mg/kg/day in equal doses q 8 h IV	Carbenicillin, 20 to 30 gm daily in equal doses q 4 h IV (adults); 300 to 500 mg/kg/day in equal doses q 4 h IV (children)

*Variation in dosage may be required in the presence of renal or hepatic impairment. DOSES GIVEN FOR ADULTS UNLESS OTHERWISE NOTED.

†If drug allergy or intolerance occurs, or if therapeutic response is inadequate.

‡Add gentamicin, 3.0 to 5.0 mg/kg/day in equal doses q 8 h IV, if trauma, predisposing underlying disease, or malignancy is present.

§Cephalosporins are useful as alternative agents in the absence of major idiosyncratic reactions to penicillin, such as angioneurotic edema, exfoliative dermatitis and anaphylaxis.

¶In neonates, chloramphenicol dose should not exceed 25 mg/kg/day.

‖Regional variations in susceptibility of Hemophilus influenzae to ampicillin have been described.

of sensitivity studies, and (4) therapy based on a presumptive diagnosis of septic arthritis when no offending organism can be identified following all appropriate microbiologic studies. Specific recommendations for therapy in all age groups are given in Table 18-1. The high frequency of infection with Hemophilus influenzae in children under age three is reflected in the programs outlined for this patient population.

Initial therapy is given by parenteral routes in order to rapidly establish high serum and synovial fluid drug concentrations. The daily dose of IV drugs is divided into equal doses, which are administered intermittently. This technique provides high peak activity of the drug. Intra-articular administration is not required because effective concentrations in the synovial fluid are achieved following parenteral administration of most antibiotics.[24] In addition, direct instillations of the drug into the joint may result in a complicating chemical synovitis. A fall in body temperature, drop in the peripheral leukocyte count, and decrease in joint swelling indicate clinical response. Therapeutic response is further monitored by periodic synovial fluid analysis and culture and roentgenologic examination. Paired samples of serum and synovial fluid should be tested for bactericidal activity against the responsible pathogen to monitor dosage requirements. Oral administration of drugs is substituted for parenteral therapy when clinical evidence of synovitis diminishes and inflammatory changes in joint fluid revert toward normal. Antibiotic treatment is continued for a minimum of one to two weeks after clinical and laboratory cure appears to have taken place. Usually, at least four to six weeks of therapy are required. Close observation of the patient is indicated for another several weeks after cessation of antibiotic therapy to detect signs of relapse.

Joint drainage by needle aspiration is performed daily or every other day if synovial fluid rapidly reaccumulates. This procedure keeps the joint cavity relatively free of destructive enzymes elaborated by bacteria and leukocytes. If needle aspiration does not control reaccumulation of fluid, or if clinical response is slow, open surgical drainage is indicated. Open drainage should be instituted even earlier in the course of management if gross pus is observed on initial synovial fluid studies, since repeated aspirations may be inadequate to remove the highly destructive bacteria and proteolytic enzymes. Open drainage should also be utilized early in septic arthritis involving the hip, since aspiration is difficult and incomplete. Early consideration of open drainage is advised for septic arthritis in children, no matter which joint is involved.

The involved joint should be placed at complete rest until significant signs of improvement are noted. Use of infected joints may result in more rapid breakdown of cartilage by the addition of mechanical stress. Pain relief is aided by immobilization in a splint. Physical therapy with gentle range-of-motion exercises is instituted when clinical remission allows.

ACUTE OSTEOMYELITIS

Osteomyelitis is most often due to infection with Staphylococcus aureus. Intravenous use of a semisynthetic penicillinase-resistant penicillin is the treatment of choice for initiation of therapy until positive organism identification and sensitivity studies have been completed. Aqueous penicillin G, given intravenously, can then be substituted if the organism is susceptible to this agent. In the presence of infection by other bacterial agents, other antibiotics specifically directed to the offending organism are utilized. Oral therapy can be substituted when the infectious process begins to respond. Periodic roentgenograms, leukocyte counts, erythrocyte sedimentation rates, and blood cultures should be performed in disease followup. As with septic arthritis, antibiotic treatment should be continued for several weeks following clinical and laboratory evidence of cure. Although many patients will respond to a four- to six-week course of therapy, the need for more prolonged antibiotic administration is not uncommon. Close observation for signs and symptoms of relapse is indicated. The erythrocyte sedimentation rate is a particularly useful parameter in evaluating the therapeutic response both during active therapy and in followup observation. Surgical drainage should be initiated in patients who do not respond to a conservative program of management.

The foregoing programs of therapy are suggested methods of management. Alternative programs are effective if based on sound principles of antibiotic usage. Specific recommendations will change as new, more effective antibiotics become available. Drug dosage may have to be lowered to avoid toxicity if renal or hepatic disease cause higher effective drug levels.

ADDENDUM

Ibuprofen (Motrin), a nonsteroidal, analgesic anti-inflammatory agent, has recently been made available for treatment of rheumatoid arthritis and degenerative joint disease. Doses of 300 to 400 mg TID or QID have been recommended, with a maximal total daily dose not to exceed 2400 mg. It has been suggested that doses at the upper end of the recommended range are required for maximal effect in patients with rheumatoid arthritis. Associated adverse reactions include gastrointestinal intolerance, occasional peptic ulceration, skin rash, dizziness and eye complaints. Leukopenia and mild decreases in hematocrit have been described. This drug may be considered for use in patients who do not respond to properly prescribed salicylates. Thorough familiarity with precautions and adverse reactions is essential before the drug is prescribed.

As with all new drugs, a period of time and observation will be required before the usefulness of this agent can be adequately delineated, and judiciousness in its use is indicated.

REFERENCES

1. Wolfe, J. D., Metzger, A. L. and Goldstein, R. C.: Aspirin hepatitis. Ann Int Med 80:74, 1974.
2. Burns, C. A.: Indomethacin, reduced retinal sensitivity and corneal deposits. Am J Ophth 61:825, 1968.
3. Carr, R. E. and Siegel, I. M.: Retinal function in patients treated with indomethacin. Am J Ophth 75:302, 1973.
4. Percival, S. P. B. and Meanock, I.: Chloroquine: ophthalmological safety and clinical assessment in rheumatoid arthritis. Brit Med J 3:579, 1968.
5. Research Subcommittee of the Empire Rheumatism Council: Gold therapy in rheumatoid arthritis. Report of a multicenter controlled trial. Ann Rheum Dis 19:95, 1960.
6. Sigler, J. W. et al.: Gold salts in the treatment of rheumatoid arthritis. A double-blind study. Ann Int Med 80:21, 1974.
7. Carter, M. E. and James, V. H.: Effect of alternate day, single dose, corticosteroid therapy on pituitary-adrenal function. Ann Rheum Dis 31:379, 1972.
8. Cooperative Clinics Committee of the American Rheumatism Association: A controlled trial of cyclophosphamide in rheumatoid arthritis. N Eng J Med 283:883, 1970.
9. Levy, J. et al.: A double-blind controlled evaluation of azathioprine treatment in rheumatoid arthritis and psoriatic arthritis. Arth Rheum 15:116, 1972.
10. Black, R. L. et al.: Methotrexate therapy in psoriatic arthritis. JAMA 189:743, 1964.
11. Baum, J. et al.: Treatment of psoriatic arthritis with 6-mercaptopurine. Arth Rheum 16:139, 1973.
12. Merlin, H. E.: Azoospermia caused by colchicine. Fertil Steril 23:180, 1972.
13. Ferreira, N. R. and Buoniconti, A.: Trisomy after colchicine therapy. Lancet 2:1304, 1968.
14. Steinberg, A. D., Decker, J. L. and Aptekar, R. G.: Completed ten week trial of cyclophosphamide or azathioprine or placebo in lupus nephritis. Arth Rheum 16:572, 1973.
15. Hayslett, J. P. et al.: The effect of azathioprine on lupus glomerulonephritis. Medicine 51:393, 1972.
16. Steinberg, A. D. et al.: Cyclophosphamide in lupus nephritis: a controlled trial. Ann Int Med 75:165, 1971.
17. Epstein, W. V. and Grausz, H.: Favorable outcome in diffuse proliferative glomerulonephritis of systemic lupus erythematosus. Arth Rheum 17:129, 1974.
18. Benson, M. D. and Aldo, M. A.: Azathioprine therapy in polymyositis. Arch Int Med 132:547, 1973.
19. Sokoloff, M. C., Goldberg, L. S. and Pearson, C. M.: Treatment of corticosteroid-resistant polymyositis with methotrexate. Lancet 1:14, 1971.
20. Mitchell, M. S., Malawista, S. E. and Bertine, J. R.: Successful therapy of disseminated vasculitis by methotrexate despite severe renal involvement. Arth Rheum 14:175, 1971.
21. Norton, W. L., Suki, W. and Strunk, S.: Combined corticosteroid and azathioprine therapy in two patients with Wegener's granulomatosis. Arch Int Med 121:554, 1968.
22. Novack, S. N. and Pearson, C. M.: Cyclophosphamide therapy in Wegener's granulomatosis. N Eng J Med 284:938, 1971.
23. Capizzi, R. L. and Bertino, J. R.: Methotrexate therapy of Wegener's granulomatosis. Ann Int Med 74:74, 1971.
24. Parker, R. H. and Schmid, F. R.: Antibacterial activity of synovial fluid during therapy of septic arthritis. Arth Rheum 14:96, 1971.

Chapter 19

PHYSICAL THERAPY, OCCUPATIONAL THERAPY AND SUPPORTIVE DEVICES

PHYSICAL THERAPY

Patients with connective tissue disorders require careful evaluation by the physical therapist. Joint motion, muscle strength and functional level should be assessed in detail, so that overall goals of treatment can be determined. The specific procedures selected by the therapist to achieve these goals will vary according to the specific problems under consideration.

Joint limitation is treated by a combined program of rest, heat and programmed exercises. Moist heat is generally more beneficial than dry heat due to its greater conductive properties. Deep heat is especially effective in treating periarthritis of the shoulder. Simple measures such as warm soaks, tub baths and Hydrocollator packs are effective and can be readily used at home on a day-to-day basis. Paraffin applications (Fig. 19-1) are beneficial in the treatment of arthritis of the hand and wrist. Hydrotherapy allows greater ease of movement during exercise because it eliminates the effects of gravity. Hubbard tank therapy is useful when multiple joints are involved.

Although heat therapy is used more commonly, cryotherapy should be considered in certain situations. The temporary anesthetic effect of cold applications is especially valuable in managing patients following reconstructive surgery, since it allows a more pain-free range of motion for exercise.

Heat, followed by exercise, is directed toward maintaining and improving joint mobility. When knees are involved, isometric exercises are generally associated with less pain than isotonic exercises. Isometric exercises are performed by contracting the muscle without moving the joint through its range of motion. During isotonic exercises, the joint moves actively through its range of motion.

Assessment of muscle strength is often difficult in patients who have limited joint range of motion or inflammatory muscle disease. In patients with polymyositis, frequent re-evaluations of muscle strength and function and careful grading of exercise programs are required.

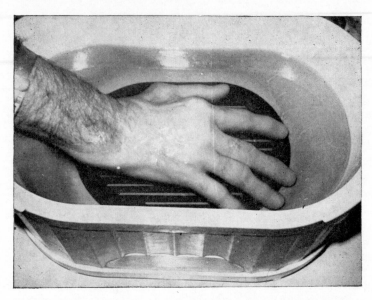

Figure 19-1. Application of paraffin to hand of patient with rheumatoid arthritis.

Maintenance of functional independence in patients with chronic disease requires careful planning with the patient in order to set realistic goals. Shoulder and knee mobility and good quadriceps strength are especially important. Adaptive equipment and appliances should be selected with care. Canes, crutches or walkers may be used to reduce stress on weight-bearing joints. Improper use of such devices can be not only ineffective but unsafe; instructions regarding their use varies with the disability. In general, a cane should be used in the hand opposite the joint to be protected. Although walkers are ordinarily one of the most stable appliances, they are unsafe on sidewalks and stairs. Modification of hand grips on appliances is often necessary for patients whose hands and wrists are affected by disease.

Cervical or pelvic traction is utilized when a distraction force is indicated. Application can be either intermittent or static; the specific method varies with the individual patient's problem.

OCCUPATIONAL THERAPY

The major goal of occupational therapy in the management of patients with arthritis and related disorders is the attainment of maximal independence in daily activity. Physical capabilities, self-care needs, and psychosocial background are evaluated. Identification of problem areas allows individualization of treatment programs and the setting of realistic goals.

Purposeful activities and exercise are utilized to overcome limitations in joint range of motion and muscle weakness. Craft activities, such as painting, loom weaving and woodworking, provide exercise for specifically involved joints. Strengthening is achieved through antigravity positioning of involved extremities or use of weighted cuffs. Small finger weights, light rubber bands and pliable plastic media are used for similar purposes.

For patients with increasing physical disability, an important aspect of the occupational therapy program is instruction in self-care.[1] The levels of function in bathing, feeding, dressing and hygienic activities are evaluated. Necessary training and assistive devices are then provided to help the patient maintain or regain maximal independence.[1]

For the arthritic patient, bathing is made easier and safer through instructions in transfer and the use of low tub stools, shower seats, nonskid rubber mats and grab rails. Special hydraulic lifts are effective in transferring patients into and out of tubs and showers, but their usefulness is limited by cost factors. Long-handled sponges and brushes are helpful for

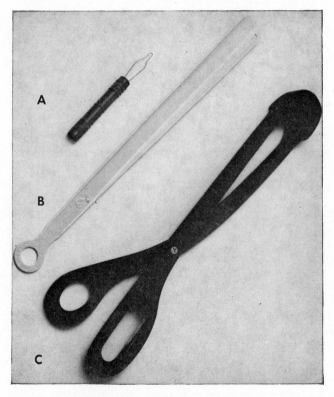

Figure 19-2. Supportive aids used in occupational therapy. (A) Button hook. (B) Long-handled shoe horn. (C) Long-handled wooden scissors (reachers).

bathing the lower extremities, particularly when hip and knee flexion is limited.

Various commercial devices are available to facilitate ease in dressing. Velcro fasteners and button aids (Fig. 19-2A) are useful for patients with limited finger movement. When arthritis or proximal girdle weakness prevents normal function of the lower extremities, long-handled shoe horns (Fig. 19-2B), stocking aids, and shoelaces that do not require tying are particularly useful. Long reachers (Fig. 19-2C) to pick items off the floor are valuable. Elevated toilet seats help patients with weakness or limitation of motion in the lower extremities.

Patients can be taught to maintain their general activity level through the use of joint protection and work simplification techniques. These techniques are prophylactic in the early stages of the disease process when deformity is minimal. Kitchen activities, for example, can be made easier with the use of wide-handled utensils (Fig. 19-3A), specially designed knives, forks and spoons (Fig. 19-3B), and lightweight pots and pans. Where possible, sitting instead of standing is encouraged, and work surfaces with adjustable heights should be used. Patients should be shown how to organize their work, daily living, and leisure time to maintain an adequate balance of rest and activity.

Throughout the treatment course provided by the occupational therapist, emotional and motivational factors are primary considerations. The patient may require a period of adjusting to his disability before he is ready to participate in purposeful activities or self-care training.

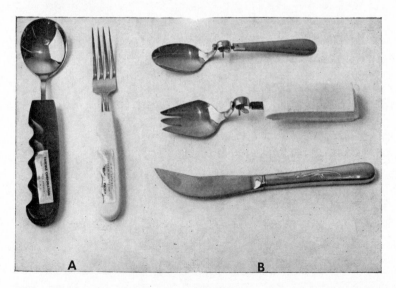

Figure 19-3. Special eating utensils. (A) Wide-handled spoon and fork to facilitate grasp. (B) Hinged spoon and fork; curved knife allows cutting with rocker motion.

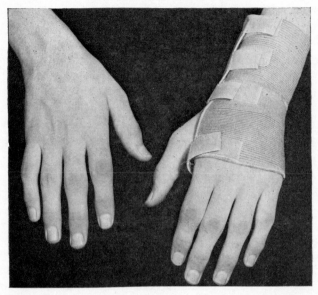

Figure 19-4. Elastic wrist splint with Velcro fasteners. Stabilization of the wrist is aided by a volar metal insert.

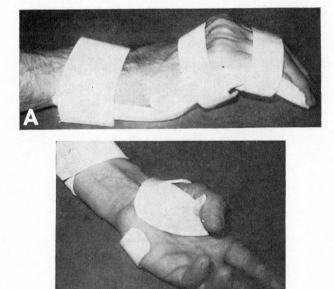

Figure 19-5. Specially designed splints. (A) Volar splint for relief of joint pain and maintenance of normal wrist and hand position. (B) Thumb opponens splint.

SUPPORTIVE APPLIANCES

Splints

For arthritic patients, resting and dynamic splints can be effective in providing pain relief, support, and the proper positioning of affected muscles and joints. They are most often applied to wrists, hands and knees and are usually worn at night. Splints of various types and sizes are available from commercial sources (Fig. 19-4) or can be individually fabricated by the occupational therapist using thermal plastic materials or plaster bandage (Fig. 19-5).

Foot Appliances

Foot pain can often be partially alleviated by various simple appliances. Transverse metatarsal pads, which take the weight off the metatarsophalangeal joints, are indicated when these joints are symptomatic. They can be built into the longitudinal arch of the shoe or may be inserted as a separate appliance. When metatarsal pads do not provide adequate relief, metatarsophalangeal joint pain may be effectively relieved by placing transverse metatarsal bars on the outer sole of the shoe. Longitudinal arch

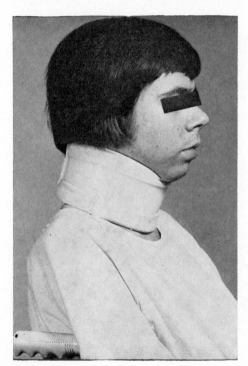

Figure 19-6. Plastic cervical collar used for treatment of neck pain in patient with juvenile rheumatoid arthritis.

supports help to prevent pronation deformities of the foot. Lifts are used to correct disparities in leg length. Inversion and eversion deformities of the foot may benefit from the use of appropriate wedging. Molded Space Shoes are helpful in the presence of severe multiple deformities.

Cervical Collars

Collars for partially immobilizing the cervical spine are indicated in the management of various neck disorders. Soft collars are available in many sizes. Rigid plastic collars should be utilized when more complete immobilization is required (Fig. 19-6). Duration of use depends upon the specific problem being treated. In patients who have significant involvement of the cervical spine with rheumatoid arthritis, the collar should be worn as often as possible. Use of the collar is especially important when riding in an automobile, since severe neck injury may occur with relatively slight trauma in case of accident.

Back Supports

Disease of the lumbosacral or dorsal spine may require the use of supportive corsets or braces; well-fitting lumbosacral or lumbodorsal corsets respectively are usually sufficient for the treatment of most such disorders. These garments require individualized tailoring by experts familiar with their use. Semirigid stays are added as required. More intensive immobilization may require use of spinal ortheses (braces).

REFERENCE

1. Klinger, J. L. (ed.): Self-help Manual for Arthritis Patients. Prepared by the Allied Health Professions Section of the Arthritis Foundation. (Available from The Arthritis Foundation, New York, New York 10036.)

Chapter 20

LOCAL INJECTION THERAPY

INTRA-ARTICULAR THERAPY

Intra-articular therapy is a valuable adjunct to general therapeutic programs in the treatment of arthritis. It is particularly useful in the management of patients with monoarticular or oligoarticular arthritis, or in the management of patients with generalized disease in whom one or two joints are "out of pace" with the clinical progress. In these situations, local therapy allows effective control of a limited number of joints and diminishes the hazard of side reactions associated with more aggressive use of potent systemic medications. Corticosteroid preparations are the most commonly used agents for intra-articular therapy. Immunosuppressive drugs and radioactive substances have also been used in an attempt to provide longer periods of effectiveness.

Corticosteroids

In addition to the general indications outlined above, this therapeutic procedure is valuable in several other clinical situations. It is useful as adjunct therapy while awaiting a response to recently-initiated gold or antimalarial treatment. Physical therapy and rehabilitation may be made more effective by its use in reducing acute or subacute inflammation. Similarly, this procedure is effective in diminishing joint pain and increasing patient cooperation when orthopedic procedures such as serial casting are utilized.

Local steroid injection therapy is not without hazard. Corticosteroids have a direct deleterious effect on cartilage.[1] In addition, the chance for joint destruction is enhanced when pain relief promotes joint overuse; too frequent use may actually promote joint deterioration. Joint infection is a serious complication that fortunately is uncommon when appropriate aseptic technique is utilized. Other complications are usually minimal. Occasionally local joint inflammation results when the crystalline steroid in suspension causes a crystal-induced synovitis. Some patients experience several days of weakness and malaise. An occasional patient may complain of increased warmth and flushing of the skin. Urticarial reactions are probably caused by allergy to components of the suspending vehicle.

As noted, a strict aseptic technique is required to avoid infection. Excess hair should be removed. Cleansing of the injection site with a germicidal soap such as hexachlorophene is followed by copious cleansing with alcohol and the application of tincture of iodine. The latter is allowed to dry for several minutes. Alternatively, one may use Betadine or Amphyl. Gloves and sterile drapes are usually not necessary if the procedure is performed by a physician experienced in injection technique. The area to be injected should not be touched after cleansing, except with alcohol sponges. All necessary materials should be available prior to beginning the injection (Fig. 20-1). Disposable syringes and needles are valuable to avoid transmission of infectious agents. A 20-gauge needle is usually satisfactory for larger joints; a 25- or 26-gauge needle is used for small joints. An 18-gauge needle may be required if the synovial fluid is especially viscous. One percent lidocaine is used for local anesthesia and for mixing with the local steroid for injection. In patients with a history of allergy to local anesthetic agents, ethyl chloride spray may be used for surface anesthesia and the steroid may be diluted in sterile normal saline.

Contraindications to corticosteroid therapy should be kept in mind before using it. Local infection in or around the joint is an absolute contraindication. It is inadvisable to use local steroid therapy to treat acute dis-

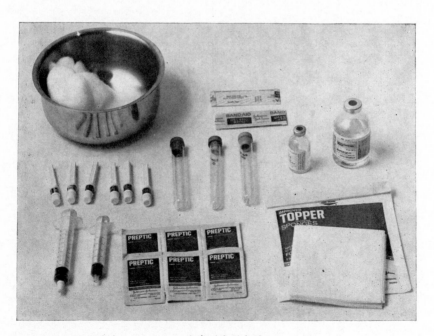

Figure 20-1. Materials for use in intra-articular joint injections.

TABLE 20-1. Average Doses of Steroid Preparations Used in Local Therapy of Musculoskeletal Disorders

Corticosteroid Preparations (Strength of Preparation in mg/ml)	Average Recommended Doses in ml								
	Shoulders, Knees, Ankles	Wrists, Elbows	PIP, MCP, First CMP, MTP*	Tendinitis, Bursitis	Epicondylitis	Costo-chondritis	Trigger areas	Ganglion	Carpal tunnel
Long-acting									
Dexamethasone acetate 8 mg/ml	1.0–1.5	1.0–1.2	0.3–0.4	1.0–1.2	0.6–1.0	0.3–0.5	0.3–0.5	0.3–0.5	1.0–1.2
Hydrocortisone acetate 25 mg/ml	0.6–1.5	0.6–1.0	0.2–0.4	0.6–1.0	0.6–0.8	0.4–0.6	0.4–0.5	0.5	0.6–1.0
Hydrocortisone tertiary butylacetate† 25 mg/ml	0.6–1.5	0.6–1.0	0.2–0.4	0.6–1.0	0.6–0.8	0.4–0.6	0.4–0.5	0.5	0.6–1.0
Methylprednisolone acetate 40 mg/ml	0.6–1.0	0.5–0.75	0.2–0.3	0.6–0.8	0.4–0.5	0.3	0.3–0.4	0.3–0.5	0.5
Prednisolone acetate 25 mg/ml	0.8–1.2	0.8–1.0	0.3–0.4	0.8–1.2	0.4–0.5	0.3–0.4	0.3–0.4	0.4–0.6	0.6–0.8
Prednisolone tertiary butylacetate† 25 mg/ml	0.8–1.2	0.8–1.0	0.3–0.4	0.8–1.2	0.4–0.5	0.3–0.4	0.3–0.4	0.4–0.6	0.6–0.8

Triamcinolone diacetate 25 mg/ml	0.6–0.8	0.6	0.3	0.6–0.8	0.4–0.5	0.3–0.4	0.3–0.4	0.3–0.4	0.6
Triamcinolone acetonide 10 mg/ml	1.0–2.0	1.0–1.5	0.3–0.5	1.0–2.0	0.75–1.0	0.5–0.6	0.5–0.6	0.5–0.6	1.0
Triamcinolone hexacetonide† 20 mg/ml	0.6–1.0	0.6–0.8	0.3	0.6–1.0	0.3–0.4	0.3	0.3	0.3	0.6
Short- and long-acting									
Betamethasone sodium phosphate 3 mg/ml plus / Betamethasone acetate 3 mg/ml	1.0–2.0	0.5–1.0	0.3–0.5	1.0	0.4–0.5	0.3–0.4	0.5	0.5–0.75	
Short-acting									
Dexamethasone sodium phosphate 4 mg/ml	0.5–1.0	0.5–0.75	0.2–0.3	0.5–0.8	0.3–0.5	0.3–0.4	0.3	0.3–0.5	0.5

*PIP = proximal interphalangeal joint; MCP = metacarpophalangeal joint; CMP = carpometacarpophalangeal joint; MTP = metatarsophalangeal joint

†Hydrocortisone tertiary butylacetate, prednisolone tertiary butylacetate, and triamcinolone hexacetonide are somewhat longer lasting in effect than their respective acetate and acetonide derivatives.

ease that involves a large number of joints; it usually does not provide adequate relief, and often only complicates the therapeutic program. Local steroid therapy should be avoided in severely damaged joints that are the site of little or no active inflammatory disease. It should be used with caution, if at all, in areas of fracture because it may impede healing.

Almost all diarthrodial joints may be approached for injection. Injection into some of these joints is difficult and intra-articular therapy should be left to the more experienced rheumatologist or orthopedist. On the other hand, injection into certain commonly involved joints can be accomplished without much difficulty or hazard. Knowledge and experience in this form of therapy adds a most useful procedure to the armamentarium of the physician treating arthritis.

The specific technique for intra-articular injection varies somewhat with the joint involved. If feasible, synovial fluid should first be aspirated to provide fluid for analysis and to lessen joint swelling and distension. However, a small amount of fluid should be allowed to remain to lessen the risk of dislodging the needle from the joint space before the injection itself is completed. In addition, a small amount of fluid allows better diffusion of

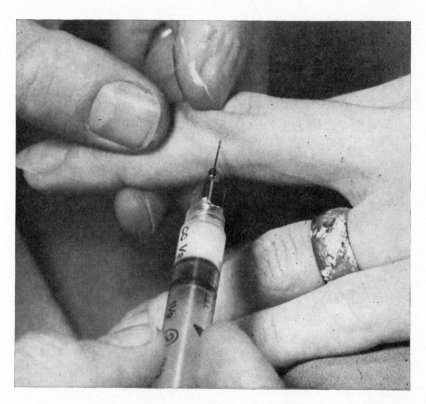

Figure 20-2. Injection into proximal interphalangeal joint. (Courtesy, Dr. A. Mackenzie)

the therapeutic agent throughout the joint. The amount of steroid injected varies with the agent used and the size of the joint to be treated (see Table 20-1). Preparations containing acetate, acetonide or hexacetonide are long-acting; the therapeutic effect begins after 24 to 48 hours and lasts for weeks to months. Phosphate derivatives have a rapid onset of action and a therapeutic effect lasting 24 to 48 hours. Some preparations contain a combination of short- and long-acting components so that the effect begins rapidly followed by prolonged improvement. Only preparations that are hydrocortisone derivatives are effective for intra-articular use. Unless contraindicated, 1% lidocaine, in a volume equal to the steroid used, is mixed and injected at the same time. This allows better dispersion of the steroid and also allows immediate evaluation of the success of the injection. Specific techniques for injection into commonly treated joints follow.

Interphalangeal and Metacarpophalangeal (MCP) Joints. A small needle is used to avoid unnecessary injury. Usually a 25- or 26-gauge needle is satisfactory. The needle is inserted from a medial or lateral approach on the dorsal aspect of the hand (Fig. 20-2). Although the joint can often be entered readily, it may be possible to inject only a small amount of the steroid into the joint. Periarticular infiltration is added for maximal benefit.

First Carpometacarpal (CMP) Joint. The needle for injection is placed at the dorsal-radial aspect of the hand in the area of the first CMP joint.

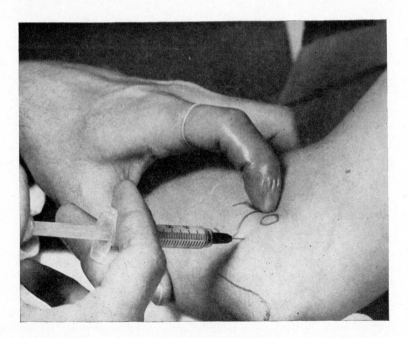

Figure 20-3. Injection into lateral aspect of elbow joint. (Courtesy, Dr. A. Mackenzie)

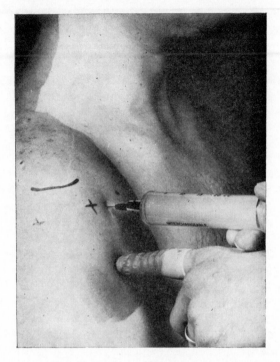

Figure 20-4. Injection into shoulder joint, anterior approach. (Courtesy, Dr. A. Mackenzie)

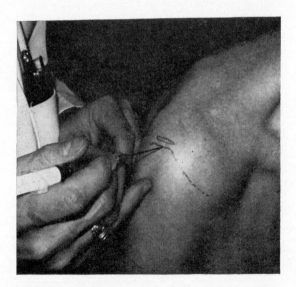

Figure 20-5. Injection into shoulder joint, lateral approach, between acromion process of the scapula and head of humerus.

Once again, it may be difficult to inject the total amount of medication within the joint. Suitable relief can usually be obtained by periarticular injection of some of the agent as well.

Wrist. Injection into the wrist is best performed from a dorsal approach. The needle is directed perpendicularly into the depression normally present at the radiocarpal indentation. The radial styloid is a helpful marker to determine the level for needle insertion. The needle is inserted for a distance of 1 to 2 cm for injection.

Elbow. Injection into the elbow may be difficult unless moderate swelling is present. A lateral approach is generally recommended to avoid injury to the ulnar nerve. With the elbow held at a 90° angle, the needle is inserted just below the lateral epicondyle and outside the olecranon process (Fig. 20-3).

Shoulder. Intra-articular injection of the shoulder joint may be performed from either an anterior or lateral approach. In the anterior approach, the needle is inserted just medial to the head of the humerus below the tip of the coracoid process (Fig. 20-4). In the lateral approach, the needle is inserted between the acromion process of the scapula and the humeral head (Fig. 20-5). Swelling of the shoulder joint usually protrudes anteriorly and the anterior approach is the simpler technique.

Knee. Aspiration and injection into the knee is usually easy when the knee is inflamed and contains increased joint fluid. Injection into osteoarthritic knees is somewhat more difficult because they usually contain little or no excess fluid, and osteophytic spurs that distort the joint margins make it difficult to insert the needle. Injection is usually performed with the pa-

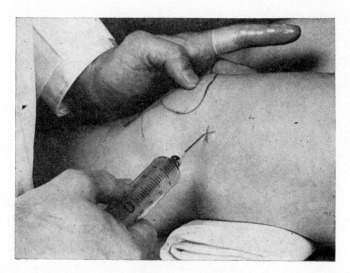

Figure 20-6. Lateral approach for injection, left knee. Note relationship of needle to outline of patella above. (Courtesy, Dr. A. Mackenzie)

tient lying on his back with the knees fully extended. If possible, injection should be made into the suprapatellar pouch to avoid inserting the needle between closely apposing cartilaginous surfaces. The superior tip of the patella is identified and used as a landmark for injection. The injection is made into either the medial or the lateral aspect of the knee. The lateral aspect is usually preferred because it can be approached more conveniently. The needle is inserted ¾ to 1 inch below the superior aspect of the patella and is directed slightly cephalad to enter the suprapatellar pouch (Fig. 20-6). If no fluid is obtained, the needle is redirected between the posterior surface of the patella and the patellar groove of the femur. An alternative approach may be considered in patients in whom deformity prevents complete knee extension. In these cases, aspiration and injection are accomplished by inserting the needle in an anteroposterior direction lateral or medial to the inferior patellar tendon (Fig. 20-7). The needle passes through the fat pad into the knee joint space between the condyles of the femur and the tibial plateaus.

For popliteal cysts of the knee, aspiration and injection may be performed directly through a posterior approach. Great care must be taken to avoid the popliteal artery. Small popliteal cysts usually respond to intra-articular injection directly into the knee; direct injection into the cyst usually is not required.

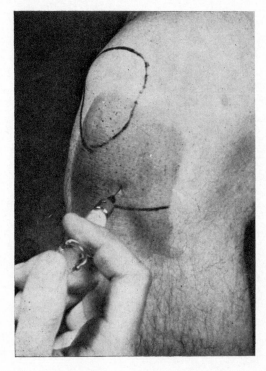

Figure 20-7. Anterior approach for knee injection. (Courtesy, Dr. A. Mackenzie)

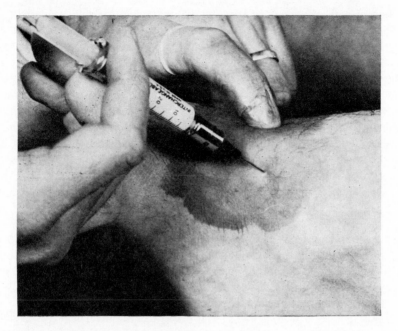

Figure 20-8. Injection into ankle. (Courtesy, Dr. A. Mackenzie)

Ankle. Intra-articular therapy of the ankle may be difficult if swelling is not great. However, the technique can usually be mastered with experience. The anteromedial approach is the most common. The needle is directed horizontally toward the tibiotalar articulation just above and lateral to the medial malleolus and medial to the extensor hallucis longus tendon (Fig. 20-8). It is well to mark the location of the dorsalis pedis artery so that it can be avoided during injection. Although this artery is usually located lateral to the extensor pollicis longus tendon, its course may be aberrant in some patients. Abrupt entrance of the needle through the capsule and into the joint is usually less obvious as compared to the knee. When joint swelling is greatest laterally, an anterolateral approach should be utilized: the needle is directed toward the tibiotalar articulation from a point 1 to 2 cm medial to the lateral malleolus.

Metatarsophalangeal (MTP) Joints. The MTP joints are readily accessible to local injection therapy. Injection is made from a dorsal or ventral approach, depending on the site of maximal pain and swelling. A 25- or 26-gauge needle is advisable. When direct injection into the joint is difficult or incomplete, injection into surrounding periarticular tissues usually provides effective symptomatic relief.

Immunosuppressive Agents

Intra-articular therapy with alkylating agents, such as nitrogen mustard or triethylenethiophosphoramide (Thio-tepa),[2] has been used to produce a prolonged anti-inflammatory effect on the synovitis of rheumatoid arthritis. Unfortunately, results have been variable and inconsistent. Nitrogen mustard is rarely used any longer for intra-articular injection because it is very irritating to periarticular soft tissues if not injected directly into the joint. Thio-tepa has minimal hazard in this regard. Thio-tepa is usually mixed with corticosteroid and 1% lidocaine prior to injection to obtain a more immediate response. Approximately 2.5 to 3.5 mg is used in the treatment of small joints such as the knuckles; 7.5 to 15.0 mg is used in large joints such as the knee. This agent seems most effective when small joints are treated, such as the proximal interphalangeal and metacarpophalangeal joints of the hands.

Radioactive Agents

Long-term suppression of synovial inflammation has been described with the intra-articular use of radioactive substances such as colloidal ^{198}Au,[3] colloidal ^{32}P and ^{90}Yttrium.[4] ^{90}Yttrium is somewhat preferable to the other agents because it drains less to regional lymph nodes and systemic areas. The use of these agents should be avoided in women of childbearing age and also in men who anticipate having more children. Their use may be considered in patients with monoarticular arthritis or in patients who have one joint out of pace with the clinical progress.

EXTRA-ARTICULAR THERAPY

Local steroid therapy is frequently used in the treatment of disorders involving periarticular soft tissues. The results are often dramatic and associated with minimal hazard. The steroid to be injected is usually mixed with 1% lidocaine in a volume one to two times that of the steroid suspension. This technique allows treatment of a wider area of involvement and also lessens the deleterious effect of high concentration of steroid on the tissue. The amount of steroid used varies with the specific agent utilized and the site to be injected (see Table 20-1). Specific techniques of injection for various disorders follow.

Shoulder area. Local steroids are therapeutically beneficial for shoulder area bursitis, supraspinatus tendinitis, periarthritis, tenosynovitis of the long head of the biceps, and rotator cuff tears. The injection should be made into the points of maximal tenderness. Inflamed subacromial and subdeltoid bursae are injected directly, aiming the needle into the areas of maximal tenderness. For treatment of supraspinatus tendinitis, the needle is inserted just at the anterior aspect of the greater tuberosity of the shoulder. Approximately one-third of the medication is placed at this point. The needle is then redirected posteriorly and anteriorly, where the remainder of the agent is injected. A successful injection is often attended by almost immediate relief of pain and increased range of shoulder motion. Specific sites of inflammation may be difficult to localize and a general periarthritis may be present; local steroid injections into sites similar to those described for supraspinatus tendinitis frequently give relief. Injection into the sheath of the long head of the biceps is made immediately over the tendon at the anterior aspect of the shoulder, as it passes through the bicipital groove of the humerus. Approximately one third of the medication is inserted at the site of maximal tenderness. The needle is then redirected in a superior and inferior direction to complete the injection. Small rotator cuff tears may be associated with pain and secondary inflammation. Local steroids injected into the site of pathology provide symptomatic relief.

Several areas of inflammation may be present in the same patient; injection should be made into all areas for maximal success. It is well to caution the patient to avoid overexerting the joint when injections have been made into areas of tendinitis, since steroid-induced atrophy may decrease the tensile strength of the tendon and predispose it to rupture. This complication is uncommon but does occur, especially in athletes.

Epicondylitis of the Elbow. Inflammation in the area of tendon origins at the lateral or medial epicondyle of the elbow secondary to chronic stress is common. Local injections are first made into the site of maximal tenderness of the involved epicondyle. The needle is then redirected into several areas peripheral to the site of maximal tenderness in order to achieve an effective result.

Tendinitis of the Fingers. Tenosynovitis of the flexor tendons of the hands is common and produces the so-called "trigger finger" (see Chapter 14). Although the patient often complains that the finger itself is the site of difficulty, the pathologic changes are usually located in the area of the distal palmar crease. Local steroids should be injected into this latter area at the site of maximal tenderness, crepitus or nodule formation.

Stenosing Tenosynovitis at the Wrist (DeQuervain's Disease). Inflammation of the abductor pollicis longus and extensor pollicis brevis tendons is usually secondary to chronic trauma. Symptoms include pain in the area of the radial styloid and weakness of grip. Local steroid injection is made directly into the tendon sheath at the site of maximal tenderness, followed by injection along the tendon sheath in a proximal and distal direction.

Olecranon Bursitis. Inflammation and swelling of the olecranon bursa occurs in various connective tissue diseases, in gout and following nonspecific trauma. Treatment includes direct aspiration of the bursa followed by the local introduction of steroids.

Greater Trochanteric Bursitis. Inflammation of the bursa over the greater trochanter of the hip is a common cause of pain in this area. The patient complains of tenderness in a localized region and symptoms are accentuated by pressure when the patient is lying on the involved side. Injection therapy is simple and effective. The needle is placed directly into

the area of maximal tenderness and local steroid with lidocaine is intro-
duced. Steroid should also be injected circumferentially to the site of maximal tenderness.

*Anserine Bursitis and Medial Collateral Ligament Inflammation at the
Knee.* Bursitis of the anserine bursa at the medial aspect of the knee is
common. Tenderness is noted at the edge of the medial tibial plateau; steroid injection is made directly into the area of tenderness just beneath the
medial collateral ligament. Inflammation of the medial collateral ligament
itself may produce similar symptoms; steroid injection is directed somewhat more superficially into the area of ligamentous inflammation.

Ischial Tuberosity Bursitis. Pain and tenderness at the base of the but-
tock are symptoms of ischial tuberosity bursitis. Pain is aggravated by
sitting. Relief is usually obtained with local steroid injection over the bony
prominence of the ischial tuberosity.

Bursitis at the Bunion Joint. Acute inflammation of the bursa at the
medial aspect of the first metatarsophalangeal joint may simulate symptoms of acute gout or rheumatoid arthritis. Treatment involves aspiration
of fluid followed by injection of local steroid into the bursal sac.

Trigger Areas of Spasm. Tender areas of muscle spasm frequently can
be palpated in patients with localized or diffuse primary fibrositis. Relief of
symptoms with local steroid injection is often good to excellent. Steroid
with lidocaine is injected directly into the site of maximal tenderness.
Further injections are made circumferentially to the site of maximal pain.
Injections may be required in several trigger areas at the same time in
order to obtain maximal relief.

Costochondritis (Tietze's Syndrome). Inflammation of the costal cartilages may cause severe, annoying chest pain. Tenderness is usually localized to specific areas of involvement. Swelling due to cartilaginous hypertrophy may be present. Injections of local steroid with lidocaine provide
effective relief. A 20- or 22-gauge needle is directed at a 45° angle down
to the rib at the site of maximal tenderness. A perpendicular approach is
hazardous because injection deep to the rib is more likely if the patient
moves inappropriately. Although injection close to the rib surface is desirable, good results are usually obtained even with more superficial injections, since the steroid-lidocaine suspension diffuses sufficiently for an
effective result. Repeat injections at intervals of days or weeks may be required for permanent relief. As noted, great care must be taken to avoid
visceral structures deep to the rib cage.

Ganglia. A ganglion is a cystic swelling in the area of a tendon sheath
or joint capsule, from which structures they appear to be derived. They
occur most commonly on the dorsum of the wrist, but may be seen elsewhere. Most ganglia are asymptomatic but tenderness may be bothersome.
Spontaneous disappearance is common. Specific treatment may be required
for relief of tenderness or for cosmetic reasons. Most cases respond to as-

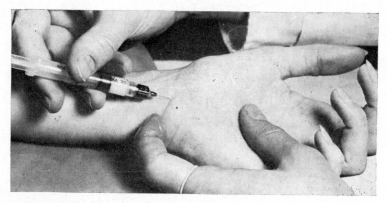

Figure 20-9. Injection for carpal tunnel syndrome. (Courtesy, Dr. A. Mackenzie)

piration of the cyst contents through a large-bore needle followed by injection of local steroid.

Carpal Tunnel Syndrome. Compression of the median nerve may be secondary to inflammatory or infiltrative diseases at the wrist. Temporary relief usually can be obtained by local steroid injection. The landmarks for injection include the palmaris longus tendon medially and the flexor carpi radialis tendon laterally. The median nerve runs in the groove between these two tendons or lies just under the palmaris longus. Injection is made over the median nerve at the wrist, just proximal to the palm (Fig. 20-9). A 22-gauge needle is usually satisfactory and is less likely to cause inadvertent damage than larger needles. One and a half to 2 cc of steroid-lidocaine mixture is a satisfactory volume for injection. The initial injection is made at a 45° angle directed away from the palm, parallel and superficial to the nerve. The remainder of the material for injection is then placed distally under the transverse carpal ligament after appropriate redirection of the needle. The needle should be withdrawn immediately if radiation of nerve pain is noted, to avoid injection into the nerve itself. Proper injection is often, but not always, associated with a lidocaine-induced nerve block in the distribution of the median nerve.

REFERENCES

1. Moskowitz, R.W. et al.: Experimentally induced corticosteroid arthropathy. Arth Rheum 13:236, 1970.
2. Ellison, R. W. and Flatt, A. E.: Intra-articular Thiotepa in rheumatoid disease. Arth Rheum 14:212, 1971.
3. Ansell, B. M. et al.: Evaluation of intra-articular colloidal gold [198]Au in the treatment of persistent knee effusions. Ann Rheum Dis 22:435, 1963.
4. Bridgman, J. F., Bruckner, F. and Bleehan, N. M.: Radioactive yttrium in the treatment of rheumatoid knee effusions. Ann Rheum Dis 30:180, 1971.

Chapter 21

STEROID MANAGEMENT IN STRESS SITUATIONS

Clinical manifestations of adrenal insufficiency may develop during stress situations in patients who are receiving or who have received corticosteroid therapy. Among the more common situations in which this complication arises are surgical procedures, obstetric delivery and intercurrent infection. The availability of rapidly-acting steroid preparations allows effective management of this untoward reaction. On the other hand, prevention of this complication by appropriate prophylactic supplementation of steroids is desirable when possible.

Several different methods of steroid supplementation can be utilized. Effective use depends upon a working knowledge of the pharmacology of available agents. The rapidity and duration of clinical action varies not only with the chemical nature of the steroid used, but also with the route of administration.[1-6] The following programs represent general methods of management of stress situations in patients with a history of steroid therapy; other procedures can be safely substituted if based on knowledgeable application of the various steroid agents available for therapeutic use.

SURGICAL STRESS

Prophylactic steroid supplementation is indicated prior to surgery in patients who are presently receiving corticosteroids or who have received suppressive doses of corticosteroids within three months of the operative procedure. Prednisone, 5 to 7.5 mg (or an equivalent dose of another steroid agent), given daily for 10 to 14 days or longer by mouth, should be considered a potentially suppressive dose. Steroids administered intermittently by intramuscular or intra-articular routes should also be considered as potentially suppressive when given frequently or in high doses. Prolonged steroid administration in the nine-month period prior to surgery should also be considered as an adrenal suppressive dose, even if the medication has been discontinued for some time. Patients with residual evidence of hypercortisonism may be susceptible to adrenal insufficiency, regardless of the interval since prior steroid administration.

These are only general guidelines to which patients should be considered for steroid supplementation at the time of surgical stress. The final decision regarding use of such therapy also involves certain variables, such as the extent of the planned surgical procedure and contraindications to steroid use. Although relatively few patients receiving prior low-dose steroids for short intervals are likely to develop adrenal insufficiency under stress, it is generally safer to err in the direction of overuse of supplementation. Complications are minimal and the support against unanticipated stress is reassuring.

Major Surgery

In patients for whom extensive, prolonged major surgery is planned, cortisone acetate, 100 mg IM, is administered every 12 hours beginning 48 hours before surgery. Cortisone acetate administered intramuscularly achieves therapeutic effectiveness only after 18 to 24 hours; this program allows a reasonable period to attain an effective parenteral depot of the drug. An intravenous infusion of hydrocortisone sodium succinate, 100 mg per liter, may be added at the time of surgery, but it usually is not necessary. However, it should routinely be administered when the full 48-hour administration of intramuscular cortisone acetate has not been carried out. Postoperatively, cortisone acetate, 100 mg IM, is given the night of surgery. On the first postoperative day, 100 to 150 mg of cortisone acetate IM is administered; on day two, 75 mg; and on day three, 25 mg. The original preoperative oral dose of steroids is re-instituted when the patient is able to tolerate oral medications. When oral intake is delayed, parenteral administration of steroids in an equivalent daily dose is continued until the oral preparation can be substituted.

In patients undergoing major surgery on an emergency basis, more rapid steroid supplementation is required. An intravenous solution of saline or glucose containing 100 mg of hydrocortisone sodium succinate is begun immediately. Cortisone acetate, 100 mg IM, is also administered. Intravenous steroids are maintained until the patient can be switched to adequate intramuscular or oral steroid support.

Hydrocortisone sodium succinate has a rapid onset of action when given intramuscularly; effective levels are achieved in 30 to 60 minutes. This route of administration can be substituted for the intravenous program outlined above. One hundred milligrams IM is given immediately preoperative, followed by 50 mg IM at four- to six-hour intervals.

Minor Surgery

Minor surgical procedures do not require extensive steroid supplementation. For short operative procedures, such as dilatation and curettage or cystoscopy, hydrocortisone sodium succinate, 100 mg IM is administered one to two hours before surgery. This dose is followed by 50 mg IM at four-hour intervals for several doses. A satisfactory alternative program is to administer the same agent intravenously, in a dose of 100 mg per liter of saline or glucose, just prior to and during surgery. The intravenous infusion is discontinued when the patient is stable and back on oral intake.

Patients undergoing dental extractions under short analgesia can be satisfactorily managed by administration of two to three times the usual oral dose of steroid several hours before extraction.

OBSTETRIC DELIVERY

Similar precautions and procedures for steroid supplementation should be considered at termination of pregnancy in patients receiving steroids for various illnesses. Although experimental studies in animals have shown some association between corticosteroid therapy and congenital abnormalities, clinical studies have demonstrated no definite hazard with respect to fetal development.[7,8] Increased doses of steroids should be utilized when indicated during the stress of normal or surgical delivery.

INTERCURRENT INFECTION

Steroid supplementation should also be considered at times of nonsurgical or obstetric stress, such as might occur in the presence of severe infection. Steroid supplementation to levels equivalent to twice the prior daily intake is adequate if the infection is mild. In the presence of severe infection, more intensive steroid supplementation may be required. Appropriate antibiotics should be utilized to treat the infectious process.

As noted earlier, the availability of steroid preparations with rapid onset of action has diminished the threat imposed by unexpected adrenal insufficiency. However, prevention of clinical adrenal insufficiency when possible is preferable to treatment of this complication. In patients in whom acute adrenal insufficiency intervenes, high doses of rapidly-acting steroid agents should be administered intravenously in whatever dosage is required to maintain corticosteroid support.

REFERENCES

1. Melby, J. C. and Silber, R. H.: Clinical pharmacology of water-soluble corticosteroid esters. Am Pract Digest Treat 12:156, 1961.
2. Melby, J. C. and St. Cyr, M.: Comparative studies on absorption and metabolic disposal of water-soluble corticosteroid esters in healthy subjects. Metabolism 10:75, 1961.
3. Buhler, D. R., Thomas, R. C., Jr. and Schlagel, C. A.: Absorption, metabolism and excretion of 6α-methylprednisolone-^{3}H, 21-acetate following oral and intramuscular administrations in the dog. Endocrinology 76:852, 1965.

4. Melby, J. C. and Dale, S. L.: Comparison of absorption, disposal and activity of soluble and repository corticosteroid esters. Clin Pharmacol Therap 10:344, 1969.
5. Christy, N. P.: The Human Adrenal Cortex. New York, Harper & Row, 1971.
6. Cope, C. L.: Adrenal Steroids and Disease. 2nd Edition. Philadelphia, J. B. Lippincott Co., 1972.
7. Bongiovanni, A. M. and McPadden, A. J.: Steroids during pregnancy and possible fetal consequences. Fertil Steril 2:181, 1960.
8. Popert, A. J.: Pregnancy and adrenocortical hormones. Brit Med J 1:967, 1962.

Part IV
APPENDIX

TEXTBOOK REFERENCES

Beetham, W. P., Jr., et al.: Physical Examination of the Joints. Philadelphia, W. B. Saunders Co., 1965.

Boyle, J. A. and Buchanan, W. W.: Clinical Rheumatology. Philadelphia, F. A. Davis Co., 1971.

Brewer, E. J., Jr.: Juvenile Rheumatoid Arthritis. Philadelphia, W. B. Saunders Co., 1970.

Cohen, A. S.: Laboratory Diagnostic Procedures in the Rheumatic Diseases. 2nd Ed. Boston, Little, Brown & Co., 1974.

Copeman, W. S. C.: Textbook of the Rheumatic Diseases. 4th Ed. London and Edinburgh, E and S Livingston Ltd., 1969.

Daniels, L. and Worthingham, C.: Muscle Testing. Techniques of Manual Examination. 3rd Ed. Philadelphia, W. B. Saunders Co., 1972.

Dubois, E. L.: Lupus Erythematosus. 2nd Ed. Los Angeles, University of Southern California Press, 1974.

Ehrlich, G. E.: Oculocutaneous Manifestations of Rheumatic Diseases. Basel, S. Karger, 1973.

————: Total Management of the Arthritic Patient. Philadelphia, J. B. Lippincott Co., 1973.

Forrester, D. M. and Nesson, J. W.: The Radiology of Joint Diseases. Philadelphia, W. B. Saunders Co., 1973.

Harris, E. D.: Rheumatoid Arthritis. New York, Medcom Press, 1974.

Hollander, J. L.: The Arthritis Handbook. West Point, Pa., Merck Sharp and Dohme, 1974.

Hollander, J. L. and McCarty, D. J., Jr.: Arthritis and Allied Conditions. 8th Ed. Philadelphia, Lea & Febiger, 1972.

Hollingsworth, J. W.: Local and Systemic Complications of Rheumatoid Arthritis. Philadelphia, W. B. Saunders Co., 1968.

Krusen, F. H., Kottke, F. J. and Ellwood, P. M.: Handbook of Physical Medicine and Rehabilitation. 2nd Ed. Philadelphia, W. B. Saunders Co., 1971.

Licht, S. L.: Arthritis and Physical Medicine. Baltimore, Waverly Press Inc., 1969.

Mason, M. and Currey, H. L. F.: Clinical Rheumatology. Philadelphia, J. B. Lippincott Co., 1970.

Preston, R. L.: The Surgical Management of Rheumatoid Arthritis. Philadelphia, W. B. Saunders Co., 1968.

Ropes, M. W. and Bauer, W.: Synovial Fluid Changes in Joint Disease. Cambridge, Mass., Harvard University Press, 1953.

Rotstein, J.: Simple Splinting. Philadelphia, W. B. Saunders Co., 1965.

Steinbrocker, O. and Neustadt, D. H.: Aspiration and Injection Therapy in Arthritis and Musculoskeletal Disorders. Hagerstown, Md., Harper & Row, 1972.

Talbott, J. H.: Gout. 3rd Ed. New York, Grune & Stratton, 1967.

Walton, J. N.: Disorders of Voluntary Muscle. 3rd Ed. Edinburgh and London, Churchill Livingstone, 1974.

309

HISTORY AND PHYSICAL EXAMINATION FORMS

NAME: _____   Occupation: _____

ADDRESS: Age___ Sex___ Race___ Birthdate___

      Home: _____

      Business: _____   Referred by: _____

PHONE:

      Home: _____   Hospital #: _____

      Business: _____   Insurance: _____

Date:

Chief Complaint:

_____

History of Present Illness:

_____

_____

_____

_____

_____

Systems Review:

Weight loss

Appetite

Fever, chills

Head

Eyes, ears, nose, throat

Cardiorespiratory

Gastrointestinal

Genitourinary

Menses

Bruising, bleeding

Pleurisy

Hair loss

Psoriasis

Sun sensitivity

Skin rash

Dry mouth (eyes)

Canker sores

Iritis

Urethritis

Colitis

Heel pain

Back pain

Sciatica

Raynaud's

Drug allergy: _____

_____

_____

Contraceptive pills:

Past Medications (arthritis)	Response	Present medications
Aspirin	_____	_____
Indomethacin	_____	_____
Phenylbutazone	_____	_____
Antimalarials	_____	_____
Gold	_____	_____
P.O. Steroids	_____	_____
I.A. Steroids	_____	_____
Immunosuppressives	_____	_____
Analgesics	_____	_____
Other	_____	_____

Past Medical History—Illness: Diabetes ﹘﹘﹘﹘﹘ Hypertension ﹘﹘﹘﹘﹘

Other ﹘﹘﹘﹘﹘﹘﹘﹘﹘﹘﹘﹘﹘﹘

Surgery (where, surgeon)

Fx (Fracture):

Past x-rays and where done:

Rheumatic fever:

Pregnancies:

Family History:

M﹘﹘﹘﹘﹘ Age﹘﹘﹘ Illnesses﹘﹘﹘﹘﹘

F ﹘﹘﹘﹘﹘ Age﹘﹘﹘ Illnesses﹘﹘﹘﹘﹘

Siblings: ﹘﹘﹘﹘﹘﹘﹘﹘﹘﹘﹘﹘﹘

Arthritis history: ﹘﹘﹘﹘﹘﹘﹘﹘﹘﹘﹘

Social History:

Home﹘﹘﹘﹘﹘﹘ Apartment﹘﹘﹘﹘﹘﹘

Lives with ﹘﹘﹘﹘﹘﹘﹘﹘﹘﹘﹘﹘

Occupational activity ﹘﹘﹘﹘﹘﹘﹘﹘Disability (date)﹘﹘

Tobacco ﹘﹘﹘﹘﹘﹘﹘﹘﹘﹘﹘﹘﹘

Alcohol ﹘﹘﹘﹘﹘﹘﹘﹘﹘﹘﹘﹘﹘

Physical therapy ﹘﹘﹘﹘﹘﹘﹘﹘﹘﹘﹘

﹘﹘﹘﹘﹘﹘﹘﹘﹘﹘﹘﹘﹘

﹘﹘﹘﹘﹘﹘﹘﹘﹘﹘﹘﹘﹘

ADL (Activities of daily living): ﹘﹘﹘﹘﹘﹘﹘﹘

﹘﹘﹘﹘﹘﹘﹘﹘﹘﹘﹘﹘﹘﹘

Physical Examination:

Temp. _____ Pulse _____ BP_____

Ht. _____ Wt. _____ Chest expansion_____

General:

  Skin:

  Lymph:

  Head:

  EENT:

  Neck:

  Heart:

  Lungs:

  Abd:

  Pelvic:

  Rectal:

  Neurologic:

  Muscles:

  Pulses:

  Nodules:

  Tophi:

Musculoskeletal: (S=swelling, T=tenderness, L=limitation)

Cervical spine: LS spine:

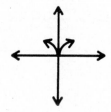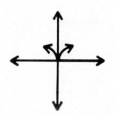

	Rt.				Lt.	
	S	T	L	S	T	L

Hands:

Wrists:

Elbows:

Shoulders:

TMJ (Temporomandibular):

AC (Acromioclavicular):

SC (Sternoclavicular):

Hips:

Knees:

Ankles:

Subtalar:

Feet:

Miscellaneous:

Diagnostic
Impressions:

Proposed study and management:

Roland W. Moskowitz, M.D.

INDEX

Page numbers in *italics* indicate illustrations; page numbers followed by "t" indicate tables; page numbers followed by "h" indicate case histories.